Surviving Vietnam

Surviving Vietnam

Psychological Consequences of the War for U.S. Veterans

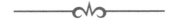

Bruce P. Dohrenwend

Nick Turse

Thomas J. Yager

Melanie M. Wall

OXFORD
UNIVERSITY PRESS

Oxford University Press is a department of the University of Oxford. It furthers
the University's objective of excellence in research, scholarship, and education
by publishing worldwide. Oxford is a registered trade mark of Oxford University
Press in the UK and certain other countries.

Published in the United States of America by Oxford University Press
198 Madison Avenue, New York, NY 10016, United States of America.

CIP data is on file at the Library of Congress
ISBN 978–0–19–090444–9

1 3 5 7 9 8 6 4 2

Printed by Sheridan Books, Inc., United States of America

The war ended, and then it really ended, the cities "fell," I watched the choppers I'd loved dropping into the South China Sea as their Vietnamese pilots jumped clear, and one last chopper revved it up, lifted off and flew out of my chest.

Michael Herr, *Dispatches,* New York: Avon Books, 1977, p. 277

CONTENTS

PREFACE

Officially, the era of U.S. involvement in the civil war in Vietnam began on August 5, 1964, and ended on May 7, 1975. During this 11-year period, about 58,000 U.S. troops were killed in action, as were an estimated 254,000 personnel from the military forces of South Vietnamese allies of the United States. In contrast, an estimated 1,000,000 North Vietnamese fighting forces were killed and about 300,000 were missing, according to North Vietnamese government sources. Despite the overwhelming military superiority of U.S. forces that these figures suggest, this is the first war in our history in which our involvement ended in defeat. This crucial, puzzling fact is part of the historical context for our focus in this monograph on the psychological consequences of service in Vietnam for U.S. veterans. The historical background of the war is described in detail in Part I of this monograph.

At the center of the psychological consequences, which we investigate in Part II of this monograph, is the relatively new diagnosis of post-traumatic stress disorder (PTSD). The formulation of PTSD that we use in much of this research is summarized in Chapter 2, as is its origin in attempts to describe the readjustment problems of substantial numbers of returning Vietnam veterans. From its beginnings, the diagnosis of PTSD has stirred controversy. Much of the controversy centered on a major report in 1990 of what numerous critics regarded as unrealistically high rates of this disorder in U.S. veterans. We describe our attempt to resolve this controversy in Chapter 2. In this chapter and throughout the monograph, we utilize interview and questionnaire data from the National Vietnam Veterans Readjustment Study (NVVRS), military histories of the war, and record data from various national archives. These sources, and the main measures we have developed from them, are described in Chapters 2, 3, and 4.

The most important information about the onset and course of war-related PTSD in the NVVRS is contained in the rigorous diagnoses conducted by experienced, doctoral level clinicians of a small subsample of the veterans. Among our monograph's most distinctive features are a sustained focus on these clinical diagnoses, an emphasis on the historical context of this war, and our unique use of military records in one of our main measures of combat exposure.

PTSD is unusual in that, unlike the large majority of psychiatric diagnoses, it includes the putative main cause—in this case, exposure to traumatic events—among the criteria required for the diagnosis. There has been controversy, however, about whether exposure to one or more traumatic events is in fact primary as compared, especially, with pre-exposure personal vulnerability factors, such as prior psychiatric disorder.

Our attempt to resolve this controversy as it applies to war-related PTSD is set forth in Chapter 5. In this chapter, we analyze not only the roles of severity of exposure to combat and personal vulnerability, but also the major part played by the involvement of some veterans in harming civilians or prisoners. We inquire further into the role of such involvement in Chapter 6.

While the large majority of U.S. Vietnam veterans are males from non-Hispanic white backgrounds, substantial minorities of males from black and Hispanic backgrounds also fought in Vietnam. And a small minority of women, mainly nurses, served in Vietnam as well. There are pronounced differences in the rates of war-related PTSD in these subgroups. In Chapters 7 and 8, we investigate the reasons for these differences.

Most of the U.S. veterans were young men when they went to Vietnam. They were usually single and did not yet have children. By the time the NVVRS was conducted 10 to 11 years after the war, substantial numbers were married and had children. This provided an opportunity to investigate the question of whether there was intergenerational transmission of psychiatric problems from veterans to their children. Our investigation of this question is described in Chapter 9.

In Part III, we explore in detail veterans' post-war adjustment. As reported here, the Vietnam war lasted 11 years, beginning in 1964. In the early years, a large majority of the U.S. public was in favor of U.S. involvement. As the war dragged on, these attitudes began to change from favorable to unfavorable. Parallel to the change in public attitudes were differences in the attitudes of soldiers who went to Vietnam later in the war compared with those who served earlier. Did such changes in public attitudes increase vulnerability of veterans to PTSD? Our answer to this question is contained in Chapters 4 and 10.

The war in Vietnam had long since ended when veterans were interviewed in the NVVRS research conducted between 1986 and 1988. Looking back, as they were asked to do in this study, how did they appraise the impact of the war on their present lives? Was its valence positive or negative? What about its salience—did it have a great or small effect on them these many years later? What were the factors that affected the valence and salience of the impact of the war on their post-war lives—especially the role of war-related PTSD? Chapter 11 sets forth our initial attempt to answer these questions.

Chapter 12 of this monograph continues the exploration of the long-term impact of veterans' service in the Vietnam war. In this chapter, we investigate new data from a follow-up concluded in 2013 of the NVVRS called the National Vietnam Veterans Longitudinal Study. We draw on the work presented in the preceding chapters and conduct new analyses to investigate whether and how well U.S. veterans and their subgroups have survived what we call "the Vietnam War" and what those we fought call "the American War"—a war whose outcome was very far from anything that could be called a triumph of American forces.

Finally, in Chapter 13, we underline research findings from previous chapters that provide useful background for developing future policies for post-Vietnam wars.

ACKNOWLEDGMENTS

The data for our research come from military histories and records and from two major congressionally mandated epidemiological studies: The National Vietnam Veterans Readjustment Study (NVVRS) and a follow-up of the NVVRS respondents called the National Vietnam Veterans Longitudinal Study (Longitudinal Study). My first contact with the idea that there was an urgent need for something like the NVVRS came when I was asked in the early 1980s by the Veterans Administration (VA) to join a scientific advisory board (SAB) composed of a small group of scholars charged with developing guidelines for a request for proposals (RFP). We did this, and the RFP was put out for bids from research organizations and groups. The NVVRS contract was awarded to researchers at the Research Triangle Institute (RTI), and I continued to serve on an enlarged SAB that met frequently with the RTI investigators. The NVVRS took four years to complete and culminated in a final report by RTI to Congress and the VA in 1988. More recently, I served on the SAB that advised the VA on the Longitudinal Study, in which the NVVRS respondents were followed up in 2012 and 2013.

Richard Kulka and William Schlenger were the RTI principal investigators for the NVVRS. I learned a great deal from them and other members of their research team over the course of the study. I also learned much from fellow members of the SAB, especially from its chairman, the late Stanislav Kasl. Charles Marmar joined Kulka and Schlenger as a third principal investigator in the follow-up research.

The RTI investigators, together with the help of the SAB and numerous colleagues and consultants, made the NVVRS an incredibly rich source of data on the psychological effects on U.S. veterans of the Vietnam war. Aspects of these data have attracted a number of other investigators—myself and my colleagues included. A three-year National Institute of Mental Health (NIMH) grant (MH 59627) from 1999 to 2002 and continuing grants from The Spunk Fund, Inc., have made it possible to conduct the research reported in this volume. I am especially grateful to Marianne Gerschel and Leonard Lamm, the president and vice-president of The Spunk Fund, not only for their continuing financial support, but also for their questions and suggestions throughout the research. For example, they are responsible for suggesting that we obtain historical accounts and record information about the war that have made our work so distinctive in the field.

Also distinctive of our work is the collaboration of an interdisciplinary group of researchers. My three coauthors and I, for example, come from social psychology and epidemiology (Bruce Dohrenwend), history (Nick Turse), sociology (Thomas Yager), and biostatistics (Melanie Wall). Contributors to the main articles around which half of our chapters are built include, especially, a sociologist (Blake Turner) who was a co-investigator on our NIMH grant; clinical psychologists (Ben Adams, Karestan Koenen, and Yuval Neria); psychiatrists (Roberto Lewis-Fernández and Randall Marshall); and a college psychology undergraduate (Nicole Gerszberg). In addition, a clinical psychologist (Eleanor Murphy) and a sociologist and epidemiologist (Stephani Hatch) made substantial contributions to two chapters. The extremely valuable contributions of all these individuals are acknowledged in the relevant chapters.

My long-term colleague Patrick Shrout provided valuable input and critical ongoing advice on the data analysis. I am also grateful to faculty and fellows in Columbia's Research Training Program in Psychiatric Epidemiology and my co-members of the Social Psychiatry Division in the New York State Psychiatric Institute and Columbia University Department of Psychiatry, whose criticisms of my seminar presentations kept me from going down at least some of the wrong paths that at one time or another seemed attractive.

Throughout our work, William Schlenger was an invaluable guide to the complex NVVRS data set. Terry Keane and the late Thomas Murtaugh from the VA also provided valuable help with the NVVRS data. Timothy O'Leary of the VA made it possible for me to have access to data from the Longitudinal Study follow-up that is essential to the analyses in Chapter 12. Without the Longitudinal Study data, this monograph would be like a play that needed, but was missing, a third act.

I served on active duty in the Navy for a brief period toward the end of World War II. I did not see combat. None of my coauthors of this monograph or collaborators in the articles on which much of it is based served in the U.S. military. Fortunately, a group of veterans—David Alcaras, Joan Furey, Daniel King, Linda King, and Erwin Parsons—met with us for several days early in our research. Three served in combat (Alcaras, D. King, and Parsons); two were nurses, one of whom served in Vietnam (Furey) and the other, Stateside (L. King). They provided much-needed education, and I am most grateful.

Special thanks go to my wife, Catherine Douglass, for editorial assistance and endless support that has included more valuable advice and criticism than she realizes.

Finally, and far from least, I would like to thank the veterans who spent hours answering NVVRS and Longitudinal Study interviews and questionnaires. I hope that what we have learned will help them, the larger population of Vietnam veterans they represent, and future policy makers, planners, and fighters of U.S. wars.

Bruce P. Dohrenwend

CONTRIBUTORS

Ben G. Adams, PhD
Staff Psychotherapist, Mayor's Office to
    Combat Domestic Violence
NYC Family Justice Center
Staten Island, New York
Clinical Psychologist, Behavioral Health
    Services
NYC + Hospitals/Coney Island
Brooklyn, New York

Bruce P. Dohrenwend, PhD
Chief of Research, Division of Social
    Psychiatry
New York State Psychiatric Institute
New York, New York
Professor of Social Science, and Foundations
    Fund for Research in Psychiatry
    Professor, Department of Psychiatry
Professor of Epidemiology, Department
    of Epidemiology
Mailman School of Public Health
Columbia University
New York, New York

Nicole Gerszberg, BA
Graduate with Honors in Psychology
Wesleyan University

Stephani L. Hatch, PhD, SFHEA
Reader in Sociology and Epidemiology,
    Department of Psychological Medicine
Institute of Psychiatry, Psychology and
    Neuroscience
King's College, London
London, England

Karestan C. Koenen, PhD
Professor, Department of Epidemiology
Harvard T. H. Chan School of
    Public Health
Boston, Massachusetts

Roberto Lewis-Fernández, MD
Professor of Clinical Psychiatry
Columbia University
New York, New York
Director, New York State Center of
    Excellence for Cultural Competence
New York State Psychiatric Institute
New York, New York
Director, Hispanic Treatment Program
New York State Psychiatric Institute
New York, New York
Co-Director, Anxiety Disorders Clinic
New York State Psychiatric Institute
New York, New York

Randall Marshall, MD
Chief Medical Officer
President, Research and Development
ArTara Therapeutics
New York, New York

Eleanor Murphy, PhD
Assistant Professor of Clinical
    Psychology (in Psychiatry), Division
    of Epidemiology
New York State Psychiatric Institute
New York, New York

Yuval Neria, PhD
Professor of Medical Psychology,
  Department of Psychiatry
Columbia University
New York, New York
Director, PTSD Treatment and Research
  Center
New York State Psychiatric Institute
New York, New York
Director, Columbia-New York
  Presbyterian Military Family
  Wellness Center
Columbia University Medical Center
New York, New York

J. Blake Turner, PhD
Assistant Professor of Social Science
  (in Psychiatry), Division of Child and
  Adolescent Psychiatry, Department
  of Psychiatry
Columbia University
New York, New York
Research Scientist
New York State Psychiatric Institute
New York, New York

Nick Turse, PhD
Historian and Journalist
The Nation Institute
New York, New York

Melanie M. Wall, PhD
Director, Mental Health Data Science,
  Department of Psychiatry
Columbia University
Research Foundation for Mental
  Hygiene, and
New York State Psychiatric Institute
New York, New York
Professor of Biostatistics,
Department of Biostatistics
Mailman School of Public Health
Columbia University
New York, New York

Thomas J. Yager, PhD
Research Scientist, Department of
  Epidemiology
Mailman School of Public Health
Columbia University
New York, New York

PART I

Historical Context

CHAPTER 1

୶

Prelude, War, and Aftermath

NICK TURSE

PRELUDE

The first official U.S. combat troops arrived in Vietnam in 1965, but the roots of the conflict stretch back many decades earlier. In the nineteenth century, France expanded its colonial empire by taking control of Vietnam as well as neighboring Cambodia and Laos, rechristening the region as French Indochina. French rubber production in Vietnam yielded such riches for the colonizers that they called the latex oozing from rubber trees "white gold." The ill-paid Vietnamese workers, laboring on the plantations in harsh conditions, had a different name for it: "white blood" (Murray, 1992, p. 60). The exploitation extended to coffee and rice plantations as well as mining operations, and this, along with decades of military conquest, the disenfranchisement of local elites, and economic policies that plunged peasants into crushing debt and forced them to pay onerous taxes, helped to fan the flames of Vietnamese discontent (Bradley, 2009).

"The hope of seeing the country one day liberated and caring for its own people stirs within every [Vietnamese] who has not been corrupted by gold or the symbolic titles of the current masters of Indochina," wrote 23-year-old Saigon-based intellectual and radical journalist, Nguyen An Ninh, in 1923. "Is revolution possible?" he asked (Schiffrin, 2014, p. 81). He didn't live to see it, but it certainly was—and its leaders found inspiration in Russian Bolshevism and Lenin's call for national revolutions in the colonial world. During World War II, the country's main anticolonial organization—officially called the Revolutionary League for the Independence of Vietnam, but better known as the Viet Minh—launched a campaign of guerrilla attacks against occupying Japanese forces and French administrators running the country. Under the leadership of Ho Chi Minh, the Vietnamese guerrillas aided the American war effort in Asia. In return, they received arms, training, and support from the U.S. Office of Strategic Services (OSS), a forerunner of the Central Intelligence Agency (CIA).

In 1945, with Japan defeated, Ho proclaimed Vietnam's independence. "All men are created equal," he told a crowd of half a million Vietnamese (and several OSS advisors) in Hanoi:

> The Creator has given us certain inviolable Rights; the right to Life, the right to be Free, and the right to achieve Happiness. . . . These immortal words are taken from the Declaration of Independence of the United States of America in 1776. In a larger sense, this means that: All the people on earth are born equal; All the people have the right to live, to be happy, to be free. (Young, 1991, pp. 10–11)

During the speech, two U.S. military planes streaked overhead. The crowd interpreted it as an endorsement of Vietnamese independence (Appy, 2003).

Ho Chi Minh hoped to obtain American support for his vision of a free Vietnam but, in the aftermath of World War II, the United States was focused on rebuilding and strengthening a devastated Europe as the chill of the Cold War began to spread. In an increasingly bipolar world dominated by two superpowers, the United States and the Soviet Union both set about consolidating their spheres of influence. The Americans saw France as a necessary ally against any Soviet designs on Western Europe, and thus had little interest in sanctioning a Communist-led independence movement in a French colony.

Ho sent letter after letter to U.S. President Harry Truman appealing for an endorsement of his country's independence and stressing that it was the Vietnamese, not the French, who had fought the Japanese in Indochina. He was ignored and, instead of support for Vietnamese self-determination and a growing independence movement, U.S. ships helped transport French troops to Vietnam to reimpose colonial rule. In November 1946, French warships bombarded the unprotected city of Haiphong, killing 6,000 and wounding another 25,000. The next month, Viet Minh forces struck back against the French beginning, in earnest, the Indochina War (Young, 1991).

After China was "lost" to Communism and with the outbreak of the Korean War, U.S. policymakers viewed the Vietnamese struggle not as an anticolonial, nationalist fight for self-determination, but as a dangerous "domino" that might set off a chain reaction of Communist victories throughout Southeast Asia. This understanding was fundamentally shaped by the development of a doctrine of "national security," which held that containment of, confrontation with, and intervention against "Communism" anywhere in the world was absolutely vital to American political, economic, and military interests (Yergin, 1977).

Soon the United States was dispatching equipment and even military advisors to Vietnam, and by 1953, was shouldering almost 80% of the bill for the French war against the Viet Minh. The conflict progressed from guerrilla warfare to a conventional military campaign, and in 1954, a well-fortified Gallic garrison at Dien Bien Phu was pounded into surrender by Viet Minh forces under General Vo Nguyen Giap. The French had finally had enough. At an international peace conference in Geneva, they agreed to a temporary separation of Vietnam into two placeholder regions, north and south of a demilitarized zone (DMZ), which were to be rejoined as one nation following a reunification election in 1956 (Appy, 1993; Bradley, 2009; Young, 2002).

The United States was present at the conference, too, but refused to sign the Geneva agreement. It instead began sending military and economic aid (by 1956, $270 million annually), covertly funneling arms, and sending advisors into a provisionally constituted southern Republic of Vietnam, whose capital was located in Saigon (Appy, 1993; Appy, 2003; Mackenzie, 1997). After American officials determined that 80% of the Vietnamese would have voted for Ho Chi Minh, the 1956 elections were permanently scuttled. Instead, the United States threw its support behind the leadership of Catholic, anti-Communist exile Ngo Dinh Diem, who held his own plebiscite in which he won 98% approval. (In Saigon, where 450,000 people were registered, Diem received 605,000 votes [Farber & Foner, 1994]). In the North, Ho Chi Minh became the leader of the Democratic Republic of Vietnam (DRV).

Diem quickly instituted repressive taxes and a return of property to landlords who had oppressed the people under the French colonial regime. He utilized authoritarian tactics against both Communist and non-Communist critics of the government, and his preferential treatment of Catholics in an overwhelmingly Buddhist nation sparked protests and widespread discontent. Many were tortured and executed by Saigon's security services during anti-Communist purges, and 50,000 or more were jailed. Former Viet Minh were especially targeted by Diem's terror campaign, and Communist Party chapters in some villages were nearly wiped out. In response, the survivors sought to strike back militarily, but comrades in Hanoi, the capital of the DRV, counseled against it and instead advocated political activism to topple Diem. U.S. support, however, continued to prop up the Saigon regime, prompting Hanoi to finally give the go-ahead for compatriots in the South to form the revolutionary-minded National Liberation Front of South Vietnam (NLF) (Chanoff & Doan, 1986; Gibson, 2000; Mackenzie, 1997; Prados, 2009; Sheehan, 1988; Young, 1991).

When John F. Kennedy was elected U.S. President in 1960, the year the NLF was established, there were roughly 700 American military personnel in Vietnam. By the end of 1961, the number of advisors (a loose definition that included Special Forces teams, fighter pilots, and full helicopter companies) had increased to 3,200, and the next year it climbed to 11,300. By the close of 1963, American troop strength reached 16,700 (Gibson, 2000). Still officially listed as advisors involved in the training of the South Vietnamese army—officially known as the Army of the Republic of Vietnam, or ARVN—the Americans increasingly took part in combat operations against southern guerrillas bent on unifying the country (Appy, 1993; Gibson, 2000).

Even with abundant U.S. support, the South Vietnamese fared poorly against the revolutionary forces. In January 1963, a battle at Ap Bac in the deep south of the Republic of Vietnam's Mekong Delta threw the situation into broad relief (Prados, 2009). Despite its armored personnel carriers, outnumbering its foes by as much as four to one, and support from American fighter-bombers and helicopters, Saigon's troops were soundly defeated by their lesser-equipped foes, suffering as many as 450 casualties to 57 of the revolutionary forces. American advisors on the scene were deeply critical of the ARVN, especially their reluctance to fully engage the guerrillas. The language of a U.S. after-action memorandum was damning, peppered with talk of "failure," "unwillingness," and "futility." One of the Americans, John Paul Vann, charged senior South Vietnamese commanders with incompetence, but Ngo Dinh Diem refused to sack them (Bradley, 2009; Prados, 2009; Sheehan, 1988).

Diem also rankled his American advisors by ignoring their counsel on other key issues, like refusing to implement land reforms and presiding over a government that allowed millions in U.S. aid to be siphoned into the coffers of top regime officials (Farber & Foner, 1994). In 1963, with South Vietnam in a state of turmoil, Kennedy took steps to undercut Diem's strength and bolster that of generals aligning against him. U.S. officials also approved a plot by members of the ARVN to overthrow him. That November, South Vietnamese officers put their plan into action, and South Vietnam's first leader was killed by members of his own military. While the U.S. had not approved Diem's murder, America did pay for it—handing over $42,000 to the Vietnamese generals to pay their troops on the morning after the coup. Just three weeks later, Kennedy was also assassinated.

America's new president, Lyndon Johnson—previously a powerful Democratic senator from Texas—found himself in a position to spearhead sweeping domestic reforms. In January 1964, Johnson announced an "unconditional War on Poverty in America," and in May, with an eye toward the presidential election in the fall, Johnson put forth a vision for the creation of a

> Great Society . . . [which] demands an end to poverty and racial injustice . . . a place where every child can find knowledge to enrich his mind . . . where leisure is a welcome chance to build and reflect, not a feared cause of boredom and restlessness . . . where the city of man serves not only the needs of the body and the demands of commerce but the desire for beauty and the hunger for community. (Isserman & Kazin, 1999, p. 112)

While Johnson spoke of beauty, community, and a battle to right social and economic wrongs, he was escalating America's undeclared war in Southeast Asia. In January 1964, Chairman of the Joint Chiefs of Staff General Maxwell Taylor sent a memo to Secretary of Defense Robert McNamara endorsing covert operations (which had been approved by Johnson a month earlier) by South Vietnamese forces against North Vietnam. In June, a new military commander, General William Westmoreland, took charge of the war effort in Southeast Asia as head of Military Assistance Command, Vietnam (MACV), and a short time later, Taylor was sent to Saigon as the new U.S. ambassador (Lewy, 1981).

Just as the United States was redoubling its support for South Vietnam, the nascent nation plunged into a succession of coups. And as the military situation rapidly deteriorated, with Saigon's troops deserting in the tens of thousands and the revolutionary forces growing in strength, Johnson's Pentagon advisors urged bombing North Vietnam despite the fact that high-level CIA and Defense Department officials had already determined that such attacks would be of limited use since "the primary sources of Communist strength in South Vietnam are indigenous" (Farber & Foner, 1994, p. 135).

WAR

In late July and early August, U.S. Navy ships *Maddox* and *C. Turner Joy*, operating in the Gulf of Tonkin, were engaged in an intelligence gathering operation in conjunction with a covert CIA-directed series of attacks on North Vietnam (known as OPLAN 34A). A few days later, President Johnson took to the television airwaves to tell Americans that the ships had, without provocation, been the object of "open aggression on the high seas" and that U.S. war planes were already attacking North Vietnamese targets in retaliation (Appy, 2003; Gibson, 1986).

"We seek no wider war," Johnson told the American public (Farber & Foner, 1994, p. 136). But the president then asked Congress to pass the Gulf of Tonkin Resolution, which empowered him to "take all necessary measures to repel any armed attack against the armed forces of the United States" (Appy, 2003, p. 112). The resolution passed by a vote of 88 to 2 in the Senate and 441 to 0 in the House of Representatives, in essence giving Johnson a blank check by which to escalate the conflict in Vietnam without a formal congressional declaration of war and the uncomfortable debate such a proposal would undoubtedly produce. What neither Congress nor the American public knew was that the Gulf of Tonkin Resolution was based on a series of misleading claims: U.S. ships were not innocently sailing through the Gulf of Tonkin as the President implied; a claim of two separate attacks on U.S. Navy ships turned out to be untrue; and the resolution itself was not drafted in the wake of the supposed attacks but had been written months before, in anticipation of an opportune incident that would ensure its passage. Deceived by the President and his top officials, the American people rallied around military action, with 85% of those surveyed supporting Johnson's response (Appy, 2003).

The real story of the Gulf of Tonkin incident was just one the many truths withheld from the American people as the White House ramped up the war. Behind closed doors, Johnson was remarkably candid about the conflict. Speaking to his Special Assistant for National Security Affairs, McGeorge Bundy, the President said: "I don't think it's worth fighting for. . . . What is it worth to this country?" (Johnson Library, Recordings and Transcripts, Tape 64.28 PNO111; Young, 2002). But the American people were kept in the dark. So, too, were they clueless that Ambassador Maxwell Taylor privately admitted that the American "soldier, armed, equipped and trained as he is [is] not a suitable guerilla fighter for Asian forests and jungles. [The] French tried . . . and failed; I doubt that US forces could do much better" (Farber & Foner, 1994, p. 144). Nor were Americans aware that General Earle Wheeler, the Chairman of the Joint Chiefs of Staff, estimated that it would take some 700,000 to 1,000,000 American troops fighting for seven years to completely pacify Vietnam (Farber & Foner, 1994). Despite all of it, Johnson intensified the war, and by the end of 1964, U.S. troop strength in Vietnam had risen to 23,310. As a result, North Vietnam responded by sending 12,000 troops south-ward in an effort to offset U.S. escalation (Appy, 2003; Clodfelter, 1995).

Johnson's War

Despite the military acceleration in Southeast Asia, Johnson ran in the 1964 presiden-tial election as a "peace candidate" and won a landslide victory over Barry Goldwater, the hawkish Republican Senator from Arizona. The next year, in addition to signing Medicare, Medicaid, and the Clean Water Act into law, Johnson launched Operation Rolling Thunder, a sustained bombing of North Vietnam, and deployed a large contingent of combat troops to South Vietnam. With that escalation, the fiction of "advisors" was fi-nally dropped, and the American War, as it is known in Vietnam, entered a new phase. In a televised speech, Johnson insisted that the United States was not inserting itself into a faraway civil war, but taking steps to contain a Communist menace. The war, he said, was "guided by North Vietnam. . . . Its goal is to conquer the South, to defeat American power, and to extend the Asiatic dominion of communism" (Young, 1991, p. 85).

As the United States saw it, the Vietnamese revolutionary forces were composed of two distinct groups: members of the North Vietnamese army, and indigenous South Vietnamese fighters of the National Liberation Front. The NLF's combatants, officially known as the People's Liberation Armed Forces, included guerrillas in peasant clothing as well as uniformed troops organized into professional units. The U.S. Information Service invented the moniker "Viet Cong"—that is, Vietnamese Communists—as a pejorative term to cover anyone fighting on the side of the NLF. American soldiers, in turn, often shortened this label to "the Cong" or owing to the military's phonetic Alpha-Bravo-Charlie alphabet, to "Victor Charlie," "V.C.," or simply "Charlie."

As the war heated up, the U.S. military turned huge swaths of the South Vietnamese coun-tryside, where most of South Vietnam's population lived, into battered battlegrounds. By June 1965, U.S. B-52 bombers were punishing targets in South Vietnam with 27 tons of explosives per airplane per mission. The next month, in the face of a series of crushing defeats of the ARVN at the hands of the revolutionary forces, Johnson announced that he was deploying another 50,000 Americans to Vietnam, but neglected to mention that he had also privately authorized sending an additional 100,000 troops by the end of the year (Appy, 2003).

The American Way of War

By the mid-1960s, the American military had turned war-making into a highly corporatized, quantitatively oriented system that sociologist James William Gibson calls "technowar." The philosophy behind it was simple: combine American technolog-ical and economic prowess with sophisticated managerial capacities, and the Pentagon was guaranteed success on the battlefield. The country's unmatched military capability would allow it to impose its will anywhere in the world with the war machine functioning as smoothly and predictably as an assembly line (Gibson, 2000).

This mindset was most embodied by Robert McNamara, the Secretary of Defense from 1961 to 1968. A Harvard Business School professor, McNamara had designed statistical methods of analysis for the military during World War II, systematizing the flight patterns and improving the efficiency of the bombers that decimated Japanese and German cities. Before answering President John Kennedy's call to return to government service, he had been a top executive of the Ford Motor Company (Gibson, 1986; McNamara & VanDeMark, 1995; "The Fog of War," 2003).

As Pentagon chief, he brought in a corps of "computer jockeys" who were to transform the military, allowing it to, as historian Tom Engelhardt put it, "be managed in the same 'scientific' and 'efficient' manner as a business" (Engelhardt, 1995, p. 208). McNamara relied on numbers to convey reality and processed whatever information he was given with exceptional speed, making instant choices with little worry that such rapid-fire decision-making might result in grave errors (Sheehan, 1988). Instead, McNamara and his "whiz kids" were sure that, given enough data, warfare could be made completely rational, comprehensible, and controllable.

In Vietnam, the statistically minded war managers focused on the notion of achieving a "crossover point": the moment when American soldiers would be killing more enemies than their Vietnamese opponents could put into the field. After that, the Pentagon expected that the revolutionary forces would give up the fight. It was, in their estimation, the rational thing to do. What McNamara and others in Washington failed to consider was that Vietnamese nationalists who had battled the Japanese and then the French for their independence might not see warfare as a simple exercise in benefit maximization to be abandoned when their ledger sheet showed more debits than credits (Gibson, 2000).

The crossover point proved to be elusive if not illusory. And, as years went by, the conflict only escalated (Young, 1991). Yet, while the Pentagon's expectations were never realized on the battlefield, America's war managers failed to question the basic assumptions behind them. Instead, officials launched countless studies to refine the tenets of technowar. Statistical analyses of enemy attacks and activity rates, measurements of the security status of every South Vietnamese hamlet, and reams of other data poured from the battlefields of Southeast Asia into the Pentagon (Gibson, 2000; Thayer, 1975, vol. 3; Thayer, 1975, vol. 4; Thayer, 1975, vol. 9). But at the most basic level, everything came down to the "body count"—the preeminent statistic that served in those years as both the military's scorecard and its *raison d'être*. How else could you tell if the "crossover point" was within reach unless you totted up the enemy dead? The Pentagon, however, gave little thought to what this strategy—basing the entire American military effort on producing Vietnamese corpses—might mean for Vietnamese civilians.

General William Westmoreland later attempted to distance himself and the military from the term "body count." In his post-war memoir, he claimed that before he arrived in Vietnam, the United States had been forced to add the phrase to its lexicon to appease the press, although he personally "abhorred" it (Westmoreland, 1976, p. 273). In reality, however, the body count concept had been employed as early as 1951 in the Korean War. There, too, "KIAs"—enemies killed in action—became the primary indicator of success (Gartner, 1995).

While prior wars had been predicated on the taking enemy territory or the capture of an enemy capital, the guerrilla conflict in Vietnam demanded a statistic that would serve as a proxy for such progress. As a result, the body count would become, in the words of Assistant Secretary of Defense Alain Enthoven, *"the* measure of success" (Gartner & Meyers, 1995, p. 380; McNamara & VanDeMark, 1995, p. 238).

The pressure to produce high body counts flowed from the Pentagon down through the chain of command and out to the American patrols in the Vietnamese countryside. As James Gibson notes:

> Producing a high body count was crucial for promotion in the officer corps. Many high-level officers established "production quotas" for their units, and systems of "debit" and "credit" to calculate exactly how efficiently subordinate units and middle-management personnel performed. Different formulas were used, but the commitment to war as a rational production process was common to all. (Gibson, 2000, p. 112)

As a result, low-level officers, who generally had six months in the field to prove their mettle and earn a promotion, and the young combat troops they led were under constant pressure to produce enemy "kills" (Gibson, 2000).

The emphasis on body counts was evident everywhere: from the early 1960s through the early 1970s, from the Mekong Delta to the DMZ, soldiers and marines experienced the same sort of pressures. "The term 'body count' kept popping up whenever officers talked to each other," Robert Peterson of the 25th Infantry Division recalled. "It seemed that securing or pacifying an area was secondary to 'getting some kills.'" "We were always pressured for a body count," said John Beitzel, who served in the 23rd Infantry Division ("Anti-War Group Hears of 'Crimes,'" 1970, p. A15). According to Rion Causey, of the 101st Airborne Division, "It was all about body count. Our commanders just wanted body count" (Sallah & Weiss, 2006, p. 312). Gary Nordstrom, a combat medic with the 9th Infantry Division, said it was a constant drumbeat: "Get the body count. Get the body count. Get the body count. It was prevalent everywhere. I think it was the mindset of the officer corps from the top down" (Nordstrom, 2008).

Whether you achieved or surpassed what were essentially killing quotas had a major impact on the tenor of your tour of duty in Vietnam. An insufficient body count meant fewer comforts. It meant, for example, less support in the form of airlifts—resulting in sweltering, dangerous hikes through treacherous terrain instead of helicopter rides to or from base (Taylor, Jr., 1975). Under pressure from commanders, low-level officers who hadn't met body count expectations would keep their troops in the field longer, risking exhaustion, and exposing themselves and their men to a greater chance of death or injury. "I knew," recalled an officer from the 9th Infantry Division, "if I went in without a body count or at least a prisoner I'd be on the shitlist, so I kept the patrol out" (Gibson, 2000, p. 120).

While officers sought to please superiors and chased promotions, the "grunts" in the field also had a plethora of incentives to produce dead bodies. These ranged from "R&R" (rest and recreation) passes, which might allow a soldier several days at a beach resort, to medals, badges, extra food, extra beer, and light duty at base camp (Appy, 2003; Caputo,

1996; Daly & Bergman, 2000; Emerson, 1976; Herr, 1977; Puller, 1991; Turse, 2013). James Daly of the 196th Infantry Brigade recalled the rewards system: "A three-day pass for every Vietnamese you kill. And it didn't seem to matter why or who—just as long as he was Vietnamese and he was dead" (Daly & Bergman, 2000, pp. 54, 63). As another veteran recalled:

> They would set up competition. The company that came in with the biggest body count would be given in-country R and R or an extra case of beer. Now if you're telling a nineteen-year-old kid it's okay to waste people and he will be *rewarded* for it, what do you think *that* does to his psyche? (MacPherson, 2001, p. 52)

In 1970, a candid report commissioned by the Army's acting general counsel analyzed whether the pressure for kills encouraged troops "to inflate the count by violating established rules of engagement" (Turse, 2013, p. 47). The findings were damning. The report found that there was "a certain inescapable logic" to claims that emphasizing the body count led to violations of the laws of war:

> It is common knowledge that an officer's career can be made or destroyed in Vietnam. A command tour there is much sought after and generally comes only once to an individual, who may have anywhere from six months to a year to prove himself in the "crucible of combat." The pressure to excel is inevitably tremendous. . . . A primary indication of such excellence has in the past been the unit's enemy body count. One reason for this has probably been the difficulty of developing other concrete indices. Under such circumstances——and especially if such incentives as stand-downs, R&R allocations, and decorations are tied to body count figures——the pressure to kill indiscriminately, or at least report every Vietnamese casualty as an enemy casualty, would seem to be practically irresistible. (Hersh, 1972, pp. 220–226)

One of the worst effects of the body count was the fostering of what came to be known as the "mere gook rule" (MGR), which held that all Vietnamese—northern and southern, adults and children, armed enemies and innocent civilians—were something less than human, "mere gooks" who could be abused or even killed without consequence (Knightley, 1975). The MGR enabled soldiers to mistreat children for amusement; it allowed officers sitting in judgment at courts-martial to let off murderers with little or no punishment; and it paved the way for officers to willfully ignore atrocities by their troops while racking up "kills" to win favor from superiors (Turse, 2013).

Even high-ranking officers, who might never actually use the slur "gook" in public, operated with an MGR mindset (Lifton, 1973). General Westmoreland told filmmaker Peter Davis: "The Oriental doesn't put the same high price on life as does the Westerner. Life is plentiful, life is cheap in the Orient. As the philosophy of the Orient expresses it, life is not important" ("Hearts and minds," 1974). And this dismissive attitude influenced many aspects of military policy, specifically the use of heavy firepower on populated areas (Turse, 2013).

As Vietnam War correspondent Frances FitzGerald incisively notes in her classic book *Fire in the Lake*, the Americans' "bombing and artillery practices would have been unthinkable for U.S. commanders in occupied France or Italy during the Second World War" (FitzGerald, 1972, p. 375). As a result of this profligate use of firepower, "the soldier and the junior officer observed the lack of regard his superiors had for the Vietnamese," wrote war correspondent and Pulitzer prize–winner Neil Sheehan. He continued:

> The value of Vietnamese life was systematically cheapened in his mind. Further brutalized by the cycle of meaningless violence that was Westmoreland's war of attrition, and full of hatred because his comrades were so often killed and wounded by mines and booby traps set by the local guerrillas and the peasants who helped them, he naturally came to see all Vietnamese of the countryside as vermin to be exterminated. (Sheehan, 1988, p. 690).

The MGR mentality encouraged troops to kill without compunction and excused abuses. "Shouldn't bother you at all, just some more dead gooks. The sooner *they* all die, the sooner *we* go back to the World," one Marine explained to another (Warr, 1997, p. 56). At the top, pursuit of the "crossover point" demanded body counts; in the field, that meant Vietnamese KIAs; and the MGR promised that any dead Vietnamese would do.

On September 1, 1969, for example, members of the 196th Infantry Brigade in Quang Tin Province spotted a group of Vietnamese in the far distance. After observing them for around 10 minutes, Captain David Janca ordered his machine gunners to open fire and called in artillery. A small patrol was then sent forward. "Upon arrival," assistant machine gunner Robert Gray testified, "we found dead and wounded Vietnamese children." Unit member Welkie Louie recalled: "I observed about four to six Vietnamese children lying in one pile, dead. About five meters from this position were two or three wounded Vietnamese children huddled together." Artillery forward observer Robert Wolz told Army investigators that he later saw an official document in which "the dead were listed as VC". Another report even referred to them as "NVA"——members of the North Vietnamese Army. In death, this group of children had been transformed into guerrillas and then uniformed enemy soldiers (Turse, 2013, p. 46).

Sometimes prisoners or detainees were simply executed when units were short of "kills." On September 22, 1968, members of the 82nd Airborne Division captured a Vietnamese in Thua Thien Province. "I got on the radio and told the CO [commanding officer] that the man was wounded, unarmed and had surrendered," Lieutenant Ralph Loomis told Army criminal investigators. According to Loomis, his superior officer, Captain John Kapranopoulous, replied, "Dammit, I don't care about prisoners, I want a body count." Although Loomis ordered his men not to execute the prisoner, his radioman, Specialist Joseph Mattaliano, "opened up with a burst of automatic fire from his M-16 killing the Vietnamese instantly," according to Army documents (Turse, 2013, p. 46).

A second Vietnamese man, a civilian, was also detained, tied up, and then forced to kneel. The unit's forward observer recalled that Sergeant Alexander Beard:

called the CPT [captain] on the horn and told him the man had no papers and the CPT replied that the man was a gook or dink "and you know what to do with him." The group of GI's left the prisoner and walked away about 5–6 yards and then I heard one weapon fire a burst and I saw the prisoner fall. . . . I then saw the group approach the dead prisoner, remove the rope from his arms and roll him over into a ditch. (Turse, 2013, pp. 46–47)

Unit member Johnny Brinson told Army investigators that it had been a standing order for months not to take prisoners (Turse, 2013, p. 47).

Similar cold-blooded killings went on in unit after unit, all over Vietnam, for the sake of the body count. The practice of counting all dead Vietnamese as enemy kills became so pervasive that one of the signature phrases of the war was: "If it's dead and Vietnamese, it's VC" (Gibson, 2000, p. 182).

American Fighting Men

In World War II, the average American soldier was 26 years old. Most U.S. troops who served in Vietnam, by contrast, were in their teens or barely out of them. Whether they had been drafted or had volunteered (often to avoid the uncertainty of the draft), they had gone off to basic training as little more than boys.

The boot camp experience was specifically structured to reduce recruits to a psychological state akin to early childhood. Their previous 18 or so years of learning were to be stripped away through shock, separation, and physical and psychological stress, creating a *tabula rasa* for the military. For eight weeks of up to 17-hour days, every detail of their lives was prearranged, every action relearned, all stringently enforced by the omnipresent authority of the drill instructor (Appy, 1993; Ebert, 2004; MacPherson, 2001). As historian Joanna Bourke put it, a deft combination of "depersonalization, uniforms, lack of privacy, forced social relationships, tight schedules, lack of sleep, disorientation followed by rites of reorganization according to military codes, arbitrary rules and strict punishment" was employed to accomplish the task (Bourke, 1999, p. 67; Bray, 2010; Duncan, 1967; Kovic, 2005).

Frequent punishments, meted out for even minor infractions, such as not beginning and ending every sentence with "sir," were vital to the process. They consisted of both psychological debasement and physical suffering—everything from being forced to eat garbage to being exercised to the point of collapse. Even everyday training could be agonizing. "Simple exhaustion," as historian Christian Appy points out, was a "key factor in explaining the willingness of recruits to follow orders" since they quickly "learned that disobedience of any kind only brought more pain" (Appy, 1993, pp. 89–90; Ball, 1998).

Recruits were also indoctrinated into a culture of violence and brutality, which emphasized a readiness to kill without compunction (Appy, 1993; Bourke, 1999; Grossman, 1996; Lifton, 1973; MacPherson, 2001). Like many soldiers, Vietnam-era draftee Peter Milord told Appy that at first he only mouthed the violent chants during his Army training—"Kill! Kill! Kill! To kill without mercy is the spirit of the bayonet!"—but later found himself being overtaken by the ethos. "I didn't become a robot," Milord recalled, "but you can get so close to being one it's frightening" (Appy, 1993, p. 95). A West Point graduate agreed:

> Over and over and over again, you got that attitude: the spirit of the bayonet is to kill. If I've said that one time, I've said it a hundred times in my life.... "What's the spirit of the bayonet? To kill, Sir." Over and over again. And when you're that young, you're pretty impressionable. After a while you begin to believe it. You think the thought, you talk the talk. And then you walk the walk.... (Sterba, 1970, p. 15)

Another veteran recalled, "They trained us to kill without it bothering you and to do it under command without a question" (MacPherson, 2001, p. 77). Still another said that after chanting "kill, kill, kill" through basic training, advanced infantry training, and long-range reconnaissance patrol instruction, he felt completely "brainwashed" (Barnes, 2009). The constant repetition of these themes, military historian Gwynne Dyer posits, helped to desensitize recruits "at the same time they are being indoctrinated in the most explicit fashion (as previous generations were not) with the notion that their purpose is not just to be brave or to fight well; it is to kill people" (Grossman, 1995, p. 252).

Vietnam-era basic training was striking not only due to its deification of killing, but also for new tactical training methods that enabled American soldiers to kill as never before. Research conducted during World War II by Brigadier General S. L. A. Marshall and his team of historians demonstrated that, in the heat of combat, only 15–20% of infantry soldiers would actually fire their weapons at the enemy (Grossman, 1995, pp. 3–4). While his survey methods are now regarded with some skepticism, Marshall's findings are bolstered by the work of Gwynne Dyer, which indicates that, during World War II, just 1% of American Army Air Corps pilots accounted for 40% of all kills (Grossman, 1996, p. 181).

Additional research indicates that throughout history, as psychologist and former infantry officer Dave Grossman has observed, "resistance to the close range killing of one's own species is so great that it is often sufficient to overcome the cumulative influences of the instinct for self-protection, the coercive forces of leadership, the expectancy of peers, and the obligation to preserve the lives of comrades" (Grossman, 1996, p. 87). Therefore it is of little surprise that R. L. Swank and W. E. Marchand, in their pioneering work on combat soldiers during World War II, found that just 2% of all troops showed a lack of the normal human resistance to killing (Grossman, 1996, p. 180).

Through a concerted effort, however, World War II's apparently low firing rates were erased. By the Korean War, U.S. soldiers boasted a 55% firing rate. During the Vietnam War, the figure stood at 90–95% (Grossman, 1996, pp. 181, 251). As Grossman has noted, "[T]he American soldier in Vietnam was ... psychologically enabled to kill to a far greater degree than any other soldier in history" (Grossman, 1996, p. xxix). This was no mere accident. The new methods of training employed by the military in the wake of World War II utilized the tenets of Pavlovian conditioning and Skinnerian operant conditioning as a method of behavioral engineering to remake civilian men into professional soldiers/killers. Grossman notes U.S. Army and Marine Corps training during the Vietnam era, unlike earlier conflicts, utilized "conditioning techniques to develop a reflexive 'quick shoot' ability" (Grossman, 1996, p. 253).

The utilization of such methods appears to have been far from mere happenstance. As the twentieth century progressed, Joanna Bourke points out, behavioral scientists, utilizing the theories of social psychology, were actively engaged in developing methods that better enabled men to kill (Bourke, 1999). Psychological theories, which began being introduced into military training regimens, drew many adherents—including future MACV commander William Westmoreland (Bourke, 1999).

From about 1967 onward, U.S. soldiers were trained in "quick kill" or "instinctive" weapons firing techniques (Bourke, 1999). This new system was part of an evolution from World War II–era training—which consisted of a recruit lying prone, calmly firing at a stationary bullseye target—to a more realistic combat experience in which, at intermittent intervals, human-shaped targets, at various ranges, would pop up into view ("Fit to Kill," 2003; Grossman, 1996).

Soldiers who immediately fired on their targets and hit them were given the instant positive feedback of watching the target fall, instead of only later checking a piece of paper with holes in it. They then received added encouragement from instructors who rewarded them for their skill. Those, however, who failed to "engage"—that is, shoot—their targets suffered punishments and opprobrium, if not psychological or even physical abuse (Grossman, 1996, p. 253). According to Grossman:

> It made a tremendous difference, because . . . conditioned stimulus with a man-shaped silhouette pops up in the field of view. Conditioned response, you have a split second to engage the targets. Stimulus feedback, you hit the target, the target drops, stimulus response, stimulus response. What we've done is, we've made killing an unthinking, conditioned reflex. (Fit to Kill, 2003)

Moreover, by the time of the Vietnam War, safeguards that may have encouraged controlled fire that had been built into an earlier post–World War II training protocols had been eradicated because the "inclusion of specially marked 'friendly' targets" were said to have introduced a "hesitancy factor of questionable value" (McFann & Hammes, 1955, p. 23). As one Army "quick kill" instructor explained in 1968: "The student learns that the first man to fire and hit is the winner—it's a lesson that is crucial in Vietnam" (Kaufman, 1968, p. 18).

When it was suggested to an Army colonel that operant conditioning was the reason for the increase in firing rates in Vietnam, he replied: "Two shots. Bam-bam. Just like we had been trained in 'quick kill.' When I killed, I did it just like that. Just like I'd been trained. Without even thinking" (Ebert, 1993, p. 275; Grossman, 1996, p. 257). Some units continued this type of drilling even after troops were in Vietnam. "By repetition," the two top commanders of the 9th Infantry Division wrote, "this became an automatic reflex action" (Ewell & Hunt, 1974, p. 125).

A West Point graduate who served in Vietnam was explicit about linking the killing of civilians to formal instruction. "I've been through the training," he said. "And I think some of the techniques and attitudes that come through in the training could lead to what happened in Sonmy" (the massacre of more than 500 civilians by U.S. troops in the village of My Lai) (Sterba, 1970, p. 15). In fact, the impact of training methods was evident during that massacre as soldiers exhibited proper rifle-firing form and combat maneuver techniques as they gunned down villagers, even though the need to do so while firing amidst a group of unarmed and defenseless people was superfluous (Bourke, 1999; Lifton, 1973).

Remorseless killing was additionally legitimized by the explicit racism that suffused formal training. As Army veteran Wayne Smith remembered, "The drill instructors never ever called the Vietnamese, 'Vietnamese.' They called them dinks, gooks, slopes, slants, rice-eaters, everything that would take away humanity.... That they were less than human was clearly the message" (Smith, 2008). Similarly, veteran Haywood Kirkland described his experience this way:

> As soon as [you] hit boot camp ... they tried to change your total personality.... Right away they told us not to call them Vietnamese. Call everybody gooks, dinks. Then they told us when you go over in Vietnam, you gonna be face to face with Charlie, the Viet Cong. They were like animals, or something other than human.... They wouldn't allow you to talk about them as if they were people. They told us they're not to be treated with any type of mercy.... That's what they engraved into you. That killer instinct. (Terry, 1984, p. 90)

While "gooks" were an obvious "external enemy," Christian Appy notes that boot camp drill instructors often "also directed hostility at a variety of civilian targets" (1993, p. 105). Women, hippies, draft dodgers, demonstrators, and average civilians; that is, all persons non-military, were also singled out as undisciplined, corrupting, and dangerous. Immediately upon arrival at Marine Corps boot camp, for example, Ron Kovic recalled the angry shouts of the sergeants who confronted them. "I want you to take off everything that ever reminded you of being a civilian," one of them yelled, directing the men to place their belongings in a wooden box. When a recruit asked about a medal around his neck that his mother had given him, the drill instructor exploded. "Don't talk back to me," screamed one sergeant. "You fucking maggot. Don't you ever talk back to me!" The sergeants descended upon him shouting in his ears, cursing at him, and punching him until he doubled over. Afterward, the recruits were roughly shorn of their hair and then shoved and herded, naked, down a hall into the showers. "Wash all that scum off!" one of the sergeants screamed. "I want you maggots to wash all that civilian scum off your bodies forever!" (Kovic, 2005, pp. 85–88).

This anti-civilian attitude was reinforced once soldiers arrived "in-country" (Downs, 1978, p. 18). Many recall being told that, official policy aside, all Vietnamese were suspect, that even a woman or a small child were possible foes or outright enemies—a particularly sinister attitude in the context of a war that was supposedly being fought to protect Vietnamese civilians from Communist aggression (Appy, 1993; Ball, 1998; Bergerud, 1991). A child, GIs believed, might throw a grenade, while an elderly woman could construct booby traps. Although official military publications aimed at troops headed for Vietnam stressed differentiating between civilians and guerillas, some of them still suggested that everyone in a conical hat or the loose-fitting Vietnamese clothes was a potential adversary (Appy, 1993; Lifton, 1973). One veteran noted that his training made it clear that the "enemy is anything with slant eyes who lives in the village. It doesn't make any difference if it's a woman or child" (Barnes interview, 2009). Another American summarized the prevailing mindset: "So a few women and children get killed. . . . Teach 'em a damned good lesson. They're all VC or at least helping them. . . . You can't convert them, only kill them" (Duncan, 1967, p. 169).

Among the many reasons for this suspicion was that, in village after village in Vietnam, U.S. patrols regularly encountered women, children, and a few old men, but almost no military-age males. "You go into a village, and there was never a man in a village. Never," said one veteran (Henry interview, 2005). "All through the whole entire time that I spent out in the field, I could literally count the amount of men or boys that we saw," recalled another who spent a year in combat (Barnes interview, 2009). To the Americans, the "missing" men, all the village's sons and husbands, were Viet Cong guerrillas. This was, of course, one definite possibility. But it was also possible that the men were off working in a distant rice paddy, market, or town, trying to eke out a living; were serving in the U.S.-allied South Vietnamese military; or were draft dodgers, hiding from the armies of both sides. In any case, older boys and young men knew to flee on the arrival of U.S. or South Vietnamese troops since they were prime targets for conscription, arrest, or even execution. Women with young children and elderly people couldn't move as fast and stood a somewhat better chance of being spared abuse, so they were often left behind.

U.S. troops also had difficulty sorting out just who was who. They often saw only brief glimpses of figures dressed in the loose-fitting "black pajamas"—which, in the countryside, were worn by men and women, young and old, civilians and guerrillas alike. From a distance, a black-clad female farmer holding a hoe could be indistinguishable from a male fighter with a rifle. Unable to readily tell friend from foe, and often unwilling to take the risk to do so, many troops simply made the decision to fire at anyone they saw. And they often did so with the tacit support or on explicit orders from superiors.

It was illegal to order the killing of unarmed Vietnamese, no matter whom they supported in the war. But illegal orders were hardly uncommon, and how soldiers ought to react to them was, at best, murky. During basic training or in-country instruction, many soldiers were given a short lesson—generally an hour long—on the laws of war, but it paled in comparison to weeks of training that suggested a very different standard operating procedure (Lewy, 1981). As psychiatrist and war crimes expert Robert Jay Lifton notes, there was "a striking contrast between the formal instruction (given rotely if at all) to kill only military adversaries, and the informal message (loud and clear) to kill just about everyone" (Bourke, 1999, p. 177; Lifton, 1973, p. 42).

Basic training stressed that obedience to commanders was paramount. Using an instructional outline in the Army's field manual, a chaplain would often advance an Orwellian-sounding concept: "The freest soldier is the soldier who willingly submits to authority." Invoking honor and self-interest, a chaplain would tell recruits: "When you obey a lawful command you need not fear, nor worry" (Appy, 1993, pp. 92–93). But no clear definition of an *un*lawful order was offered, and recruits were pressed to exhibit simpleminded obedience (Anderson, 2007; Appy, 1993; Turse, 2013, p. 30).

The young officers whom troops were to unquestioningly obey were themselves often poorly educated in the laws of war. A 1967 Army report noted that even after receiving instruction on the proper treatment of prisoners, half the students in a class of officers-in-training about to graduate from the Army's Officer Candidate School (OCS) at Fort Benning, Georgia, told officials they would mistreat a prisoner of war to obtain information—a clear violation of the laws of war (Training in the Geneva Conventions Pertaining to Prisoners of War, n.d.). More troubling still, another study discovered that more than 96% of the Marine Corps second lieutenants surveyed would resort to torture to obtain information. The report found that troops in Vietnam "stated they would maltreat or kill prisoners, despite having just received instructions" on the laws of war. "In many cases," according to the study, "they felt they were at liberty to substitute their own judgment for the clear provisions of the [Geneva] Convention" (Hersh, 1998; Training in the Geneva Conventions Pertaining to Prisoners of War, n.d.)."

In addition to inadequate leadership and slipshod instruction, the military failed to provide troops with any specialized training on the additional responsibilities and moral complexities of fighting a guerrilla war in villages filled with civilians (Appy, 1993). Often, there was no relevant training in the laws of war as they related to the way Americans actually fought in Southeast Asia. One of the crimes detailed in the U.S. military's formal investigation of the My Lai massacre was "the burning of dwellings" (Peers, 1976, p. 315). But for years before and after the massacre, homes, hamlets, and whole villages were regularly torched by U.S. troops, generally on the orders of officers. Sometimes Americans burned homes where they found hidden war materiel or enemy propaganda literature. At other times they burned houses or hamlets in reprisal for a nearby booby trap, sniper fire, or simply because they were angry, upset, and looking to strike back at any Vietnamese people they could find.

When they did actually locate enemy forces, American troops held a distinct technological advantage. As the U.S military faced off against guerrillas armed with old rifles and homemade grenades fashioned out of soda cans or North Vietnamese troops with AK-47 assault rifles and rocket-propelled grenade launchers, it had at in its arsenal more advanced technology, destructive force, and killing power than any military in the history of the world (Bibby, 1999; Turse, 2013). American forces roared into battle with fighter jets and helicopter gunships. They shook the earth with howitzers and mortars. In a country of pedestrians and bicycles, they rolled over the landscape in massive tanks. They had armored personnel carriers for the roads and fields, Swift boats for the brown water of canals and rivers, and battleships and aircraft carriers for the blue waters off shore. The Americans unleashed millions of gallons of chemical defoliants, endless canisters of the jellied gasoline known as napalm, high explosive shells, cluster bombs, anti-personnel rockets, incendiary rockets, high explosive rockets, grenades by the millions, and myriad types of landmines.

Even average infantrymen wielded weapons of astounding power, including M-16 automatic rifles, M-60 machine guns, and M-79 grenade launchers. The M-79, for example, allowed a soldier to kill from 430 yards away. Later in the war, even the standard

M-16 could be outfitted with a semiautomatic grenade launcher, a modification that, as military psychiatrist William Gault put it, made "every soldier a miniature artilleryman" (Gault, 1971, p. 453; Stanton, 1987, pp. 298–299).

Advanced military technologies also encouraged GIs to fire their weapons for the simple thrill of it; the "hedonism of destruction . . . attested to by countless veterans," as historian Christian Appy puts it (Appy, 1993, p. 262). Veteran William Broyles, for example, wrote of the intoxicating allure of a "grunt's Excalibur"—the M-60 machine gun—while Gault called attention to the "formidable technology of arms whereby a solitary man's destructiveness is preternaturally magnified" (Bourke, 1999; Gault, 1971, pp. 451–452). The M-16, for example, was not only potent—you could fire up hundreds of rounds in a minute, and tear off a limb at 100 yards—but exceedingly compact and lightweight (Appy, 1993; Prokosch, 1995; Stanton, 1987; Thompson, 1990). The young soldiers called it "rock and roll" when they fired it on full automatic, and the rifle resembled a child's plaything to such an extent that it came to be known as the "Mattel toy" (Appy, 1993). Given all this, it's hardly surprising that the amount of ammunition fired per soldier was 26 times greater in Vietnam than during World War II.

The childlike elation elicited by the destructive power of America's weapons may have been near-universal, but the men who arrived at boot camp in their teens, who learned "quick kill" techniques, who carried the M-16s, M-60s, and M-79s through villages and rice paddies in Vietnam were not a completely representative cross-section of America. Certain types of men, it turned out, were specifically channeled into military service, into the combat arms, and sent to war in Southeast Asia. The way that "the draft," as it was known, was run had much to do with this.

Who Served and Why

During World War II, 10 million American men were drafted into military service. While student deferments existed, increasing manpower needs saw to it that only those preparing for employment in the fields of engineering, science, and medicine—jobs deemed critical to the war effort—were eligible (Baskir & Strauss, 1978). Beginning in 1948, the government implemented its first permanent peacetime draft by which all American men between ages of 18 and 26 were subject to military service. Pentagon planners calculated the number of men needed to fill the ranks of the armed services, and the Selective Service System assigned goals to 4,000 local draft boards, which summoned individuals for induction (Baskir & Strauss, 1978; Prados, 2009).

Of the 27 million men who came of draft age during the conflict, 40% went into the military, but only 10% went to Vietnam (Appy, 2015). Overall, about one-third of the American men who served in Vietnam over the course of the war were drafted, and roughly another third enlisted to avoid the draft. A 1968 Department of Defense survey found that 47.2% of volunteers said draft motivations (such as attempting to exercise some measure of control over the timing of their tour or their service branch) were their most important reason for enlisting. Patriotism, by comparison, was cited by 6.1% of enlistees (Appy, 1993).

During World War II, as historian and Vietnam veteran Andrew Bacevich notes, "the draft took black and white, rich and poor, the famous and the obscure, Ivy Leaguers and high school dropouts." The number of Harvard men killed during the war was 453—just 35 fewer than the total number of graduates of the U.S. Military Academy at West Point. The sons of top elected officials like President Franklin Roosevelt and multimillionaires like Joseph Kennedy distinguished themselves in combat. Matinee idols like Clark Gable, Henry Fonda, and Jimmy Stewart served in uniform, as did baseball stars including Ted Williams and Joe DiMaggio. The war claimed the lives of 19 players from the National Football League (NFL) (Bacevich, 2013, p. 20).

During the Vietnam war, in contrast, NFL teams made special arrangements to protect players from the draft by shuttling them into the National Guard and Reserves, which, except for one instance in 1968, were never called up during the conflict. "We have an arrangement with the Colts," Major General George Gelson, Jr., of the Maryland National Guard said of Baltimore's professional football franchise. "When they have a player with a military problem, they send him to us." In Detroit, 50-yardline tickets at Lions games helped to secure a place for two star players in an Army reserve unit. The Dallas Cowboys had 10 players assigned to a National Guard division at one time. When the Miami Dolphins were about to lose a key player to the draft, a front office official contacted Selective Service headquarters in Washington, D.C., to secure a temporary deferment until a National Guard spot could be arranged (Baskir & Strauss, 1978, p. 49).

Professional football players were no anomaly. Throughout the war, men of privilege found sanctuary from the draft, and possible service in Vietnam, through a wide variety of means. The Guard and Reserves, for their part, took on a disproportionate number of college-educated men. In 1969–1970, researchers Lawrence Baskir and William Strauss (1978, p. 49) note, "28,000 more college-trained men entered the National Guard or Reserves than were enlisted or inducted into all active forces combined." Due to Selective Service manpower "channeling" efforts, draft deferments were also automatically available for those in graduate school (until 1968) and college (until 1973). Deferments were also available to teachers, engineers, scientists, and other college-educated professionals. Local draft-boards, overwhelmingly white and white-collar, also wielded a tremendous amount of discretionary power in deciding who would be inducted into the military.

The affluent, well-educated, and those with ample financial means found many ways to avoid service (Appy, 1993). Around 3.5 million men, for example, received medical exemptions. As Christian Appy notes, one might expect the poorest Americans, with the least access to high-quality healthcare, to have received the bulk of such exemptions. In reality, these men were forced to rely on military doctors for their physicals, while affluent men could visit private physicians and obtain letters to excuse them for even the most minor injuries, such as skin rashes or high school football injuries. One study found that 90% of men with the means to press such claims were successful even if they were in good health (Appy, 2015).

While the U.S. force that deployed to Vietnam in 1965 was a highly professional one, the number of draftees quickly rose. The last quarter of 1965 saw 170,000 young men called up. The next year, draft calls jumped from 10,000 to 30,000 a month

(Prados, 2009). At the same time, the U.S. military also began to radically lower its admissions standards. Men whose scores on the military's entrance exam, the Armed Forces Qualification Test (AFQT), would have led to rejections from service in the pre-Vietnam era were channeled into the military. Many of these men were poor, half had IQ scores of less than 85, and 80% were high school dropouts. As a result of the new AFQT standards, the overall rate of rejection from military service fell from 50% to 34% between 1965 and 1966.

Even the new standards weren't sufficient to meet America's demand for soldiers, which prompted Secretary of Defense Robert McNamara, on August 23, 1966, to announce the establishment of Project 100,000—a program designed to merge the Great Society's "War on Poverty" with the war in Vietnam. "The poor of America have not had the opportunity to earn their fair share of this nation's abundance. They can be given the opportunity to return to civilian life with skills and aptitudes which will reverse the downward spiral of human decay," said McNamara as he announced that the armed services would annually admit 100,000 men who had scored low on mental aptitude tests. These men would be provided with education and training that would that would allow them to rise from the ranks of the "subterranean poor" (Appy, 1993, p. 32; Laurence & Ramsberger, 1991).

By any measure, Project 100,000 turned out to be a failure. Of the 240,000 men inducted by the program between 1966 and 1968, only 6% received the additional training they were promised, and even this proved to be little more than an attempt to raise their reading proficiency to a fifth-grade level (Appy, 1993). Instead of acquiring skills useful for the civilian job market, the "new standards men" were trained for combat at markedly elevated levels—40%, as opposed to only 25% for all enlisted men. Department of Defense estimates also found that roughly 50% of Project 100,000 men were sent to Vietnam, as opposed to 25% of men who served in the military during the era (Appy, 1993; Baskir & Strauss, 1978). These men, maligned within the military as McNamara's "moron corps," paid a heavy price, suffering a death rate twice as high as that of U.S. forces as a whole (Appy, 1993).

The "new standards men" were only one method of creating a military force to wage what David Halberstam called a "silent, politically invisible war" (Halberstam, 1972, p. 593). Instead of mobilizing the National Guard and Reserves, which might draw unwanted attention to the war and foster antiwar sentiment among politically powerful segments of the American public, Lyndon Johnson turned to the draft and active duty military personnel. He waged, in the words of Christian Appy, a "working-class war" in which about 80% of the enlisted ranks in Vietnam hailed from poor or working-class backgrounds. Appy observed:

> The Selective Service System's class-biased channeling, the military's wartime slashing of admissions standards, Project 100,000, medical exemptions that favored the well-informed and privileged, student deferments, the safe haven of the National Guard and the Reserves—these were the key institutional factors in the creation of a working-class military. But these are not the only factors that encouraged working-class boys to serve so disproportionately. In many respects [American] culture served to channel

the working class toward the military and the middle and upper classes toward college. (Appy, 1993, p. 37)

While class may be the key factor regarding the composition of the American force that fought the Vietnam War, race is still an important category for understanding marked disparities of which men served and why. Project 100,000 was a case in point. While blacks represented 10% of the entire military, they made of up 40% of the "new standards men." Outside the program, too, racial disparities were unambiguously clear. While the National Guard became a refuge for young men seeking to avoid the war, only 1% of Guardsmen were black. A 1966 study found that of the 16,638 draft board members in America, only 1.3% were black (Appy, 1993). Not surprisingly, a 1965 study found that blacks accounted for 24% of all Army combat deaths in Vietnam although they represented only 12% of the male draft-age population in the U.S. and made up only 14.8% of the Army in Vietnam at the time (Baskir & Strauss, 1978; Graham, 2003).

The Rise of the Civil Rights Movement and Black Power

Racial disparities in Vietnam were paralleled by exasperation and alienation among blacks at home. A 1965 survey showed that while 64% of whites were satisfied with their family income, only 30% of minority respondents said the same (Isserman & Kazin, 1999). That same year, the unemployment rates for non-whites was nearly double that of whites (8.1% to 4.1%) (Farber & Foner, 2001). The economic situation was even worse for minority men of or approaching draft age, with an average of 27% unemployment for black males aged 16–19 from 1965–1970. At the same time that minorities were suffering disparate economic hardship, many civil rights advocates, including prominent leaders like Dr. Martin Luther King, Jr., of the Southern Christian Leadership Council (SCLC), were growing weary of slow progress in achieving equal rights. As a result, they began carrying out high-profile protests from Washington, D.C., to rural Mississippi, but most notably in Alabama—first in Birmingham and later in Selma (Isserman & Kazin, 1999; Farber & Foner, 1994).

The civil rights movement had caught fire between the spring of 1960 and the summer of 1963 with nonviolent protests, most conspicuously in the form of lunch-counter sit-ins and "Freedom Rides" to desegregate interstate bus terminals, but progress soon began to slow (Farber & Foner, 1994). In an effort to revitalize the movement, King and the SCLC focused their efforts on Birmingham, a city that was 40% black and had seen no fewer than 50 Ku Klux Klan cross-burnings and 18 race-motivated bombings between 1957 and 1963. In May 1963, television viewers and newspaper readers saw images of police attack dogs sicced on African-American children and water-cannons knocking youngsters off their feet as the youths attempted to undertake a protest march. The vicious treatment prompted public outcry and presidential pressure that caused Birmingham's city leaders to undertake some reforms, including desegregation of public accommodations and relaxation of some employment restrictions. Building upon the success in Birmingham, 758 civil rights demonstrations followed across the country over the next 10 weeks. Not long after, President Kennedy also sent federalized

National Guard troops to safeguard the integration of the previously all-white University of Alabama (Farber & Foner, 1994).

In August, the movement received another big boost when 250,000 people gathered in Washington, D.C., in support of civil rights legislation and to call for "jobs and freedom" (Isserman & Kazin, 1999; Farber & Foner, 2001). There, Martin Luther King gave his famous "I have a dream" speech and announced that change was, one way or another, coming:

> Now is the time to make real the promises of democracy. Now is the time to rise from the dark and desolate valley of segregation to the sunlit path of racial justice. Now is the time to lift our nation from the quicksands of racial injustice to the solid rock of brotherhood. Now is the time to make justice a reality for all of God's children.
>
> It would be fatal for the nation to overlook the urgency of the moment. This sweltering summer of the Negro's legitimate discontent will not pass until there is an invigorating autumn of freedom and equality. Nineteen sixty-three is not an end, but a beginning. Those who hope that the Negro needed to blow off steam and will now be content will have a rude awakening if the nation returns to business as usual. There will be neither rest nor tranquillity in America until the Negro is granted his citizenship rights. The whirlwinds of revolt will continue to shake the foundations of our nation until the bright day of justice emerges. (King, Jr., 1963)

The next year, Robert Moses, a civil rights leader who focused on grassroots activism in the Mississippi Delta, helped organize a "Freedom Summer" program to bring white student volunteers from the North into the South to help increase black electoral turnout through voter registration drives. Over 1,000 Northern whites answered Moses' call. By the end of the "Freedom Summer," white and black volunteers had endured brutality at the hands of the Ku Klux Klan, law enforcement, and white racists; had been shot at 35 times; had suffered 30 bombings, 80 assaults, and six deaths; but made great political strides and continued to build the movement (Farber & Foner, 1994).

In early January 1965, SCLC civil rights workers launched another high profile campaign, this time in the backwater town of Selma, Alabama—a location that King said was chosen as "a symbol of bitter-end resistance to the civil rights movement in the Deep South" (Isserman & Kazin, 1999). Throughout January and February, Selma's Sheriff Jim Clark and his deputies became infamous for beating voting rights supporters with nightsticks and carrying out mass arrests of protesters. Law enforcement violence culminated in the "Bloody Sunday" battle of March 7, 1965. During the day, marchers protesting the killing of a man who had shielded his mother from a beating at a voting rights rally were attacked by Alabama state troopers and Clark's posse who were armed with billy clubs, tear gas, and lengths of rubber hose wrapped in barbed wire. That evening, television stations interrupted their normal programming to show raw footage of the violent encounter, outraging many across the nation. On March 15, President Johnson took to the airwaves and proclaimed that the violence in Selma was not a "Negro problem" or "Southern problem," but an "American problem" and federalized National Guard troops to protect civil rights activists (Isserman & Kazin, 1999).

On July 2, Johnson took his support further and signed into law the Civil Rights Act, which outlawed segregation in public facilities and racial discrimination in employment and education (Isserman & Kazin, 1999). Just over a month later, he signed the Voting Rights Act, which guaranteed African-Americans, including the South's 2.5 million disenfranchised blacks, the right to vote (Isserman & Kazin, 1999). New laws, however, could not make up for generations of injustice. On August 11, in the black community of Watts, California, racial tensions, animosity towards law enforcement, and typical urban problems like high unemployment and poor-performing schools, mixed with tales of police brutality and ignited six days of rioting, looting, and arson—all to the chant of "Burn, baby, burn!" (Farber & Foner, 1994, p. 111).

"These fucking cops have been pushin' me 'round all my life. Kickin' my ass and things like that. Whitey ain't no good. He talked 'bout law and order, it's his law and his order, it ain't mine," said one young rioter reflecting on the situation in Watts, where 98% of residents were black but 200 of 205 police officers were white (Isserman & Kazin, 1999, p. 141). In the end, it took 16,000 law enforcement personnel and National Guardsmen five days to quell the rioting, which left 34 dead, 1,000 injured, 4,000 in jail, and caused $40 million in property damage (Farber & Foner, 1994; Isserman & Kazin, 1999).

The mood of the streets soon found expression in the activist community. In the spring of 1966, Stokely Carmichael was elected chairman of the Student Non-Violent Coordinating Committee (SNCC), ushering in a new generation of civil rights leadership. SNCC had been at the vanguard of the civil rights movement of the early 1960s, leading multiracial "freedom rides" on interstate buses to desegregate bus terminals and challenging Jim Crow laws throughout the South. As the decade passed its midpoint, however, many in the SNCC had grown frustrated by the mainstream civil rights movement, typified by King's SCLC, which they saw as timid, and the old guard of the SNCC, which preached nonviolence and interracialism. Instead, Malcolm X, the Muslim African-American leader who had been assassinated in 1965 (and had embraced black nationalism and saw black adherence to nonviolence as undignified), not King, became the icon of many young black activists (Farber & Foner, 1994; Isserman & Kazin, 1999).

In June 1966, after civil rights pioneer James Meredith was shot by a white gunman on just the second day of his one-man "March Against Fear" to promote voter registration in Mississippi, prominent movement leaders, Carmichael included, vowed to continue his march. Along the route, an SNCC activist began firing up the crowd with the slogan "Black Power!" Carmichael adopted the phrase and announced to the media, "The only way we gonna stop them white men from whuppin' us is to take over. We been saying *freedom* for six years—and we ain't got nothin'. What we gonna start saying now is Black Power!" (Farber, 2001; Isserman & Kazin, 1999, p. 175).

The concept of black power found a receptive audience in two West Coast militants, Huey Newton and Bobby Seale, who formed the Black Panther Party for Self Defense in 1966. As the Black Panthers armed themselves to discourage police brutality and abuse of authority (in addition to advocating community control and black self-help), small but growing numbers of white radicals expressed solidarity with the group and embraced the rhetoric of "picking up the gun," even if few actually did. The Panthers were a different story. Between 1967 and 1969, nine police officers were killed and 56 were wounded in shootouts with members of the black militant group, while dozens of Panthers were injured and 10 killed by members of law enforcement (Farber, 2001; Isserman & Kazin, 1999).

The antiwar movement would grow alongside the civil rights movement and increasing black militancy. The 1965 escalation of the American war in Vietnam led to growing criticisms by newspapers and prominent Democratic senators as well as increased awareness on the part of the general public (Herring, 1986). In September 1965, 19% of Americans said that Vietnam was the most important problem facing the United States, second only to the 27% who cited civil rights. Three months later, civil rights had dropped to 19%, while Vietnam had jumped to 33% (Gallup, 1978). In the face of increased concern over U.S. involvement in the conflict, a burgeoning antiwar movement began to become ever more visible. In March 1965, a first ever "teach-in" about the Vietnam War on the campus of the University of Michigan attracted 3,000 people. By the end of the year, similar events had been held at around 120 colleges and universities nationwide.

The teach-ins came to typify the actions—later joined by campus revolts, draft resistance, moratoriums, and large-scale rallies—of the emerging New Left, a movement of young, largely white, college-educated Americans interested in addressing political, social, and economic inequity. In April 1965, student activists from one of the most prominent New Left groups, the Students for a Democratic Society (SDS), sponsored an antiwar march in Washington, D.C., that drew 20,000 people. That August, hundreds of protesters from the University of California (where, in the fall of 1964, the student Free Speech Movement had drawn widespread attention to the beginnings of the New Left), attempted to block the path of troop trains en route to the Oakland Army Base (Isserman & Kazin, 1999).

SDS was joined in its antiwar activities by the American Friends Service Committee, a prominent Quaker group, and the Committee for a Sane Nuclear Policy (SANE). More mainstream and conventional critics of the war, like Democratic senators Frank Church, Mike Mansfield, and George McGovern, called upon President Johnson to seek a negotiated settlement to the conflict (Addington, 2000; Herring, 1986). In 1966, Senator J. William Fulbright held hearings on Vietnam and questioned whether the Gulf of Tonkin Resolution had given Johnson the authority to escalate the war, while Senator Robert Kennedy, the brother of the slain President, joined calls for a negotiated peace (Addington, 2000). The huge protests in the fall of 1965 in Berkeley, New York City, and Washington—which drew 15,000, 20,000, and 25,000 people, respectively— looked positively tiny just two years later when hundreds of thousands marched in New York. Millions would flood the streets in the years that followed as crowds that once were typified by jackets, ties, and skirts gave way to increasing numbers of long-haired protesters wearing military surplus gear or the hippie garb favored by the growing counterculture (Addington, 2000; Gettleman, 1985). Increasingly, members of SDS, SNCC, and others in the New Left saw themselves as a repressed minority in their own country, identified with the Black Panthers, and championed revolutionary movements sweeping the Third World.

Notions of Black Power and black consciousness would eventually surface in Southeast Asia, along with a growing GI discontent, but these developments were still a long way off and would have been unimaginable to most Americans when, in the spring of 1965, President Lyndon Johnson signed off on a change in tactics for U.S. troops in Vietnam, permitting offensive action. A few days later, he would sign a hush-hush National Security Memorandum providing for a significant increase in U.S. forces, and would also approve a 12-point covert operations program to be run by the CIA (Prados, 2009). The war in Vietnam was entering a new phase.

America in Vietnam

In March 1965, the first official U.S. combat troops in South Vietnam, a contingent of Marines, waded ashore at Da Nang. More Marines arrived in the next months and soon began patrolling rural Quang Nam province, a heavily populated heartland of the Vietnamese revolution. U.S. troops continued to do so into the 1970s in an effort to pacify the region, but never succeeded (Turse, 2013). While they pursued "hearts and minds" efforts, like building cribs for orphanages, making desks for school children, and handing out school supplies, food, and clothing, American forces mainly fought a war in the villages—launching near-ceaseless search-and-destroy operations, driving large numbers of the rural villagers into shantytowns and refugee camps, burning hamlets, and taking heavy casualties in the process (Lewy, 1981; Morris & West, 1970). Lieutenant General Victor Krulak, commander of the Fleet Marine Force, Pacific, summarized the military's mindset:

> The real war is among the people and not among these mountains. . . . If we can destroy the guerrilla fabric among the people, we will automatically deny the larger [enemy] units the food and the intelligence and the taxes, and the other support they need. (Young, 1991, p. 165)

In practice, that meant the fabric of rural life in Quang Nam would be torn to shreds.

On July 12, 1965, for example, Marines entered the village of Cam Ne and met stiff resistance, suffering seven casualties. The next month, the Americans had their revenge (Lewy, 1981). With CBS correspondent Morley Safer and a cameraman in tow, the troops set out for the area in armored vehicles. "They told us if you receive one round from the village, you level it," recalled Marine Reginald Edwards (Young, 1991, p. 143). Safer heard much the same:

> I talked to a captain, trying to get some idea what the operation was about. And he said, "We've had orders to take out this complex of villages called Cam Ne." I'd never heard anything like that. I'd heard of search-and-destroy operations; I'd seen places ravaged by artillery or by air strikes. But this was just a ground strike going in. He said to "take out" this complex of villages. And I thought perhaps he's exaggerating. . . .

The troops walked abreast toward this village and started firing. They said that there was some incoming fire. I didn't witness it, but it was a fairly large front, so it could have happened down the line. There were two guys wounded in our group, both in the ass, so that meant it was "friendly fire."

They moved into the village and they systematically began torching every house—every house as far as I could see, getting people out in some cases, using flame throwers in others. No Vietnamese speakers, by the way, were among the group with the flame thrower. (Ferrari & Tobin, 2004; Safer, 1990, pp. 85–94)

About 150 homes in Cam Ne were burned; others were bulldozed, as Marines razed two entire hamlets. Artillery was then called in on the wreckage. According to reports, one child was killed and four women wounded (Safer, 1990; Turse, 2013; Young, 1991). In reality, many more may have died. Edwards remembered being ordered to fire on a fleeing Vietnamese and missing, only to see another Marine kill the man with a grenade as he was dashing through a doorway. "But what happened," Edwards said, "was it was a room full of children. Like a schoolroom. And he was runnin' back to warn the kids that the Marines were coming. And that's who got hurt. All those little kids and people." Months later, Safer learned that Cam Ne had been targeted because the Saigon government's province chief wanted to punish the village for delinquent taxes (Young, 1991, pp. 143–144).

Cam Ne was no anomaly. Day after day, hamlets were attacked as a matter of policy. On August 2, 1965, for example, U.S. artillery blasted the "Vietcong dominated" village of Chan Son with 1,000 artillery shells. After the bombardment, Marines attacked Chan Son, one of them bellowing, "Kill them. I don't want anyone moving." The Americans came upon a dead woman with a wound in her side. Next to her, a baby with an injured arm was wailing in pain. As enemy shots rang out, a Marine threw a grenade into a bunker, killing two children. In all, 25 people in the village died in the attack, according to U.S. sources. NLF reports put the total at more than 100. Afterwards, acting on orders from higher command, the Marines burned homes from which they had received enemy fire (Pickerell, 1966, p. 2; Turse, 2013, p. 112).

The next day, just three miles south of Da Nang, Marines set close to one hundred homes ablaze in response to sniper fire from a village (Turse, 2013, p. 113). Days later, Duc An, also south of Da Nang, went up in flames when Marines used incendiary white phosphorus rockets against "Viet Cong positions" in the village (Turse, 2013, p. 113). Another nearby enclave, Phu Loc, "was a prosperous hamlet of brick houses on some of Quang Nam's richest river land," wrote one reporter. It, too, was targeted and "completely burned by American bombs because the land was too rich to leave to the Communists" (Larsen, 1971). Civilians in the region suffered immensely. By the end of the year, a U.S. advisor noted that Quang Nam's main hospital needed additional supplies to cope with increasing numbers of wounded (Turse, 2013, p. 113).

The Marines were soon joined by Army troops. In May 1965, soldiers from the 173rd Airborne Brigade deployed to Vietnam. In July, elements of the 1st Infantry Division and 101st Airborne Division also arrived. In September, they were joined by the nearly 16,000-man 1st Cavalry Division. Unlike standard infantry divisions that were supported by roughly 100 aircraft and 3,000 ground vehicles, the 1st Cavalry, the Army's first "airmobile" division, was supported by 434 helicopters and light airplanes and only 1,600 land vehicles. Air mobility—the tactical doctrine of utilizing helicopters to find the enemy; transport men, weapons, and material into battle; provide ground soldiers with gunship support (in the form of machine gun and rocket fire); and position artillery, among other missions—was most famously employed by the 1st Cavalry and 101st Airborne Divisions, but it was a fundamental military concept utilized by many other U.S. and allied units throughout the war (Clodfelter, 1995).

In November 1965, General Westmoreland charged the 1st Cavalry to seek out and destroy enemy forces operating in the Ia Drang river valley. Over the course of a month, U.S. forces clashed with North Vietnamese troops in "one of the largest and most conventional campaigns of the war" (Appy, 2003, p. 129). "The 1st Battalion had been fighting continuously for three or four days, and I had never seen such filthy troops," Specialist-4 Jack Smith, a supply clerk who was nonetheless out in the field, recalled of the fighting (Smith, 1967, p. 208). Men wore tattered clothes and were splattered with blood—some of it their own, some from their wounded compatriots. After three days of heavy bombardment, he wrote in an article for *The Saturday Evening Post*, men no longer automatically dropped to the ground as artillery rained down, having become accustomed to interpreting the sound of an especially close shell from one a little farther off.

Late one morning, 100 enemy soldiers jumped up and made a headlong charge at the American lines. The Cavalry troopers answered with everything they had, and planes streaked through the skies dropping what, to Smith, looked like "green confetti." It may have resembled a ticker-tape, but it was actually antipersonnel charges that exploded on impact. "Every one of the gooks was killed," he wrote. Another group of North Vietnamese troops almost breached a weak point in the American lines, but the planes dropped napalm canisters on them. "I couldn't see the gooks," Smith recalled, "but I could hear them scream as they burned. A hundred men dead just like that" (Smith, 1967, p. 208). Afterward, his company dug in and withstood another minor attack, then took fire throughout the night.

The next morning, Smith's unit received orders to move out. "I guess our commanders felt the battle was over," he wrote (Smith, 1967, p. 209). Hiking toward a helicopter landing zone six miles away, the unit encountered four North Vietnamese soldiers who claimed to be deserters and said there were three or four diehard snipers in the trees ahead who would not surrender. Soon, bullets came whizzing past the men. Instead of three or four sharpshooters, there were reportedly more than one hundred North Vietnamese tied to high branches of the trees all around them. An officer gave the order to make a break for it and the Americans began running, not realizing that they were heading deeper into the ambush.

Smith watched as one of the unit's radiomen was shot. "I knelt down and looked at him, and he shuddered and started to gurgle deep in his stomach. His eyes and tongue popped out, and he died" (Smith, 1967, p. 210). The soldier had been hit directly in the heart. Smith had been yelling for a medic and stopped just as North Vietnamese machine gunners opened up on the surviving Americans. He remembered:

> Men all around me were screaming. The fire was now a continuous roar. We were even being fired at by our own guys. No one knew where the fire was coming from, and so the men were shooting everywhere. Some were in shock and were blazing away at everything they saw or imagined they saw. (Smith, 1967, p. 210)

Soldiers all around Smith fell victim to the withering fire from the North Vietnamese or errant shots from their brothers-in-arms. They were crying out in agony, collapsing, some of them bleeding out.

Fighting at close quarters, Smith was able to fire point blank at an enemy machine-gunner. "I saw his face disappear," was how he put it. "I guess I blew his head off, but I never saw the body and did not look for it" (Smith, 1967, p. 211). Just then, American airplanes soared over them, dropping napalm on North Vietnamese machine gunners. Smith heard the anguished cries not only of enemy troops, but also Americans who had also been hit by the brutal incendiary agent. Despite the bombing, the firefight continued. "All around me, those who were not already dead were dying or severely wounded, most of them hit several times," wrote Smith who was one of the few members of his unit who had not been wounded. "I must have been talking a lot, but I have no idea what I was saying. I think it was 'Oh God, Oh God, Oh God,' over and over. Then I would cry" (Smith, 1967, p. 212).

The enemy attack continued, and soon his unit's position was overrun and enemy troops began executing wounded Americans. Smith played dead in an effort to survive. While lying on the ground, he was wounded by an American grenade attack on the North Vietnamese who now occupied his unit's position. Finally, Smith decided he had to escape and began creeping away.

> I crawled over many bodies, all still. The 1st Platoon just didn't exist anymore. One guy had his arm blown off. There was only some shredded skin and a piece of bone sticking out of his sleeve. The sight didn't bother me anymore. The artillery was still keeping up a steady barrage, as were the planes, and the noise was as loud as ever, but I didn't hear it anymore. (Smith, 1967, p. 214)

Smith managed to crawl away and nearly reached his unit's mortar platoon just before the North Vietnamese machine gun teams set their sights on those men. It took the enemy gunners just 30 seconds to all but wipe them out. "When they opened up, I heard a guy close by scream, then another, and another. Every few seconds someone would scream. Some got hit several times," he wrote.

> It also seemed that most of them were hit in the belly. I don't know why, but when a man is hit in the belly, he screams an unearthly scream. Something you cannot imagine; you actually have to hear it. When a man is hit in the chest or the belly, he keeps on

screaming, sometimes until he dies. I just lay there, numb, listening to the bullets whining over me and the 15 or 20 men close to me screaming and screaming and screaming. They didn't even stop for breath. They kept on until they were hoarse, then they would bleed through their mouths and pass out. They would wake up and start screaming again. Then they would die. (Smith, 1967, p. 215)

Smith lay crying next to a severely wounded sergeant who shrieked incessantly, begging someone to help him or kill him. The ground had turned red and sticky as men bled out. There were no medics, no medical supplies, no relief. Several wounded men killed themselves due to the pain or the fear of being taken prisoner, though the North Vietnamese, Smith said, weren't taking captives.

At dusk, Smith watched as several helicopters attempted to land, but were driven off by heavy enemy fire. Then the North Vietnamese began mortaring his position, using American equipment they had just captured. For the second time that day, Smith was wounded. After bandaging his bleeding leg, he crawled off in search of water, finding the canteen of a dead man that was, he wrote, about one-third blood. He drank, then crawled onward and lay among the dead. Around midnight, he heard soldiers approaching and gripped a grenade, intending to use it to kill himself rather than be taken prisoner. The troops, however, turned out to be Americans sent to rescue the wounded. Since they had only four stretchers, they could take only those with the most severe injuries. Smith was left with a promise that they would return in a few hours.

As the night dragged on, Smith and the other wounded around him heard nearby North Vietnamese troops and prayed they wouldn't come closer to the almost defenseless survivors. They listened and stayed silent as other wounded Cavalrymen begged for their lives before being silenced by gunshots. An hour before dawn, Smith heard the crack of gunfire and ricochets close by. It wasn't enemy gunners shooting this time, but an advancing group of Americans. A man near Smith was hit by the friendly fire, he recalled. "He let out a long sigh and gurgled" (Smith, 1967, p. 219).

As dawn broke, Smith looked around to see a blood-soaked hellscape. He was surrounded by dead men and found he had been resting on the corpse of a friend through the night. Those bodies were, Smith wrote, "beginning to stink" (Smith, 1967, p. 220). Up above, dead Vietnamese snipers who had lashed themselves to branches hung lifeless, dangling from the trees. Unable to ascertain if the area was secure enough, medevac helicopters were still withheld by American commanders and, instead, an artillery barrage and airstrikes pummeled a landing zone throughout the morning. Finally, after about 24 hours of combat, Smith was evacuated.

When the losses were tallied, it was found that Smith's company suffered 93% casualties—an even split between those killed and those wounded. Of the 500 men in his battalion, just 84 returned to their base camp a few days later. Smith spent a week shuttling between field hospitals, before ending up at an American medical center in Japan where he underwent two operations. "They tell me I'll walk again," he wrote. "But no one can tell me when I will stop having nightmares" (Smith, 1967, p. 222).

U.S. troops suffered 300 dead during the battle for the Ia Drang, but claimed more than 3,000 enemy kills, prompting MACV commander William Westmoreland to declare the battle a victory. Still, the campaign also demonstrated that the enemy was—when it chose to do so—willing to stand firm and slug it out with U.S. forces and their colossal firepower and technological superiority. The Americans also found that while the much touted air-mobility concept was crucial in moving infantry and wounded in and out of the field, it could not make tough topography, like thick jungles or steep hills, irrelevant. Soldiers still had to be dropped into convenient landing zones (LZs) and then strike out on foot through harsh terrain. Nor could air mobility save American ground forces—as was the case for Jack Smith and his unit—from devastating ambushes that pinned them down for long stretches of time (Appy, 2003).

Fighting the War

The enemy's control of tactical initiative often meant soldiers were dropped into a landing zone (LZ) and sent out to patrol on foot for days and sometimes weeks through harsh terrain, be it jungles, mountains, or rice paddies, in an effort to search out and destroy enemy forces. Some 12.5% of the time the LZ would be "hot" and U.S. troops were attacked as they deployed. Whether hot or cold, the choppers soon flew off and left troops without the protection of their powerful weapons systems. Alone in the countryside, columns of "grunts," spaced about five yards apart, then set out in an often vain search for an elusive foe (Appy, 1993).

As Leonard Dutcher waited for a helicopter to airlift his unit ten miles north of his base camp to conduct a "search and clear" operation on a mountain suspected of being a Viet Cong sanctuary, he wrote a letter to his parents. "I've got more equipment on that I don't think I could use it all in a month of Sundays," he told them.

> I have over six hundred rounds of M16 ammo, six frag[mentation] grenades, three white phosphorus grenades and four smoke grenades. I've also got on a bayonet, entrenching tool, helmet, rifle and web gear. In my field pack there is enough C-rations to last for three days, foot powder, extra socks, flares, and cigarettes. On my web gear there is four canteens of water, first aid kit, ammo pouches, and field glasses. (Ebert, 1993, p. 163)

Some men also wore steel helmets with cloth covers that, in addition to protecting their heads, became billboards for scrawled slogans, complaints, jokes, or calendars reflecting their days left in-country. Others wore cloth "boonie hats" or "bush covers" which were more comfortable, but offered no protection (Ebert, 1993).

Throughout the war, countless "grunts" laden with 40–80 pounds of gear regularly trudged mile after mile through sweltering jungles and flooded rice paddies, through thorny hedgerows or razor-sharp elephant grass standing six feet high, up and down forested highland hills and valleys. Dirty, hungry, and dehydrated, they slogged through mud and muck and water, each step an ordeal, day after day, sometimes for weeks, until their feet swelled and the skin painfully sloughed off in chunks. They came down with bacterial infections, suffered oozing sores, "crotch rot," and other fungal infections. They burned off leeches and faced heat exhaustion, all while being bitten by fire ants and feasted on by mosquitoes.

"What the soldiers did," recalled *New York Times* correspondent Gloria Emerson in her classic book *Winners and Losers*:

> the walking, the searching, the hiding, the waiting, the ambushes and the shooting— was known as humping. Humping the boonies, they would say, hating it. To meet the enemy was to have contact, to be in a firefight. It did not matter if the boonies was elephant grass or a rubber plantation with slender, sticky trees, if it was the great tangled blotches of jungle or flat, scratchy land. It was all of these things and more. (Emerson, 1976, pp. 66–67)

Often, "humping" led to nothing but fatigue. Dwight Reiland recalled a typical sequence of waking up, getting organized, and then moving out on patrol. "You walked an hour and sweated, took your breaks. Maybe a break for lunch and send out a couple X-ray [local] patrols in different directions to see if they would find any indication of enemy activity," he remembered. "They would come back and off you went. Lots of days that is all that happened" (Ebert, 2004, pp. 207–208).

One patrol blended into the next, lulling men into complacency; and then all hell would break loose. Christian Appy, in his *Patriots: The Vietnam War Remembered From All Sides,* offers a composite vision of "contact":

> As the patrol moves off into the jungle, the silence is shattered by small arms fire. The platoon has walked into a Viet Cong ambush. . . . Twenty miles away at an airbase in Danang or offshore on an aircraft carrier in the South China Sea, word arrives that an American unit has made contact. Several F-4 Phantom jets are scrambled. Within minutes they catch sight of a small forward observation plane marking a spot in the jungle with a flare. There is a deafening roar as the jets sweep in and drop napalm and bombs on the target. The guerillas have learned to anticipate the likelihood of an air strike and may have disengaged quickly to scurry deeper into the jungle or into an underground bunker. Or perhaps they continue to "cling to the belt" of their enemy, a common guerrilla tactic. Occasionally, combatants on both sides are caught in the destruction that rains down from above, their fates entangled by forces beyond their control. Survivors are left to evacuate their wounded, the guerrillas to the nearest jungle hospitals, the Americans onto medical evacuation helicopters that often put casualties into field hospitals in a matter of minutes. (Appy, 2003, p. xxiii)

While Appy's scenario only hints at the wide range of combat-related experiences of American troops, most infantrymen were, indeed, engaged in small patrols during search-and-destroy operations. By June of 1967, in fact, U.S. battalions were spending 86% of their time on such missions, but where they might do so and whom they might encounter varied widely (Kinnard, 1991).

Some troops served in areas that were almost devoid of civilians, and predominantly faced enemy regulars. The Central Highlands, for example, were home to only 5% of the population, but the rugged terrain was perfect for enemy troops who trekked down from North Vietnam via the so-called Ho Chi Minh Trail—the enemy supply-line and troop transit highway. There, not coincidentally, U.S. forces gener-ally fought uniformed North Vietnamese (Appy, 2003). Some faced nightmare battles and, like Jack Smith and his fellow 1st Cavalry troopers in the Ia Drang valley, took heavy losses. Almost three years after that battle, another element of the 1st Cavalry Division—Company D, 2nd Battalion, 8th Cavalry—was carrying out a search-and-destroy mission in South Vietnam's National Forest. After meeting enemy resistance on May 21, 1968, the unit called in three days of artillery and airstrikes to soften up what was assumed to be a large enemy force. Finally, they moved forward. Medic Charles Dawson recalled:

> We advanced without any contact whatsoever when our lead element spotted two enemy soldiers and killed them both. As we continued on farther, Charlie had concealed himself and set up an ambush, which he let us walk right into before he sprung the trap. The enemy opened up, hitting one of our men in both legs. At this time we pulled back, but in the excitement we didn't know that we had a man laying back there wounded until we heard his shouts.
>
> At this time we couldn't get to him because the firing was so heavy, so I crawled for-ward aided the man, but I couldn't pull him back because they had me pinned down. A five-man team was sent forward to provide a base of fire for me while I carried my wounded buddy back. But those five men never made it to my position. They were all shot down and wounded. So I left the other man and began applying aid to the other wounded members of my company. Richard [Carlson, a fellow medic] crawled up to my side and began patching up the nearest man to him when he was shot in the leg. He was bleeding badly and in great pain. I applied morphine to his wound to ease the pain (Edelman, 1985, pp. 76–77).

Once the morphine took effect, Carlson rolled himself over to an officer who had been shot in the head and attempted to treat him, Dawson later wrote. In the process, Carlson was shot three more times—once in the arm and twice in the chest. Dawson scrambled over and began applying bandages to staunch the bleeding. "Doc, I'm a mess," Carlson said looking up at Dawson. "Oh God, I don't want to die. Mother, I don't want to die. Oh God, don't let me die." A helicopter swooped in to evacuate Carlson and the other wounded to a hospital for treatment, but the 20-year-old medic died before it arrived (Edelman, 1985, pp. 76–77).

Many other troops experienced short firefights that filled them with pure terror but ended without definitive resolution—no enemy bodies, no American casualties. Other times, the Americans emerged victorious, though what they had actually won, in the end, was sometimes just as uncertain. In late 1968, for instance, *Newsweek*'s Kevin Buckley accompanied the men of Company A, 1st Battalion, 28th Infantry of the 1st Infantry Division near Loc Ninh, some 70 miles north of Saigon, as they marched be-neath the shade of rubber trees. In the distance, they heard the rattle of gunfire and learned that D Company, a sister unit out ahead of them, was held up by an enemy landmine. Eventually, however, the "mine" was discovered to be nothing but one of the bowl-like containers used to collect latex from the trees of the rubber plantation.

Without drawing so much as one shot from a sniper, Company D passed through an area that had previously seen heavy fighting, evidenced by caved-in North Vietnamese bunkers and pockmarked rubber trees. When Company A got to the area, however, enemy troops opened up from the surrounding jungle with automatic weapons, causing the Americans to scramble for cover and begin returning fire. Edward Knoll, the 21-year-old company commander, strode forth, standing upright, "and started to pump round after round into the underbrush," wrote Buckley. Then, all of a sudden, he ordered a ceasefire, fearing that they were actually firing on D Company. During the lull, the enemy opened up on them again. "Screw it! Fire!" Knoll yelled. "They're gooks all right" (Buckley, 1968, p. 665).

The Americans poured gunfire and grenades into the jungle. After a while, Knoll instructed his South Vietnamese interpreter to call for the enemy troops to surrender. The interpreter was huddled behind a tree and refused to come out into the open. "Just kill them," he told Knoll, before halfheartedly calling out to the enemy and flopping back on the ground. "At this point, possibly out of disgust," wrote Buckley, "Knoll indulged in pure bravado by relieving himself against the tree in what seemed to me to be in full view of enemy troops" (Buckley, 1968, p. 665). Only once he was finished did the North Vietnamese open up again, covering a running withdrawal that saw them bolt from the jungle, to bunkers, and then a series of smaller fighting positions.

Company A pursued them and poured gunfire at the Vietnamese. As the remnants of the enemy unit fled, Knoll ordered his men forward where they found four dead soldiers—their bodies mutilated by the Americans' weapons. "OK, you mother, you tried to kill one of my buddies, didn't you," a soldier said, lifting up one of the corpses. The men of Company A then proceeded to strip the dead men—taking their belts, knives, and rifles and leaving 1st Infantry Division patches on their faces. "We let those people know who's been through here," one of the men said as they moved out (Buckley, 1968, p. 666).

Taking trophies from North Vietnamese troops was common in many units, but plenty of infantrymen and riflemen hardly ever encountered uniformed enemy soldiers. Like the Marines who began patrolling outside of Da Nang in 1965, they instead fought a war in the villages of South Vietnam with enemy farmer-fighters. Often, guerrillas withdrew shortly after an attack. And many times, the Americans encountered only their mines or other booby-traps, leaving local civilians in the path of angry American troops. When soldiers from the 1st Infantry Division entered a village, as part of a search-and-destroy operation north of Saigon in early 1966, their lieutenant ordered them to "Kill everything." One sergeant said he wouldn't kill women and children, but as the troops moved through the village, shooting animals and setting fire to homes, a soldier tossed a grenade into a bomb shelter where voices had been heard. After the explosion, ten or more women and children came out of the bunker, crying. Another soldier approached. "Oh my God!" he cried out. "They hit a little girl." The seven-year-old had a hole in the back of her skull. She clung to life for a few moments then shuddered and died (Sack, 1966).

Bob Gabriel, who served with Company B, 2nd Battalion, 12th Cavalry of the 1st Cavalry Division, recalled patrolling through the Que Son valley, on the border of

Quang Nam and Quang Tin provinces, in early 1968. The guerrillas attacked so often that his unit couldn't remain in the field at night and, during the day, B Company made it so the civilians in the area could hardly live at all. He remembered:

> We had orders to burn all the villages in the valley. We'd tell all the people to go to the little town of Que Son. We burned a lot of villages. We'd just go burn people's houses down. . . . A lot of them were holed up in bunkers and stuff and we'd tell them to come out, and they wouldn't come out and one thing leads to another and somebody will throw a hand grenade in there and people would get hurt. (Appy, 2003, p. 299)

In March 1968, West Pointer Robert Johnson began serving in the heavily populated region south of Da Nang. He testified that about "90 percent of the surrounding countryside was a free-fire zone . . . we were allowed to shoot anything that moves in that area." Artillery was, he said, unleashed in an effort to terrorize villagers into leaving the countryside, and ground operations were often just as brutal. "On one of our first major operations, we bombed, strafed, hit with artillery, a particular village complex for approximately three hours, and then moved up. . . . When I got to the village, there was nothing there but civilians," he recalled. "I guess I participated in about thirteen search-and-destroy operations. On all these operations we systematically destroyed every home. . . . If we could not burn the hootches [homes], we would blow them up with dynamite" (Dellums, 1972, pp. 40–42).

Such attacks happened time and again. On April 15, 1970, for instance, members of Company B, 1st Battalion, 5th Marines, asked their company commander whether there were "any friendlies" in the hamlet of Le Bac-2. As Sergeant Paul Cox recalled, his commander replied: "No, this is a free fire zone" (Cox interview, 2009). Immediately, there was shooting. "The first hut I got to, there was an old mama-san lying in the middle of the floor gut-shot, she was dying," Cox recalled. At the next hut, a small group of elderly villagers and mothers with children had been gunned down. Nearby, he saw yet another similar scene (Cox interview, 2009; Ostertag, 2006).

Inside the hamlet, a young girl named Ho Thi A watched in terror as the carnage unfolded. "There were three of us standing at the entrance to the bunker, me and two old women—my neighbor and my grandmother," she remembered. They had just climbed out of their bomb shelter when an American took aim and shot the two elderly women, one after the other. Ho Thi A wheeled around and scrambled back into the bunker, cowering there as the Americans tossed in grenades after her. She later emerged to find that 15 villagers had been killed in Le Bac-2 that day. All of the victims, she and other survivors of the massacre said, were civilians (Turse, 2008; Turse, 2013, p. 261).

Two provinces to the south, in Quang Ngai, 2nd Lieutenant Frederick Downs and his men from the 4th Infantry Division weaved their way through dangerous *punji* pits and "wait-a-minute" vines that entangled men and held up patrols. Like so many other infantrymen, they struggled with the heat and insects and forced themselves forward by sheer will. "It was a search-and-destroy mission," he recalled, "which meant we searched all the hootches we found and then burned them down. Whether a single farmer's hootch or a whole village—all were burnt" (Downs, 1978, p. 31).

Looking back, top U.S. commander General William Westmoreland claimed that "many Americans apparently failed to comprehend 'search-and-destroy,'" claiming that it was *not* a "brutal" policy of "aimless searches in the jungle" and the "random destroying of villages." Instead, Westmoreland insisted the tactic's meaning had been distorted by "detractors of the war" (Kinnard, 1991, pp. 39–41; Westmoreland, 1976). His troops, however, had a firm idea of what it really meant. One soldier, being questioned under oath about a massacre perpetrated by his unit, testified about how the term was understood in the field:

Q. What about this operation. . . . Were you told anything—were you given any special instructions?

A. Destroy everything.

Q. Destroy it all: village, livestock, and food stocks?

A. (Witness nods in the affirmative.) That's what a search and destroy is, isn't it?

That soldier explained that his commander didn't say "kill all the people," but instead told the men it was a search-and-destroy mission with the implication that this meant "anything there was VC and to do away with it" (Peers, 1974, pp. 9–10). Another veteran had a similar assessment, "The search-and-destroy mission is just another way to shoot anything that moves" (Appy, 2003, p. 350). As combat correspondent Michael Herr observed, search-and-destroy was "more a gestalt than a tactic, brought up alive and steaming from the Command psyche. Not just a walk and a firefight, in action it should have been named the other way around, pick through the pieces and see if you could work together a [body] count . . ." (Herr, 1977, p. 61).

Search-and-destroy also often amounted to what veteran and future senator James Webb, in his Vietnam war novel *Fields of Fire*, called "dangling the bait" (Webb, 1978, p. 130). U.S. troops were to be used as the "principal combat reconnaissance force" and "supporting fires as the principal destructive force," wrote Colonel Sidney Berry in a widely disseminated 1967 essay on the tactic. That is, Americans were a lure for the enemy because, as Brigadier General Glenn Walker put it, "You don't fight this fellow rifle to rifle. You locate him and back away. Blow the hell out of him and police up" (Gibson, 2000, p. 103).

While it looked good on paper, search-and-destroy often proved to be unworkable in the field. Enemy forces refused to do battle as Americans wished them to. They declined to fight at the time and place of the U.S. military's choosing; they recognized U.S. patterns and were not taken by surprise when loud U.S. war machinery broadcast its proximity for miles around with preparatory artillery and the sounds of roaring helicopters. Moreover, if they chose to fight, the revolutionary forces would often do so at such close quarters that heavy firepower could not be called in (Appy, 2003; Gibson, 2000).

The *rational* but illogical technowar method of "search-and-destroy" allowed Vietnamese revolutionary forces to transform the U.S. strategy from one of offensive operations to a series of defensive stands against enemy attack. According to *The Pentagon Papers*, the revolutionary forces surprised their U.S. foes and dictated the time, place, and duration of combat engagements 78% of the time. Another official report showed that the revolutionary forces initiated 73% of the firefights, and still another study revealed 88% of combat engagements were initiated by the enemy (Gravel, 1971; Thayer, 1975, vol. 4).

With the enemy in overwhelming control of tactical advantage, the U.S. technowar strategy of attrition—killing the enemy's forces faster than they could be replaced—was at the mercy of the revolutionary forces. So while they were successful in the unenviable role of bait, U.S. troops had no control over enemy losses, and furthermore, were often unable to fix the enemy in a position long enough to destroy them with heavy firepower (Gibson, 2000).

As a result of technowar's real-world failings, the overwhelming majority of U.S. patrols never resulted in a combat engagement. A CIA analysis of two years of statistics showed that less than 1% of nearly 2 million U.S. and Allied small-unit actions resulted in contact with enemy forces (Gibson, 2000). As a result, Americans spent the bulk of their time on exhausting treks up and down valleys, or through thick triple-canopy jungle, or into one hamlet after another, with nothing to show for their efforts.

Instead of attacking U.S. forces headlong, Vietnamese revolutionary forces often relied on remote methods. Over the course of the war, mines and other booby traps accounted for 11% of Americans killed and 17% of those wounded (in World War II and the Korean War, such methods accounted for only 3–4% of U.S. casualties) (Clodfelter, 1995). In a letter to his parents, Robert Ransom, a young officer, explained the terrible toll the weapons took on his men:

> We jumped off the tracks [armored personnel carriers], and one of my men jumped right onto a mine. Both his feet were blown off; both legs were torn to shreds; his entire groin area was completely blown away. It was the most horrible sight I've ever seen.... In the month that I have been with the company, we have lost four killed and about thirty wounded. We have not seen a single verified dink the whole time, nor have we even shot a single round at anything. (MacPherson, 2001, p. 408)

When the enemy did show itself, in almost one quarter of engagements, it was in the form of an ambush of a U.S. patrol—something U.S. forces, themselves, despite Westmoreland's pronouncements that his troops would "out-guerilla the guerilla and out-ambush the ambush," were able to execute less than 9% of the time, according to Department of Defense statistics (Farber & Foner, 1994, p. 144; Gravel, 1971). Another Army study revealed that American GIs were ambushed 46% of the time (Gravel, 1971; Thayer, 1975, vol. 4, pp. 7–9). "Without a front, flanks or rear," wrote Marine officer Philip Caputo, "we fought a formless enemy who evaporated like the morning jungle mists, only to materialize in some unexpected place" (Caputo, 1996, p. 95).

Of the U.S. soldiers wounded by booby traps, ambushes, firefights, or other hostile actions, some 54% received injuries to their limbs (arms, legs, or shoulders). Another 20% suffered from multi-site wounds, and 14% received head injuries. Many of those seriously wounded were "medevacked" (medical evacuation) by helicopter, sometimes within minutes of injury (although a 1968 study showed that, on average, it took 2.8 hours for those deemed "salvageable"), to the receiving ward of an American hospital where they were triaged by medical personnel.

There, military nurses and doctors worked to save the lives of exceptionally young soldiers (the average enlisted man's age was 19, and 70% of the enlisted men who died were between 18 and 21 years old). Most of the time, the medical personnel were successful in their task. "If I had been in World War II, I'd have died," recalled Max Cleland, a Vietnam veteran who lost both legs and one arm before going on to head the VA and serve as a senator (MacPherson, 2001, p. 440). In fact, the total number of wounded U.S. soldiers who lost at least one limb in Vietnam was greater than the total for both World War II and the Korean conflict combined. At military medical facilities, mortality rates were under 3%, but many who would have died in previous wars were, like Cleland, left maimed and permanently disabled (Appy, 2003; Clodfelter, 1995; Norman, 1990). "When you finally saved a life," nurse Peggy DuVall recalled, "you wondered what kind of life you had saved. We saw football-hero types with their legs blown off." Saralee McGoran, another nurse, recalled the same: "We didn't know whether to work on them or not. I couldn't bear to look at their faces" (MacPherson, 2001, pp. 439–440, 447).

Those lucky enough to survive a firefight unscathed or make it through a day of slogging through muddy rice paddies—to avoid mines seeded in the more easily traversable paddy dikes—hiking several kilometers, up and down, over hills and mountains in the highlands or searching hamlets in the coastal plains, without incident, ended the ordeal by (beginning at about 4:00 pm) setting up "night defensive perimeters." There, "grunts" dug their foxholes and cleaned their rifles as well as the bullets and magazines. Behind tripwires, flares, and claymore mines, they might write letters to family, friends, and loved ones before dining on C-rations: individual packages of canned foods to be eaten in the field. After heating the cans with a small amount of C-4 plastic explosive, they would choke down a meal of "ham and motherfuckers" (ham and lima beans) or "beans and dicks" (beans and hot dogs), accompanied by a can of crackers with a cheese spread and another of peaches (Appy, 1993; Warr, 1997).

Most troops stayed in the new position (a "night laager"), sleeping in shifts to protect against guerrilla attacks. This generally meant a few hours spent curled up on the ground—generally damp, wet, or drenched, wrapped in a poncho liner, being feasted on by mosquitoes—before being roused for guard duty. Often sounds, real or imagined, shook men awake. Disturbing thoughts did so as well. The hard earth and the stiff joints and sore muscles it produced didn't help either. Men often slept about four hours per night and seldom woke up refreshed. Vernon Janick, who served with the 4th Infantry Division from 1966–1968, recalled:

> A day seemed like a week. You walked all day and slept part of the night. You were dragged out. You were amazed that all day you humped the hills with those packs and only a little to eat. Then, if you only had a couple guys in a hole, you would be on two [hours' watch], and he would be on for two—two on, two off; two on, two off—all night. You would get half a night's sleep. Right away in the morning you were back humping again. Same

thing every night. Many times everybody just dozed off. You couldn't help it. You took a hell of a chance, but you could only put up with so much. After a while you were just in such a daze. You were tired. I don't know how in the hell we did it except that we had to! (Ebert, 2004, pp. 306–307)

In a letter to his wife, Marine Lieutenant Joseph Giannini echoed this. "My men, and sometimes myself, are drained of physical endurance," he confided. "They are so tired they can't stay awake when they know the VC are all around them. If we don't get some slack soon we might get into a real bad mess one night" (Napoli, 2013, p. 51).

Other troops were sent beyond the perimeter to a listening post to detect enemy movement. Some might head out on a night ambush. Often, it was a fruitless exercise resulting in no enemy contact. Sometimes, however, it yielded a firefight with the enemy. At other times, civilians became targets (Ebert, 1993).

On August 27, 1966, for example, a Marine platoon commander went looking for volunteers for a four-man "hunter-killer" team that was officially charged with killing armed guerrillas, or, as court-martial documents put it, "anyone found outside at night." Lance Corporal Frank Schultz, however, viewed the assignment as a means to avenge the deaths of fellow Marines. He eagerly volunteered, saying that he "knew the area and could get a VC." After the team set up an ambush near Khai Dong hamlet in the early morning hours, Schultz, according to a fellow Marine, announced that he would bust into one of the nearby hootches, grab a "gook," and kill him. Schultz later testified that after he saw a light flickering in a home:

I wanted to get to that house. I had to kill a VC for those guys, I just had to kill one. . . . I went to the house and there was a man in there. . . . I pulled him out in front of the house and he was pulling out his ID card and was showing it to me but this didn't matter to me because I had seen many VC before that I'd killed with ID cards on them identical to that. I . . . shoved him down the trail. . . . I brought my rifle to my shoulder and shot him (*United States* v. *Frank C. Schultz*, 1969).

There is no evidence that the man killed by Schultz, almost at random, was even an NLF sympathizer, let alone a guerrilla (*United States* v. *Frank C. Schultz*, 1969).

Most U.S. troops, however, never went on hunter/killer missions or ambush patrols or spent long nights in cramped, clammy, rain-flooded foxholes, week after week, month after month. Throughout South Vietnam, the United States built seven jet-capable airfields, 75 smaller tactical airfields, six deep-water ports, and 24 permanent base facilities—many of them the size of small towns—not to mention innumerable smaller firebases, LZs, and other outposts. The majority of veterans served on these firebases—relatively small installations, designed to support troops in the field with supplies and artillery fire—or larger base camps, which might house a brigade or division.

The so-called tooth-to-tail ratio of support troops to front line forces was somewhere between 5 to 1 and 10 to 1. That is, for every infantryman "humping the boonies," there were five or more truck drivers, clerk-typists, petroleum storage specialists, cooks, or mechanics, among other non-combat personnel, at a camp or firebase. Many of these rear echelon forces served at large facilities in places like Long Binh, Cam Ranh Bay, and Qui Nhon. They regularly enjoyed luxuries like electricity, hot showers, and warm meals that were generally unavailable to men serving in the field. They could frequent enlisted men's clubs to play slot machines and drink cold beer, watch movies and TV shows, and shop at the PX for everything from cigarettes and candy to cameras and stereos (Appy, 1993; Record, 1998; Sheehan, 1998).

Troops at many larger bases even had ready access to U.S.-supported "massage parlors" and "steam baths" where they could purchase sexual services at low cost. In 1966, *Time* magazine reported on the 1st Cavalry Division's "Sin City," a "25-acre sprawl of 'boom-boom' parlors" which they dubbed "the first brothel quarter built exclusively for American soldiers in Vietnam" (Appy, 2015, p. 109). "You had to go through a check-point gate, but once you were in there you could do anything. There were all kinds of prostitutes and booze," the 1st Cavalry's Jim Soular recalled of Sin City. "The [U.S.] army was definitely in control of this thing. The bars had little rooms in the back where you could go with the prostitutes. I know they were checked by the doctors once a week for venereal diseases" (Appy, 2003, p. 159).

While serving at base camps was much safer than life in the boonies, danger was never far away. Throughout the war, the Vietnamese revolutionary forces carried out a persistent campaign of rocket and mortar attacks as well as reconnaissance probes, sapper raids, and even full-scale ground assaults (Prados, 2009). On the night of October 27–28, 1965, for example, VC sappers raided the American airfield at Chu Lai. "They were barefooted and had on a loin cloth and it was kind of a John Wayne dramatic effect," recalled Colonel Leslie Brown, making reference to the fact that the attackers wore almost no clothes that could get snagged while sneaking through barbed wire. "They had Thompson submachine guns and were spraying the airplanes with Tommy guns and . . . throwing satchel charges into tail pipes." The Vietnamese destroyed two jets and damaged six others. That same night, sappers also hit a Marine base at Marble Mountain, destroying 19 helicopters and damaging 35 others—about one-third of the helicopters on the base (Wilkins, 2011, pp. 29–30).

William Nelson served as a military stevedore officer (MSO) with the 155th Transportation and Terminal Company at Cam Ranh Bay. He and his men did hard work in the tropical heat, offloading and storing hazardous material like ammunition, bombs, napalm, and jet fuel, in addition to general cargo and equipment. But that wasn't all. "Duty there was dangerous," he recalled. "The Viet Cong frequently mortared this important facility." The base came under attack by enemy forces. Once, he said, the guerrillas blew up 150 tons of napalm and killed an American soldier. Other times, Viet Cong snipers pinned down his men, halted their truck convoys, and blew up their oil pipeline. When a barge loaded with 500 tons of napalm broke loose from its mooring and floated away, he had to lead his men into "unfriendly territory" to retrieve it (Li, 2010, pp. 192–196).

The complex at Long Binh took up 25 square miles and, at its height, it housed 50,000 soldiers. It was also hit by rocket and mortar attacks throughout the war (Tucker, 1998). And it was the same all over Vietnam. Gary Panko, a Navy corpsman at the large Marine base at Da Nang, recounted a rocket attack he experienced in late July 1967. "All of a sudden I woke up to the sound of a loud whoosh," he told his mother in a letter.

Then all hell broke loose. The explosion from the first one demolished one hut and killed three guys instantly. That happened about half a block away. . . . Then before I knew it, everyone ran out of the hut [I was in], and when I got to the door I looked up and saw flames across the runway. Later on, we heard that two of the helicopters got direct hits and were all ablaze. Then we all got into the bunker . . . we sat in the bunker shaking and listening to the 31 (140-mm) rockets we received. (Edelman, 1985, p. 163)

Even if there were no casualties, there was ample fear and uncertainty. Nurse Saralee McGoran, who served at the 12th Evacuation Hospital at Cu Chi, recalled her base being "shelled a lot." Just before she left Vietnam, a special spaghetti dinner had to be rescheduled. On the original night of that celebration, the mess hall was hit by a mortar round. "If we'd had it as originally planned, we would have been killed," she recalled (MacPherson, 2001, pp. 440–441). Jimmy Bacolo, an artilleryman who served on relatively secure firebases and landing zones, expressed the same sort of fear:

I was scared enough just being over there, knowing you had 5 million people and 4.5 million hated your guts and you couldn't tell them apart because nobody had uniforms. . . . There was no battle lines; there was no secured areas. You could walk into a village one day, and the next day they're dropping rockets and mortars on you. Or at night, you know, there's a guy . . . he's cutting your hair in a village in the daytime, at night he's lobbing mortars into your position. (Napoli, 2013, p. 116)

Bases were a tempting target to enemy forces. More than 30% of all combat engagements were enemy assaults on established U.S. perimeters (Gravel, 1971). And from 1967 to 1972, U.S. positions experienced an average of more than 14,000 such "stand off attacks" per year by mortars, rockets, and artillery shells (Thayer, 1985).

By the end of 1966, 385,000 U.S. troops were deployed in South Vietnam—an increase of 201,000 from the previous year. Already, more than 6,000 U.S. soldiers had died and 37,000 had been wounded in the conflict (Clodfelter, 1995). In 1965, only 16% of battle deaths were draftees. In 1966, the number jumped to 21% (Prados, 2009). With the increase in troops and casualties, military morale began to drop while opposition to the war rose. On June 3, three privates from Texas refused to deploy to Vietnam. Several months after the "Fort Hood Three" took their stand, Army doctor Howard Levy refused to train elite Green Beret medics for service in Vietnam on the grounds that doing so would make him complicit with atrocities there (Prados, 2009). The tenor of the times was beginning to change.

Uprisings on the Home Front

The birth of GI resistance to the Vietnam War came as uprisings were occurring in America's ghettos. In the summer of 1966, 11 major riots (defined as civil disturbances lasting two or more days) and 32 minor ones rocked American cities. A year later, the unrest continued with 25 major and 30 minor riots. From July 12–17, 1967, Newark,

New Jersey, erupted in a rebellion that left 26 dead, more than 1,500 injured, and saw the streets become a war zone complete with an armored personnel carrier and National Guardsmen brandishing bayonets on their rifles. Rioting in Detroit, Michigan, ignited just days later (July 23–30, 1967) killing 43 people, injuring 2,250, causing $250 million in property damage and prompting the deployment of paratroopers and tanks in an effort to restore order (Gilje, 1996; Isserman & Kazin, 1999). From 1965 to 1967, more than 100 riots rocked American cities, from Flint, Michigan, to Memphis, Tennessee, to South Bend, Indiana. A presidential commission determined that white racism was "essentially responsible for the explosive mixture which accumulated in our cities" and set off the uprisings (Farber & Foner, 1994).

As the inner cities erupted in violence, the antiwar movement grew in strength. The April 15, 1967, Spring Mobilization to End the War in Vietnam drew more than 250,000 people to rallies in New York City and San Francisco, and in October, following a traditional rally at Washington, D.C.'s Lincoln Memorial, some 30,000 more adventurous activists crossed the Potomac and marched on the Pentagon. More than 600 protesters were arrested and 47 were hospitalized after being beaten and tear-gassed, but what made the demonstration most notable was the fact that it was the first major protest event to have in attendance a large contingent of counterculture activists, who looked, wrote novelist Norman Mailer, "like the legions of Sgt. Pepper's band" (Isserman & Kazin, 1999, p. 184).

While he had quietly spoken out against the war since 1965, it was during an April 1967 speech in Riverside Church in New York City that Martin Luther King made it clear that he opposed the conflict in Vietnam, not just because of domestic concerns, like racial disparities of the draft and money being drained from poverty programs, but because, he said, "I knew that I could never again raise my voice against the violence of the oppressed in the ghettos without having first spoken clearly to the greatest purveyor of violence in the world today: my own government" (King, 1967).

Taking a forceful tone, King told the audience that he feared for America's soul.

> Somehow this madness must cease. We must stop now. I speak as a child of God and brother to the suffering poor of Vietnam. I speak for those whose land is being laid waste, whose homes are being destroyed, whose culture is being subverted. I speak . . . for the poor of America who are paying the double price of smashed hopes at home, and death and corruption in Vietnam.
>
> This business of burning human beings with napalm, of filling our nation's homes with orphans and widows, of injecting poisonous drugs of hate into the veins of peoples normally humane, of sending men home from dark and bloody battlefields physically handicapped and psychologically deranged, cannot be reconciled with wisdom, justice, and love. A nation that continues year after year to spend more money on military defense than on programs of social uplift is approaching spiritual death. (Buckley, 2001; King, 1967)

In the midst of this culture of death, and perhaps in reaction to it, 1967's "Summer of Love" saw the blossoming of a youth culture of "hippies" and "freaks" that led thousands of young people to flock to urban youth enclaves such as San Francisco's Haight-Ashbury neighborhood. The local scene there was marked by up-and-coming rock bands like the Grateful Dead and the Jefferson Airplane, the use of recreational drugs such as mari-juana and LSD, experimental theater, and a group of anarchists known as "The Diggers" who distributed free food and clothing.

Following the lead of the "Beats" of the 1950s, an emerging hippie counterculture challenged mainstream America as well as the vision of social change offered by the New Left. For cultural revolutionaries, the means of ending repression often focused on personal self-expression, loosened sexual mores ("free love"), drug use, and the pursuit of sensual pleasures and creative activities, as opposed to those in the New Left, who embraced political or revolutionary means of governmental change. Some, however, like John Sinclair of the radical White Panthers, and Abbie Hoffman, a founding member of the Youth International Party ("Yippies"), sought to merge the New Left and the coun-terculture with only modest success (Isserman & Kazin, 1999).

Many men in the emerging counterculture embraced a vision of sexual liberation that advocated promiscuity and a diversity of partners. Emerging young feminists, how-ever, saw this new brand of "freedom" as a repackaged form of sexual subordination and discrimination. Thus it was hardly surprising that, in the fall of 1967, following the "Summer of Love," female "consciousness-raising groups" began meeting in big cities across America, issuing a call for what would become known as "women's liberation" (Farber & Foner, 1994; Isserman & Kazin, 1999).

The women's movement grew out of the criticism by activists such as Casey Hayden and Mary King of the SNCC, who in 1965 called attention to the rampant sexism and adherence to gender stereotypes within the supposedly egalitarian New Left and civil rights movements and pointed to parallels between the treatment of blacks and women in America. The movement also drew upon a renewed middle-class feminism embodied in such works as Betty Freidan's *The Feminine Mystique* (1963) and the group she co-founded in 1966, the National Organization for Women (NOW). By the 1970s, the in-fluence of the civil rights and women's movements could be seen in the burgeoning gay rights, Chicano, American-Indian, disabled American, and environmental movements (Isserman & Kazin, 1999).

Vietnam: 1967

U.S. forces in Vietnam began 1967 with a large-scale operation, code-named Cedar Falls, targeting the so-called Iron Triangle, a 60-square mile area north of Saigon that had long supported the NLF. More than 16,000 U.S. troops and 14,000 South Vietnamese forces took part in the two-and-a-half–week "hammer and anvil" attack, which was designed to destroy a major Viet Cong force and pacify locals who were dubbed "hostile civilians" by the Americans (Prados, 2009, p. 178; Schell, 2000, pp. 127, 130–150, 167–168; Tucker, 1998).

Within the Iron Triangle lay Ben Suc, which had been "liberated" by the revolu-tionary forces in 1964. From then on, the NLF was the government of the village, and the people paid their taxes (on a sliding scale, with the poor paying nothing) to it, joined its associations (Farmers' Liberation Association, Women's Liberation Association, etc.), and sent their children to its schools. The next year, U.S. and South Vietnamese forces bombed Ben Suc, killing and wounding more than 20 people, including children. As a result, the NLF resettled residents from the middle of town to its outskirts and encouraged people to dig bomb shelters. Airstrikes and artillery barrages continually increased, leaving the area pock-marked with craters. Villagers lived in a constant state of fear under falling artillery shells and bombs as well as leaflets, which read: "Do you hear the planes? Do you hear the bombs? These are the sounds of DEATH: your DEATH. Rally now to survive" (Schell, 2000, pp. 62–72).

On the morning of January 8, soldiers of the 1st Infantry Division were airlifted to Ben Suc, as speakers mounted on a helicopter blared, "Attention, people of Ben Suc! You are surrounded by Republic of South Vietnam and Allied Forces. Do not run away or you will be shot as V.C. Stay in your homes and wait for further instructions." Some sporadic enemy fire was received after U.S. troops landed, and it was answered by helicopters' rockets, artillery shells, and bombs from planes. Afterward, Americans began searching the homes and questioning the Vietnamese, in English, to no avail ("America takes charge," 1983; Prados, 2009; Schell, 2000). According to a *New York Times* report, at least 41 persons in the village were "tracked down and killed" for a variety of reasons, including: "fleeing on bicycles," crawling in a rice paddy, thrashing in a river, and being "discovered at the mouth of a cave with an assortment of surgical instruments and commercially produced drugs" (*N.Y. Times*, 1967, p. 4)." Major Charles Malloy explained to reporter Jonathan Schell, "O.K, so some people without weapons get killed. What're you going to do when you spot a guy with black pajamas? Wait for him to get out his automatic weapon and start shooting? I'll tell you I'm not" (Schell, 2000, p. 119).

Outside the village, napalm and white phosphorus bombs fell in the forest. Inside, surviving villagers were rounded up and segregated, by age, sex, and perceived suspiciousness. Some were beaten by Vietnamese interrogators as U.S. advisors stood by. Others received even worse treatment. Captain Ted Shipman, one of those advisors, told Schell:

> You see, they *do* have some—well, methods and practices that *we* are not accustomed to, that we wouldn't use if we were doing it, but the thing you've got to understand is that this is an Asian country, and their first impulse is force. . . . Only the fear of force gets results. It's the Asian mind. It's completely different from what we know as the Western mind. . . . Look—they're a thousand years behind us in this place, and we're trying to educate them up to our level (Schell, 2000, p. 112).

The next day, trucks arrived in Ben Suc, and the people, some with their belongings and animals, were jammed on board and driven away to Phu Loi, a vast field with just a few small homes belonging to local farm families who had no idea they were about to be swamped with several thousand refugees from Ben Suc and its environs (Schell, 2000). Even General Bernard Rogers, the Assistant Commander of the 1st Infantry Division, called the forced removal a "pathetic and pitiful" sight (Mangold & Penycate, 1985, p. 168). David Ross, an Army medic at Ben Suc, remembered of the locals: "They understood that they couldn't really change the situation. They were going to be taken out of their homes. I'm sure that deep down inside they knew that that was the end of Ben Suc as a village—that we were going to destroy the village" ("America takes charge," 1983).

Demolition teams arrived in Ben Suc, saturated the homes with gasoline, and lit them ablaze. Bulldozers then rolled through, pulverizing the skeletons of houses, fences, and ancestral graves. Afterward, Air Force jets screamed overhead and bombed the rubble (Schell, 2000). Ben Suc was then designated a free-fire zone (Falk & Kolko, 1971). "It was kind of sad in a way because Ben Suc was a pretty village. It was a very old village and the people there seemed to enjoy a little better standard of living than people in many of the other villages," Ross recalled. "Basically, once the people were taken out, the whole thing was just turned into a parking lot" ("America takes charge," 1983).

Meanwhile, those sent to Phu Loi arrived to find no shelter, no facilities, no latrines, nor any aid. The refugees—70% of them children, the rest mainly women—were left to sleep on the bare ground inside coils of barbed wire—along with pigs, chickens and other animals they had brought. South Vietnamese troops later began to erect nylon canopies and hand out rice to some, but many were left without (Schell, 2000).

An elderly farmer whose family had lived and farmed in Ben Suc for generations grappled with life in the camp. "How can I farm here? What work will I do?" he asked Jonathan Schell. "They have given us rice here, but I can't eat it. The American rice is for pigs. And we have no cooking oil." Another family in the camp—who had been bombed out of their home village of My Hung before taking up residence in Ben Suc and subsequently being forced from there to Phu Loi—lost their cattle, rice, carts, farming tools, and all other worldly possessions. "They gave me a ticket a day ago, but they never have enough rice. We couldn't even bring blankets or clothes. My son is naked. Look!" the wife told Schell as she gestured at her nude four-year-old boy. "It's no good for children here. Not good for their health" (Schell, 2000, pp. 181–184).

While 1967 brought increased suffering for the Vietnamese, it brought more of the same for American combat troops, as up to 90% of all company-sized firefights were initiated by the revolutionary forces. U.S. losses also skyrocketed, more than doubling the previous year's totals, with close to 9,400 combat deaths and more than 62,000 wounded (Clodfelter, 1995). The percentage of draftees dying in Vietnam was also on the rise, reaching 34% (up from just 16% in 1965) among the dead of all services—including 57% of all Army deaths. By January 1968, there were nearly 500,000 Americans in-country. That year would prove to be the costliest of the war for the United States (Appy, 2003; Clodfelter, 1995).

Despite the fact that 83% of Americans said that they expected the war in Vietnam to be a long one (up from just 54% in October 1965) according to a Louis Harris survey commissioned by *Newsweek*, 1967 had ended with rosy predictions from America's war managers ("A Nation at Odds," 1967). "I have never been more encouraged in my four years in Vietnam," said General William Westmoreland when he and Ambassador Ellsworth Bunker traveled to Washington in November to brief President Lyndon Johnson. Bunker assured Johnson and the American public that the Republic of Vietnam now held sway over 67% of the country's population while the NLF controlled only 17%. And 1968 promised even more success. Viet Cong recruitment, the ambassador reported, had dropped by as much as 50% over the course of 1967, and Saigon's military was performing better than ever. Westmoreland added that 45% of enemy forces were not fit for combat and let it slip that in two years, the U.S. might begin a "phase-out" of its troops. "We have reached an important point when the end begins to come into view," the general told the National Press Club in Washington. It was now only a matter of "mopping up" (Farber & Foner, 1994; Gibson, 2000, p. 162; Sheehan, 1988; Smith, 1967; Turse, 2013).

Tet, 1968: Fighting on All Fronts

Back in Saigon, at 3:00 am on January 31, 1968, Bunker's Marine guards woke him with startling news: the city was under attack. The ambassador only had time to throw on a bathrobe before Marines hustled him into an armored personnel carrier that quickly drove off as dawn approached. Others stayed behind at his villa to set fire to secret documents in his private study as gunfire echoed across the city.

It was *Tet Mau Than*—Tet, the Year of the Monkey; the Vietnamese lunar new year— and 6,000 revolutionary fighters, the same guerrilla forces that had been given last rites by Bunker and Westmoreland all autumn long, infiltrated the South Vietnamese capital and its suburbs, attacking some of the best fortified and highest profile landmarks, including the Independence Palace, the seat of South Vietnam's government. Guerrillas also took over the studio of the government radio station; and struck Tan Son Nhut, Saigon's mammoth air base and military complex, the nerve center of the war effort. What captured the attention of the American public, however, was the work of a tiny commando unit that had set its sights on the American embassy in Saigon, a multi-million-dollar, six-story fortress of reinforced concrete walls and solid teak doors that had been unveiled only months before (Oberdorfer, 1985; Prados, 2009; Sheehan, 1988).

It took six and a half hours for U.S. forces to finally secure the embassy compound. During the that time, guerrillas exchanged gunfire with U.S. military police, while 101st Airborne Division paratroopers landed on the embassy roof. Journalists also flocked to the scene and were shocked by what they saw. The new complex, featured in puff pieces the year before, was now a war zone. American troops and armed personnel in civilian attire were crouching for cover on the manicured lawn, huddling against decorative fountains and ornamental trees. The bodies of dead U.S. personnel lay sprawled in the street out front. Vietnamese corpses littered the compound lawn, gaping hole marred the blast wall, and buildings were bullet scarred.

The attack on Saigon was part of a coordinated strategy. The revolutionary forces struck four other major cities, 35 of 44 provincial capitals, 64 district seats, and 50 other villages and hamlets throughout South Vietnam (Prados, 2009). Hoping to spark a popular uprising, guerrillas and North Vietnamese regulars holed up wherever they could. This left the Americans with two options: fight at close quarters, house by house, to dislodge small bands of enemy fighters, or broadly target great swaths of cities and towns as they had long targeted the countryside.

John Singlaub, the commander of a clandestine U.S. special operations force known as MACV-SOG, summed up the Tet counteroffensive: "We had been trying for years to get them to come out in the open so we could slaughter them, and we slaughtered them. . . . I've never seen so many dead people stacked up" (Appy, 2003, p. 93). But revolutionary fighters weren't out in the open. They were inside cities and towns that were soon transformed into free-fire zones (Hemphill, 1999; Sheehan, 1988; Turse, 2013). As journalist Neil Sheehan observed, "saving of the soldiers' lives was not the principal reason for the lack of restraint. It was more in the nature of a reflex to turn loose on the urban centers the 'stomp-them-to-death' firepower that had brutalized the Vietnamese countryside" (Sheehan, 1988, p. 718). As a result, Tet not only revealed the United States' inability to protect even those "friendly" city-dwelling Vietnamese who were most intimately involved with the U.S. effort and the Saigon government, but also that American forces did not value their lives. Firepower was unleashed with impunity and distinctions between Vietnamese combatants and noncombatants were all but ignored.

Bombs, shells, and rockets pounded entire residential neighborhoods in Saigon, leaving nothing but smoldering rubble (Durrance, 1988; Lewy, 1981; Oberdorfer, 1985). In the capital and its environs, around 6,300 civilians died and 11,000 were wounded. Some 19,000 dwellings were destroyed, more than 125,000 people were left homeless, and 206,000 Saigon residents became refugees. According to a U.S. military inspector general's report, most of the damage in the capital was caused by U.S. forces (Gibson, 2000; Oberdorfer, 1985; Sheehan, 1988).

In the Mekong Delta, the revolutionary forces attacked 13 of 16 provincial capitals along with numerous district capitals and dug in (Oberdorfer, 1985). As Don Oberdorfer, a reporter for the *Washington Post* and author of *Tet!: The Turning Point in the Vietnam War*, observed:

> The Viet Cong, whose military means were more closely tailored to political ends, placed strict limitations on the use of their firepower. They killed for a purpose, and put a high value on the good will of the people—for example, their orders in the Mekong Delta at Tet were that "in attacking the enemy, we are required to respect the lives and property of the people, not to fire freely, and not to exploit the people's goodness in any way." The United States and the South Vietnamese government forces, on the other hand, were indiscriminate in their use of firepower, and seemed to value their own safety far beyond the political purpose (if any) for which they fought (Oberdorfer, 1985, pp. 184–185).

In Can Tho, the capital of the Mekong Delta's Phong Dinh Province, for example, aid worker John Balaban awoke to sounds of urban combat as a U.S. helicopter gunship hovering above the town fired off rockets. Later, he would watch South Vietnamese forces open fire on a slum with small arms and an armored personnel carrier. "Soon the whole village started to burn, house by house. We could hear people screaming," he remembered (Balaban, 2002, pp. 103–104).

Overhead, helicopters continued to fire rockets into the town, while Air Force jets dropped cluster bombs on the city's outskirts. "Whole families, reunited at Tet the night before, now lay about us shredded and bleeding to death in the dirt," he recalled (Balaban, 2002, p. 104). Many who survived swamped the hospital. There, Balaban saw a napalm-burned woman thrashing wildly on the floor, next to her infant daughter "who was perfectly whole except for one arm burned black." He watched as another wounded mother tried to comfort her injured children while her toddler wailed "*May bay!*" ("Airplane!") (Balaban, 2002, pp. 103–104).

In the Mekong River town of My Tho, Lieutenant Tobias Wolff, an advisor to South Vietnamese forces, participated in a similar effort. "We leveled shops and bars along the river. We pulverized hotels and houses, floor by floor, block by block. . . . I didn't think of our targets as homes where exhausted and frightened people were praying for their lives," he recalled in his 1994 memoir *In Pharoah's Army*. Following days of artillery shelling and bombings, he saw the fruits of the VC attack and the American response.

> The corpses were everywhere, lying in the streets, floating in the reservoir . . . the smell so thick and foul we had to wear surgical masks scented with cologne, aftershave, deodorant, whatever we had. . . . Hundreds of corpses and the count kept rising. . . . One day I passed a line of them that went on for almost a block, all children. . . . (Wolff, 1994, pp. 138–139)

Well to the north, Hue, South Vietnam's third-largest city and once the capital of the country, also suffered mightily. While Westmoreland had focused most of his pre-Tet attention on the Marine base at Khe Sanh, the revolutionary forces had secretly withdrawn two regiments that had been laying siege to the outpost and sent them to join in the assault on Hue. For nearly a month, the revolutionary forces held large portions of the city and carried out one of the most notorious and well-publicized atrocities of the war: pre-planned, targeted executions of officials, military personnel, and others loyal to the Republic of Vietnam. In all, 3,000 or more people may have been killed in the massacre (Braestrup, 1977; Brenner, 2005; Clodfelter, 1995; Laurence, 2002; Sheehan, 1988; Tucker, 1998; Valentine, 1990; Young, 1991).

As part of the U.S. counteroffensive, Navy ships fired 7,670 shells into Hue, and Marine Corps aircraft flew dozens of sorties, dropping napalm and 500-pound bombs on residential neighborhoods. U.S. forces unleashed an astounding 600 tons of bombs, plus barrages from artillery and tank cannons, flattening swaths of the city while ground troops fought street to street (Clodfelter, 1995). "We used everything but nuclear weapons on this town," said one Marine (Braestrup, 1977, p. 277). At least 3,800 of Hue's citizens were killed or reported missing as a result of the bombardment and battle, and 116,000 people were made homeless. More than three-quarters of the city's homes were seriously damaged or destroyed (Clodfelter, 1995; Laurence, 2002; Warr, 1997; Young, 1991). "Nothing I saw during the Korean War or in the Vietnam War so far has been as terrible, in terms of destruction and despair, as what I saw in Hue," wrote correspondent Robert Shaplen (Brenner, 2006, p. 112).

The cities were only a fraction of the story. In already battered rural areas, the Tet counteroffensive became an orgy of brutality. On February 8, 1968, a day after General Westmoreland flew to Quang Nam for a "head knocking" session with top U.S. commanders in the area and barked orders for them to "take some risks," B Company, 1st Battalion, 35th Infantry of the 4th Infantry Division, which was operating in the countryside not far away, received new and blunt operation orders. When they entered a tiny hamlet, B Company's Lieutenant Johnny Mack Carter reported to Captain Donald Reh that he had rounded up 19 civilians. Carter asked what should be done with them. Medic Jamie Henry later told an Army investigator: "The Captain asked him if he remembered the Op Order [Operation Order] that had come down from higher [command] that morning which was to kill anything that moves. The Captain repeated the order. He said that higher said to kill anything that moves." Within moments, four or five men around the civilians, said Henry, "opened fire and shot them. There was a lot of flesh and blood going around because the velocity of an M-16 at that close range does a lot of damage." An Army investigation later concluded that all the civilians had been killed (Turse, 2013, p. 126).

One province south, in Quang Tin, members of A Troop, 1st Squadron, 1st Cavalry Regiment used their tanks and armored personnel carriers to punish the population for the guerrillas' Tet attacks. In a letter to his wife, Staff Sergeant John Pryor hinted at the brutality: "We went out today[,] didn't see much[.] I burned three houses just because and that was about it. . . ." In another letter, he wrote: "I wish you could have seen us today[,] we real[l]y messed up a big village. Burned and ran over every dam[n] house they had. . . . Tomorrow we go out to cigar island and we'll burn and destroy every damn thing we can. . . . Meby [sic] we'll even get to shoot some V.C." Fellow unit member Thomas Anderson was equally blunt in a letter home. After lamenting about how badly prisoners were beaten, he asked, "Does it help the poor farmer when we run over his rice paddy with our tanks and armored personnel carriers? I don't think so. Anyone wearing black pajamas and running is considered VC and shot. As a result, many innocent people are killed" (Nolan, 2006, pp. 186–188).

Unit member Richard Brummett would later write a letter to Secretary of Defense Melvin Laird protesting the unit's wanton destruction. He said that A Troop

> did perform on a regular basis, random murder, rape and pillage upon the Vietnamese civilians in Quang Tin Province . . . with the full knowledge, consent and participation of our Troop Commander. . . .
>
> These incidents included random shelling of villages with 90 mm white phosphorus rounds, machine gunning of civilians who had the misfortune to be near when we hit a mine, torture of prisoners, destroying of food and livestock of the villagers if we deemed they had an excess, and numerous burnings of villages for no apparent reason. (Turse, 2013, p. 97)

On March 14, 1968, after a booby trap killed one soldier and severely wounded two others, unit members rampaged through several hamlets. They roughed up a villager on a bicycle, assaulted children, and set upon an unarmed woman. "They shot and wounded her," one GI wrote in a letter home to his father. "Then they kicked her to death and emptied their magazines in her head" (Hersh, 1970, pp. 37–38).

The next day, members of Company C were briefed by their commanding officer, Captain Ernest Medina, about a planned operation the following morning in an area they knew as "Pinkville." As unit member Harry Stanley recalled, Medina "ordered us to 'kill everything in the village.'" Infantryman Salvatore LaMartina remembered Medina's words only slightly differently: "kill everything that breathed." What struck forward artillery observer James Flynn's mind was a question one of the other soldiers asked: "Are we supposed to kill women and children?" And Medina's reply: "Kill everything that moves" (Belknap, 2002, p. 171; Bilton & Sim, 1992, pp. 381, 97–99).

The next morning, the troops were airlifted into what they thought would be a "hot LZ"—a landing zone where they would be under hostile fire. They expected to find Vietnamese adversaries spoiling for a fight, but the Americans entering My Lai encountered only civilians: women, children, and old men. Many were still cooking their breakfast rice. Nevertheless, Medina's orders were followed to the letter.

Advancing in small squads, the men of the unit shot chickens, pigs, cows, and water buffalo. They gunned down old men sitting in their homes. They tossed grenades into homes without bothering to look inside. A monk was murdered. A woman emerged from her home with a baby in her arms and was shot down on the spot. As the tiny child hit the ground, another GI opened fire on the infant with his M-16.

Over four hours, members of Charlie Company methodically killed more than 500 unarmed victims, executing some in ones and twos, others in small groups, and collecting many more in a drainage ditch that would become an infamous killing ground. They faced no opposition. They even took a quiet lunch break in the midst of the carnage. Along the way, they also raped women and young girls, mutilated the dead, and systematically burned homes (Hersh, 1972).

While members of Charlie Company were destroying My Lai, the men of Bravo Company, 4th Battalion, 3rd Infantry, were sent to the nearby coastal hamlet of My Khe-4. And like the soldiers at My Lai, Company B encountered no enemy forces as they approached. In fact, peering through heavy brush, the Americans saw only women, children, and old men going about their daily chores. Nevertheless, Lieutenant Thomas Willingham had his two machine gunners open fire on the enclave. When the machine guns stopped, the Americans entered the hamlet (Hersh, 1972).

Willingham's radioman, Mario Fernandez said that the first men to enter the hamlet indiscriminately sprayed the area with rifle fire. Then the rest of the unit entered the village, and Willingham ordered the men to destroy it (Peers, 1976). Infantryman Homer Hall said that they moved through the hamlet grenading bunkers without bothering to check if civilians were sheltering inside. "They just threw it in there without calling them out," agreed unit member Jimmie Jenkins. According to Fernandez, when Vietnamese did emerge from the bunkers, they were shot. Other villagers were gunned down while attempting to run to safety (Peers, 1976; Turse, 2013).

According to an Army report, one soldier used a baby for target practice with a .45 caliber pistol. The child was about ten feet away, said a witness, and he "fired at it with a .45. He missed. We all laughed. He got up three or four feet closer and missed again. We laughed. Then he got right up on top of him and plugged him." By this time, said a unit member, "the word was out. You know, like you more or less can do anything you like" (Hersh, 1972, pp. 15–16). One American who kept count said that 155 people were killed at My Khe, and an official U.S. Army investigation found "no reliable evidence to support the claim that the persons killed were in fact VC" (Hersh, 1972, p. 18; Peers, 1976).

This was not to say that civilians were the only ones dying in the counteroffensive. Many American units were, indeed, engaged in heavy fighting with determined foes. At Firebase Burt near Dau Tieng, troops from the 2nd Battalion, 22nd Infantry, 25th Infantry Division, a mechanized unit, were hit by a withering mortar barrage followed by a determined ground assault. Rocket-propelled grenades knocked out one armored personnel carrier and then hit another. When a "Duster," a vehicle with a quad .50-caliber machine gun, drove toward the perimeter to counter the attack, it was blown up, too. From about midnight until dawn, soldiers were engaged in a nonstop firefight. Corporal Herb Mock fired so long with his .50-caliber machine gun that he burned out two gun barrels as he and his fellow troops held off the attackers. "We got three hundred fifty or sixty of them," Mock later recalled. "The next day you just saw their bodies laying all over" (Prados, 2011, pp. 196–197).

At Khe Sanh, Marines were long pinned down under heavy fire. In early February 1968, John Wheeler of the Associated Press huddled in a sandbagged bunker with them as enemy shells and rockets rained down and red-hot shrapnel tore into those unlucky enough to be caught out in the open. During the attack, a shelter occupied by an Army communications team assigned to the base took a direct hit. "The whole Army bunker just got wiped out," a stunned survivor reported (Wheeler, 1968, p. 577). When Wheeler made his way to the casualty clearing station, he saw men hobbling in and others carried on the shoulders of friends or on stretchers. "One prayed, a few cried, some were unconscious," he wrote. "Many showed shock on their faces" (Wheeler, 1968, p. 578).

During the first two weeks of the Tet Offensive, U.S. forces suffered 920 killed in action. Throughout February and March, U.S. troops were dying at a rate of 500 per week, compared to 140 per week the year before. And from the entire period from January 29 to March 31, 1968, the U.S. lost 3,895 troops (Clodfelter, 1995). Despite it all, Westmoreland declared the Tet Offensive to be an unmitigated defeat for the revolutionary forces—citing a figure of 45,000 enemy deaths. This left the enemy with only about 200,000 troops, and employing the standard ratio of 3.5 wounded for each killed (indicating 157,500 wounded), this meant the enemy could no longer field an effective fighting force (Gibson, 2000).

Westmoreland's post-Tet actions, however, hardly suggested that the United States had utterly incapacitated the revolutionary forces. In the face of his supposed victory, Westmoreland requested an additional 205,000 personnel. While it was rejected in Washington, he was still allowed nearly 25,000 more soldiers than had been originally slated for deployment.

Despite Westmoreland's rosy assessment, it had become clear that not only could the enemy strike at will and sustain major losses, but also that it still had firm hold on combat initiative and could control the tempo and number of its casualties. It was also estimated that, despite their losses during the Tet Offensive, the North Vietnamese could fight for up to 30 years before exhausting their manpower. Thus, the attrition strategy, even with a mass influx of U.S. troops, appeared doomed without a commitment America was never prepared, willing, or able to make (Gibson, 2000; Prados, 2009).

In the end, the enemy's offensive won temporary control of 1,000 hamlets, home to 1,100,000 people, and even after the Allied counteroffensive, the revolutionary forces retained control of an area that increased the population under their control by 340,000 (Clodfelter, 1995). And while the early-year offensive received the most press coverage in the United States, it was only the first of three phases that occurred that year. The second period, beginning in May and lasting until early June, was punctuated by attacks on 119 cities, towns, and military bases on the night of May 4. The third phase kicked off in mid-August and lasted for six weeks (Young, 1991).

The manpower costs of the offensives, especially of the second and third phases, were especially grievous for the revolutionary forces (Young, 1991). However, for the Saigon government, the attacks were an overwhelming political defeat. And for their U.S. allies, the psychological import of Tet was even more staggering, as the offensive laid to rest the optimistic American reports of late 1967 and suggested that there was truly no end in sight for the war. The Tet Offensive also shattered the illusion that Saigon had effective military control over any part of South Vietnam, much less political legitimacy. America's crushed hopes were further highlighted by trusted television newsman Walter Cronkite who announced, in late February, that it was now "more certain than ever that the bloody experience of Vietnam is to end in stalemate" (Isserman & Kazin, 1999, p. 223). As historian John Prados put it:

> Tet struck at America—not South Vietnam—with shock and awe. The widespread attacks and the fight for the embassy contradicted all the press releases. Pacification was set back everywhere, as was only too obvious. The infamous photograph of General [Nguyen Ngoc] Loan shooting an NLF cadre challenged any notion that Saigon's was a government of laws. . . . The battle for Hue refuted the argument that Hanoi had no staying power. The siege of Khe Sanh negated the talk of light at the end of the tunnel. And all this happened on film, recorded by journalists throughout the land and played back every day on America's TV screens and in its print media. . . . Public opinion turned decisively. In February, one poll showed 56 percent support for U.S.-withdrawal from Vietnam. A month later a Harris poll recorded the view that Tet represented a U.S. failure to attain its objectives in Vietnam. (Prados, 2009, p. 241)

The shock of Tet, flagging support for the war, and a tepid victory in the year's first Democratic primary caused Lyndon Johnson to decide against running for a second term. On March 31, 1968, he took to television and announced his intention not to seek or accept the Democratic nomination for the presidency. Tet had brought down America's president. Within a few days, an assassin's bullet would fell another American leader and would turn many U.S. cities into veritable battlefields.

On April 4, 1968, while in Memphis, Tennessee, supporting a strike by black sanitation workers, Martin Luther King was killed by a white gunman, sparking an outpouring of grief and rage across United States. Following the assassination, more than 120 cities erupted in riots, resulting in the use of 21,000 federal troops and 34,000 National Guardsmen in addition to untold numbers of local police to quell the disturbances. In Washington, D.C., soldiers set up machine guns on the steps of the Capitol to defend it from attack, while the angry and oppressed of the city vented their frustrations in a looting spree that caused $25 million in damage (Isserman & Kazin, 1999).

As 1968 wore on, protests broke out at previously unlikely venues. On April 26, a million high school and college students took part in a one-day boycott of classes to voice opposition to the war in Vietnam. That same week, in New York City, hundreds of black and white activists engaged in a takeover of Columbia University, "liberating" and occupying several university buildings in an effort to halt the construction of a gymnasium (dubbed "gym crow") in a nearby park that many thought would be an affront to the largely black area residents; force the university to sever ties to a military research institute; and, more broadly, transform Columbia from an elitist educational institution to an exemplary training-ground for revolutionary social change.

In the end, more than 1,000 police officers swinging clubs, blackjacks, and fists cleared the occupied buildings and put down the student rebellion, arresting nearly 700 protesters and leaving 148 injured. While it failed to achieve its lofty goals, the Columbia uprising was a watershed event, and in the two years following the protests, similar incidents took place on hundreds of other campuses across the United States. Still, the events at Columbia paled in comparison to 1968's most visible and notorious unrest, which took place in Chicago. There, however, the rioters weren't student radicals, but instead Mayor Richard Daley's police force (Appy, 2003; Isserman & Kazin, 1999; Morgan, 1991; Prados, 2009).

With Lyndon Johnson out of the presidential race, the Democratic Party had split into pro- and anti-war camps. While pro-war Vice President Hubert Humphrey was poised to garner the nomination from party officials, Minnesota's antiwar senator Eugene McCarthy and charismatic New York senator Robert Kennedy made a great deal of noise in the state primaries. With his popularity surging, and following a hard-fought victory in the California primary on June 5, 1968, Robert Kennedy, like his brother before him, was killed by an assassin. That left McCarthy, and his legion of "Clean for Gene" youths, to face off against Humphrey at the Democratic National Convention in Chicago.

The two factions of the Democratic Party, however, weren't the only ones traveling to Chicago that August. The antiwar umbrella group known as the National Mobilization Committee to End the War in Vietnam (or "the Mobe") was bringing activists to town for a march; members of the SDS were coming to convince McCarthy kids that real change would come only outside of the political system; while the Yippies, led by self-professed non-leaders Jerry Rubin and Abbie Hoffman, announced plans to bring 500,000 people to Chicago for a "festival of life" which would serve as a counterpoint to the Democratic "party of death" (Isserman & Kazin, 1999; Prados, 2009).

In the end, the security forces brought to bear by Mayor Daley dwarfed the protesters in the Windy City. Not only did Daley put all 12,000 Chicago police on 12-hour shifts (with 1,000 sent undercover to infiltrate activist groups) for the Democratic National Convention, but they were supported by 6,000 National Guardsmen and 7,500 Army troops. While only about 10,000 people took part in protests at the four-day convention, millions of television viewers had a front-row seat for 17 minutes of live coverage of an August 28 police riot in which Daley's cops rampaged through downtown Chicago, clubbing, macing, and beating protesters, journalists, and bystanders alike. From the podium at the convention, Connecticut's Senator Abraham Ribicoff locked eyes on Daley and denounced the "Gestapo tactics in the streets of Chicago." While it was inaudible on TV, it was easy to read the response from Daley's lips: "Fuck you, you Jew son-of-a-bitch, you lousy motherfucker! Go home!" (Appy, 2015, p. 185).

Following the sordid scene at the convention, nominee Hubert Humphrey fell far behind Republican candidate Richard Nixon in the polls. Humphrey eventually took a more critical stance on the war, which, coupled with Lyndon Johnson's decision to participate in peace negotiations in Paris, buoyed the vice president's standing. The Nixon campaign, however, dispatched an envoy to Saigon to encourage the government, who refused to negotiate with the revolutionary forces, that a Nixon presidency would be highly favorable to them. Without South Vietnamese support of the peace negotiations, no end of the war was forthcoming, stifling the Democratic candidate's surge. In November, Nixon received only half a million more votes than Humphrey, but he handily won the electoral college and the presidency on a "law and order" platform and a promise of swiftly ending the war in Vietnam via a "secret plan" that would bring "peace with honor" (Appy, 1993; Appy, 2003; Hunt, 1999; Isserman & Kazin, 1999; Nguyen, 2012, p. 131; Young, 1991).

Nixon's War

Shortly after coming into office, Nixon put the "Vietnamization" plan of turning the battle for the future of South Vietnam over to the ARVN (which was initiated by previous Defense Secretary Clark Clifford) into high gear, with the aim of reducing American casualties. The primary role of U.S. forces would now be, in Nixon's words, "to enable the South Vietnamese forces to assume the full responsibility for the security of South Vietnam" (Lewy, 1981, p. 146). In June 1969, the president announced that 25,000 U.S. troops would be withdrawn by the end of the summer, and by the beginning of 1970, some 69,000 Americans had left Vietnam (Isserman & Kazin, 1999; Lewy, 1981).

To an increasingly war-weary American public and its soldiers, the new policy suggested disengagement, a lessening of the combat burden, and an end to the American ground war. In reality, U.S. troops continued to fight and die, and Vietnamese civilians continued to suffer mightily, especially in the deep south of the Mekong Delta where an operation launched during the waning days of Lyndon Johnson's presidency would develop into nothing short of a bloodbath.

During the summer of 1968, planning began for a large-scale offensive in the region to, as an Army report put it, "maximize the opportunity presented during the dry season for ground, air-mobile, and water mobile operations" (Turse, 2013, p. 208). Codenamed "Speedy Express," the operation would run from December 1968 through May 1969, with 9th Infantry Division troops conducting missions across much of the Mekong Delta—most notably Kien Hoa and Dinh Tuong—in conjunction with other U.S. ground, air, and naval assets, as well as South Vietnamese forces. It would be carried out under the command of General Julian Ewell, a West Point grad and World War II hero whose obsession with high body counts was almost as legendary as his abuse of subordinates who didn't kill what he deemed to be sufficient numbers of Vietnamese (Appy, 2003, p. 323; Krepinevich, 1986, p. 204; Turse, 2013, p. 208).

Ronald Bartek, a fellow West Pointer who attended a briefing by Ewell, said the general had simple formula for the conflict: "He wanted to begin killing '4,000 of these little bastards a month,' and then by the end of the following month wanted to kill 6,000," and so on from there (Dellums, 1972, p. 65). To achieve his aims, Ewell regularly hurled invective and sacked commanders. "What the fuck are you people doing down here, sitting on your ass? The rest of the brigades are coming up with a fine body count. . . . If you can't get out there and beat 'em out of the bushes, then I'll relieve you and get somebody down here who will," was how William Taylor, then a major assigned to division headquarters, recalled the general's typical threats to subordinates. Battalion commander David Hackworth remembered Ewell screaming: "Jack up that body count or you're gone, Colonel" (Hackworth & England, 2002, p. 98; Hackworth & Sherman, 1989, pp. 485, 501). It didn't take long for Ewell to become known as "The Butcher of the Delta" (Appy, 2003, p. 323; Emerson, 1976, p. 154; Hackworth & England, 2002, p. 99; Krepinevich, 1986, p. 203; Nolan, 2006, p. 156; Turse, 2013, p. 207).

As the planning for Speedy Express progressed, politics intervened to give the hard-charging Ewell a mandate for more military resources and an even freer hand in employing them. With the U.S. presidential election looming in the fall of 1968, Lyndon Johnson had jump-started stagnant peace talks with the North Vietnamese and the NLF in Paris. This gave Speedy Express added importance, as the Pentagon sought to bring the rice-rich region and its large population under Saigon's control before any peace deal was struck. With the military eager for rapid results, Ewell became the wrong man in the wrong place at the wrong time for the Vietnamese of the Mekong Delta. The United States brought to bear almost every option in its arsenal: heavily armed helicopter gunships, bomb-laden B-52s, F-4 Phantoms dropping canisters of napalm by the ton, massive Navy ships stationed off the coast that could hurl Volkswagen-sized shells at targets miles inland, Swift Boats patrolling the Delta's waterways with machine guns, elite teams of commandos, large numbers of snipers, and, of course, regular infantry by the thousands.

"All of these efforts jelled in the winter and spring of 1968–1969, greatly increasing the combat power and flexibility of the division," Ewell and his deputy Ira Hunt later wrote in their history of the 9th Division's operations in the Delta (Ewell & Hunt, 1974, p. 16). The statistics bear this out. During the first month of Speedy Express, the 9th Infantry Division logged a 24:1 kill ratio. It would jump to 68:1 in March 1969 and an astounding 134:1 in April (Turse, 2013). For the first quarter of 1969, the 9th Division had doubled the kill ratio of the next most prolific U.S. division. By April 1969, the Pentagon noted that of eight U.S. divisions then being tracked for statistical analysis, the 9th Infantry Division accounted for fully one-third of the enemy KIAs (Thayer, 1975, vol. 4).

As Ewell demanded, Vietnamese were dying all across the Delta. In many cases, however, they weren't enemy troops. The guerrillas were well-armed but incapable of going toe-to-toe with Ewell's war machine, so they generally avoided combat when faced with the full might of the Americans (Elliott, 2007; Hunt, 2010; Turse, 2013). And while

Ewell's heavy firepower certainly killed many guerrillas, it wasn't difficult for the revolutionary forces to replenish their ranks with new recruits and replacements. The Army's own estimates indicated that the number of enemy forces in the region never dipped during Speedy Express and may have actually increased (Elliott, 2007; Turse, 2013).

For civilians in the Delta, Speedy Express made an already perilous existence even more dangerous. Many villagers who lived through that period recall, in particular, the relentless threat of American helicopters. A villager from Dinh Tuong Province summed up the Vietnamese perception of American helicopters in the Delta: "If a gunner saw anyone, even a woman or a small child or a water buffalo, he blew them apart" (Borton, 1995, pp. 38–39). From January through April of 1969 alone, the 9th Division's aviation battalion flew a total of 4,338 gunship sorties. In addition to the destruction inflicted by the 9th Division's own helicopters, the Delta was also hit hard by the newly arrived Cobra helicopter gunships of the Phantom III program (Ewell, 1969, pp. 7–8).

As one 9th Infantry Division veteran observed, "A Cobra gunship spitting out six hundred rounds a minute doesn't discern between chickens, kids and V.C." (MacPherson, 2001, p. 22). U.S. advisor Louis Janowski echoed this assessment. In his official end-of-tour report, he called Phantom operations a form of "non-selective terrorism." Most missions, he wrote, consisted of attacks on houses, sampans, and bunkers, carried out with no knowledge or concern about who was in them. If any enemy forces were killed, it was almost entirely by random chance. "I have flown Phantom III missions," he wrote, "and have medivacked enough elderly people and children to firmly believe that the percentage of Viet Cong killed by support assets is roughly equal to the percentage of Viet Cong in the population. That is, if 8% of the population [of] an area is VC about 8% of the people we kill are VC" (Turse, 2013, pp. 90–91).

December 1968, the first month of Speedy Express, also saw the beginning of "night search" hunter-killer missions. In these operations, spotters—using primitive night-vision devices—identified targets with a burst of tracer fire, which then signaled accompanying helicopter gunships to rake the area with machine guns (Ewell, 1974; Ewell, 1979; Lewy, 1981). When top advisor John Paul Vann flew on some of these missions, he found the helicopters simply targeted any and all people, homes, and water buffalo they saw. Once anyone or anything had been sighted, the information was relayed to the flight commander, and the helicopters attacked. No attempt was made, Vann said, to determine whether the people or structures were civilian, and large numbers of innocents were killed and wounded as a result. Ewell admitted as much in a post-war interview, noting that, at night, "anybody that was out there was fair game." If any "peasants" were killed during nighttime curfew, he said, that was just "tough luck" (Turse, 2013, p. 210).

Americans hovering in their heavily armed helicopter gunships weren't the only threat to Vietnamese civilians during Speedy Express. According to the military, almost 6,500 tactical air strikes were carried out in support of the operation, dropping at least 5,078 tons of bombs and 1,784 tons of napalm (Buckley, 1972; Turse, 2013). Air Force Captain Brian Willson carried out bomb-damage assessments in free-fire zones throughout the Delta and saw the results firsthand. "It was the epitome of immorality," he later told an interviewer. "One of the times I counted bodies after an air strike—which always ended with two napalm bombs which would just fry everything that was left—I counted sixty-two bodies. In my report I described them as so many women between fifteen and twenty-five and so many children—usually in their mothers' arms or very close to them—and so many old people." When he later read the official tally of dead, he found that it listed them as 130 VC killed (Valentine, 1990, p. 216).

Ewell, for his part, claimed that the 9th Division stressed "discriminate and selective use of firepower," and that some of the region actually appeared "unharmed from the air." Still, even he admitted that in "other areas, where this emphasis wasn't applied or wasn't feasible, the countryside looked like the Verdun battlefields" (Ewell, 1969, p. 12; Thayer, 1975, vol. 4, p. 27; Turse, 2013, p. 213).

The carnage was evident even in official U.S. statistics, which note that more than 13,000 civilians were wounded in IV Corps in just the first half of 1969. This may even have been a significant undercount. One American general wrote that during Ewell's tenure, the workload of provincial hospitals and foreign medical field teams was approximately "12,000 admissions monthly, 100,000 outpatient visits, and 1,000 major operations" (Turse, 2013, pp. 213–214). If just half of these were war victims, the total casualty count would be staggering. But it may have been an even greater percentage.

An American medical team that carried out a fact-finding mission in the Delta during Speedy Express found that both Phong Dinh's 500-bed provincial hospital at Can Tho and Dinh Tuong's provincial hospital at My Tho were "overflowing" with civilian war casualties. In both the Can Tho hospital and in Kien Phuong's Cao Lanh provincial hospital, the team noted, civilian war casualties accounted for up to 80% of all the patients (*Civilian Casualty, Social Welfare and Refugee Problems in South Vietnam: Hearings Before the United States Senate Committee on the Judiciary, Subcommittee to Investigate Problems Connected with Refugees and Escapees*, 1969). A separate inquiry into Speedy Express, carried out by the chief of the MACV Inspector General's investigative division, concluded that:

> While there appears to be no means of determining the precise number of civilian casualties incurred by U.S. forces during Operation Speedy Express, it would appear that the extent of these casualties was in fact substantial, and that a fairly solid case can be constructed to show that civilian casualties may have amounted to several thousand (between 5,000 and 7,000). (Turse, 2013, pp. 255–256)

Other U.S. efforts were similarly deadly for civilians and of dubious military value. The CIA organized, coordinated, and financed several projects devoted to intelligence collection and targeted killings: the most infamous was called the Phoenix program. Employing elite U.S. troops as well as South Vietnamese mercenaries known as Provincial Reconnaissance Units or PRUs, the program sought to "neutralize" members of the "Viet Cong infrastructure," as the Americans called civilians working for the NLF (McCoy, 2006; Turse, 2013, p. 190). The Phoenix program soon developed a reputation as a corrupt, informant-driven operation in which a significant number of noncombatants, some completely innocent, were captured, interrogated, or assassinated merely to meet quotas, win bounties, or settle grudges. William Colby, the program's director, even conceded that there were some "illegal killings," while Pentagon documents, distributed at the highest levels of the government, admitted that some Saigon officials were "using the program against personal enemies" (Balaban, 2002, p. 49–50; McCoy, 2006; Thayer, 1975, vol. 10, p. 80; *Colby*,1982, p. 7; Valentine, 1990, 17–171, 218–219, 264–265, 315).

In 1969, the Phoenix Program accounted for 19,534 enemy "neutralizations," including 4,832 people killed. Only 150 of those "neutralized" were, however, categorized as senior NLF cadres, and just 81 of those were classified as priority targets. The next year, neutralizations jumped to 22,341, but the number of priority targets fell to just 17 senior NLF leaders (Prados, 2009). Despite this, U.S. officials continued to cite progress, estimating a drop in enemy troop strength while pointing to large numbers of defectors as clear evidence. Still, only 368 turncoats were army deserters, and the NLF was able to launch nearly the same number of attacks it had the year before. After 1969, despite many years of combat, defections actually began dropping, and the next year Hanoi also sent 103,000 fresh forces southward (Prados, 2009).

Nixon's policy was to escalate militarily while carrying out, sometimes publicly, sometimes privately, peace negotiations. The president's ability to wage war was, however, limited by the men under his command (Gettleman, 1985). As American troop strength in Vietnam began to decline—after reaching a peak level of 543,000 in April 1969— signs of disillusionment, indiscipline, and low morale within the military were rising fast. A 1969 Nielson survey of Vietnam veterans found that only 10% supported the war's mission and the tactics embraced by commanders. Forty-four percent, a plurality of those surveyed, said the war was a mistake, and 40% said it had been fought incorrectly (Lewis, 2013). Meanwhile, their brothers still in Vietnam developed a shorthand for their efforts—the four U's: "We are the Unwilling, led by the Unqualified, to do the Unnecessary, for the Ungrateful" (Shkurti, 2011, pp. 8–9). In fact, studies commissioned by the Army in 1970 and 1971 found that 37% of soldiers surveyed admitted to engaging in "dissent" or "disobedience," one third of them repeatedly (Lewis, 2013; Lewy, 1981).

Another indicator of the troops' breakdown in discipline and the rise of disenchantment with the war was the level of drug use. In 1966, the U.S. military carried out only about 100 drug investigations in Vietnam—one investigation for each of 3,853 American soldiers. During 1969 and 1970, military police made 11,000 drug arrests (Prados, 2009), roughly one arrest for every 400 soldiers (troop levels to calculate rates of investigation and arrest are from The American War Library). This increase was mirrored in other data. In 1967, it was estimated that 29% of all U.S. troops in Vietnam smoked marijuana (Clodfelter, 1995). By 1969, a study showed that the number of users had jumped to 51%, and by 1971 approached 60% (Appy, 1993). That year, a Department of Defense-sponsored survey found that 28.5% of U.S. personnel in Vietnam had used narcotics (such as opium and heroin), and 30.8% had used various psychedelic drugs (Lewy, 1981). The Pentagon estimated about one in eight troops—30,000 men—in Vietnam used opiates or cocaine, not to mention those using amphetamines, barbiturates, LSD, and other substances (Shkurti, 2011).

Growing disillusionment was also reflected in the number of disciplinary actions, the most serious of which—general courts martial—jumped from 176 in 1966 to 377 in 1969, a period during which troop levels increased only 23%. Over the same years, non-judicial punishments—better known as Article 15s—increased 44%, from 46,392 to 66,702. While troop levels had dropped 30% in 1970, the number of Article 15s remained high—with some 64,534 administered by year's end. In 1971, when mid-year troop strength stood at less than half that of the previous year, the most serious form of punishment, general courts martial, still numbered 350 (Lewy, 1981; Prugh, 1975; troop levels are from The American War Library).

Another indication of the military's disintegration was evident in the rise of away-without-leave (AWOL) infractions and outright desertions. While Vietnam-only totals are unknown, worldwide rates reflect indiscipline across the service branches stemming from the conflict in Southeast Asia. For the Army, AWOL and desertion rates (per 1,000 average enlisted monthly strength) stood at 60.1 and 15.7, respectively, in 1965. In 1969, the rates had risen to 112.3 and 42.4, and by 1971 stood at 176.9 and 73.5 (in comparison, the highest Army desertion rate in Korea was 22.3 per 1,000). For the Marine Corps, the numbers were even more dismal. In 1970, AWOL and desertion rates reached 174.3 and 59.6 (per 1,000 average enlisted monthly strength), and by 1973, the last year of U.S. combat operations in Vietnam, the rates stood at an astounding 234.3 and 63.2, respectively (Lewy, 1981).

In Vietnam, discipline and battle-worthiness suffered. Careless units bumbled into ambushes or accidentally opened fire on fellow Americans. On bases, slack security and enemy skill led to devastating enemy attacks (Lepre, 2011). By 1969, the monetary damage of an average sapper raid was more than $1 million (Wilkins, 2011). During 1969 and 1970, enemy sappers raided bases in the 4th Infantry Division's area of operations five times without incurring a single casualty. In just one of those assaults, they killed an American and destroyed 19 helicopters. Confronted by a sapper attack in June 1970, U.S. sentries at a petroleum storage facility in Qui Nhon played dead as the revolutionary forces destroyed 450,000 gallons of fuel and the headquarters building. A year later, Americans apparently failed to fire even a single shot during an enemy raid on a different U.S. outpost at Qui Nhon. The same thing happened in 1971 when enemy forces attacked the huge U.S. base at Cam Ranh Bay and destroyed 1.5 million gallons of jet fuel (Lepre, 2011). That year, an enemy rocket also slammed into a single bunker on a base in Quang Tri Province, killing 30 soldiers and wounding 30 others. Asked why they had ignored proper procedures of dispersing during an attack, one of the survivors explained that they were all eating dinner and ran to the closest bunker (Shkurti, 2011).

As Colonel David Hackworth, on his third tour in Vietnam in 1969, put it: "Anarchy ruled. My unit was composed of 99 percent draftees. They were all good men, but none in their heart of hearts wanted to be there. They just wanted to stay alive and get the hell out" (Prados, 2009, p. 277). In fact, combat troops increasingly undertook "search and evade" or "sandbagging" missions, calling in fake coordinates and holing up in safe areas until it was time for them to return from the patrol. "By 1969," Christian Appy notes, "combat avoidance increasingly developed into direct 'combat refusals,' the military's euphemism for mutiny" (Appy, 1993, p. 245). This is evidenced by the fact that, in 1968, the official number of cases of insubordination, mutiny, and "other acts involving willful refusal to perform a lawful order" recorded by the Army alone was 94. By 1970, it had jumped to 152 despite a marked drop in U.S. troop strength in Vietnam (Appy, 1993; Lewy, 1981).

That same year, for example, Captain Brian Utermahlen of the 1st Cavalry Division told *Life* magazine that it was getting more and more difficult to convince American soldiers to fight costly battles. "The colonel wants to make contact with the enemy and so do I," he said, "but the men flat don't. It's frustrating but I understand how they feel." One of his men, Private First Class Steve Wright, underscored the point. "Two of them want to kill gooks," he said of the Captain and the Colonel, "and the rest of us never want to see any again." Joe Curry, one of Utermahlen's platoon sergeants—a man who wore beads and a peace medallion—explained their mindset. "We don't try to frustrate the captain's attempts to kill gooks, but we don't put our hearts in it," he said. "Supposedly, the mission comes first. I put the welfare of the men first" (Saar, 1970). Utermahlen's unit was no anomaly. Over the course of the year, elements of the 1st Cavalry—the elite airmobile division that had distinguished itself in the Ia Drang valley five years before— refused combat at least three dozen times (Prados, 2009).

Other soldiers did more than simply refuse to fight. As Appy observed, "by 1969– 1970, officers were fully aware that authoritarian rule posed the ultimate risk: their own men might kill them" (Appy, 1993, p. 246). The practice of killing superiors, known as "fragging" (as the preferred method was using a fragmentation grenade), markedly rose in the last years of the war. In 1969, the Army reported 126 fragging incidents, the next year it rose to 271 and stood at 333 in 1971. This represented an increase from 0.265 fraggings per 1,000 troops in Vietnam, to 0.810 per 1,000, to an astonishing 2.12 per 1,000 in 1971. For the war, the official total of fraggings stood at 1,017, although some estimates suggest that five times as many incidents went unreported or undocumented. In about 80% of officially documented attacks, victims were non-commissioned officers or officers (Appy, 1993; Clodfelter, 1995; troop levels to calculate fragging rates are from The American War Library).

Major General Melvin Zais, the commander of the 101st Airborne Division, report- edly had a $10,000 bounty placed on his head by his own troops for ordering repeated frontal assaults on the North Vietnamese–held Hill 937 (Gibson, 2000). The battle, which took place in May 1969 and became better known by the moniker "Hamburger Hill" (since the combat turned U.S. troops into veritable ground meat), lasted 10 ex- hausting days and left 56 U.S. soldiers dead and another 420 wounded. In the end, American forces achieved a body count of 505 and succeeded in taking the hill. Almost immediately, however, the U.S. abandoned the hard-won ground to be reoccupied by enemy troops (Gibson, 2000; Appy, 1993; Clodfelter, 1995).

At home, uproar over Hamburger Hill caused the Nixon administration to issue or- ders to reduce the number of U.S. casualties. But that didn't deter the president from expanding the war as he attempted to simultaneously withdraw from Vietnam and compel the revolutionary forces to accept defeat. In March 1969, Nixon and his national security advisor Henry Kissinger escalated the conflict in Southeast Asia by ordering the implementation of Operation Menu—the bombing of Cambodia. A plan so secret that even some top military officials were unaware of it, Operation Menu consisted of clandestine B-52 raids on suspected enemy targets inside the officially neutral nation of Cambodia with records falsified to preserve the fiction that the strikes took place in South Vietnam. The secret bombings continued until 1973 but failed to meet Nixon's goal of applying so much pressure that Hanoi would be "begging for peace" (Appy, 2003, p. 278). Instead, the strikes killed innocent civilians and politically, economically, and socially destabilized Cambodia and drove growing numbers to join the fledgling and ultimately auto-genocidal Khmer Rouge movement (Gibson, 2000; Prados, 2009, Young, 1991).

One of Vietnam's own killing fields was finally exposed in the fall of 1969, after freelance journalist Seymour Hersh received a vague tip about an officer who had killed some 70 or 80 people. Hersh managed to find and interview Lieutenant William Calley, at Fort Benning, Georgia, laying the foundation for a series of articles on the My Lai massacre that would eventually win him a Pulitzer prize. Despite stunning reporting of a blockbuster story, *Life* and *Look* magazines passed on Hersh's reporting (Knightley, 1975). Finding newspapers similarly uninterested, Hersh turned to Dispatch News Service, a little-known, left-leaning news agency, which finally shepherded his story into the mainstream media (Peck, 1985; Engelhardt, 1995).

On November 13, Hersh's article about the massacre by members of the 23rd Infantry Division's Charlie Company, 1st Battalion, 20th Infantry, in the village of My Lai ran in 36 newspapers, including the *Chicago Sun-Times, St. Louis Post-Dispatch*, and *Milwaukee Journal*, and soon the story was picked up elsewhere. Soon, the *Cleveland Plain Dealer* and *Life* magazine published grisly photographs of the massacre taken by Army photographer Ron Haeberle, including a heap of civilian bodies with children clearly among them. Adding fuel to the fire, Charlie Company's Paul Meadlo appeared in a confessional television interview with CBS's Mike Wallace (Bilton & Sim, 1992; Engelhardt, 1995; Knightley, 1975). He admitted that the troops had rounded up and shot hundreds of men, women, and children. "And babies?" Wallace asked repeatedly. "And babies," Meadlo replied (Wallace, 1969, p. A16).

A panel conducting an inquiry into the cover-up of the massacre concluded that 28 officers, including two generals, had committed 224 serious offenses, but just 14 officers ultimately faced charges. Of them, 12 saw their cases dismissed before trial. The other two were acquitted. More than 500 Vietnamese civilians had been killed at My Lai, but only lowly Lieutenant Calley—who nonetheless had plenty of blood on his hands—was tried, found guilty, and handed a life sentence. President Nixon intervened, freeing Calley from prison. The young veteran eventually served about 40 months, most of it under house arrest, before being paroled.

On the day that Hersh's story of the My Lai massacre broke, the second major U.S. antiwar protest of autumn 1969 began with a "March Against Death" from Virginia's Arlington National Cemetery into Washington, D.C. Over the course of four miles, in the bitter cold, demonstrators each carried a placard with the name of an American killed in Vietnam and, during the hours of darkness, a lit candle. Leading the way was 23-year-old Judy Droz, who carried the name of her late husband. She called out his name at the White House and then kept marching to the steps of the Capitol where she deposited the placard in a coffin. She was followed by 45,000 others who marched through wind and rain and thunderstorms, through two nights and into the next day.

Each read out a name of a dead American soldier and then added their placard to the coffin. On Saturday, November 15th, hundreds of thousands converged on the Mall in front of the Washington Monument for a huge demonstration while President Nixon adopted a siege mentality and literally circled the wagons, ringing the White House with bumper-to-bumper buses (Young, 1991).

The protest, carried out under the auspices of the New Mobilization Committee to End the War, was the largest in the history of the country with an estimated 500,000 to 1 million taking part in Washington, D.C., and hundreds of thousands more turning out in San Francisco. In the days leading up to the demonstration, more than 1,300 active-duty troops, including almost 200 stationed in Vietnam, signed a letter that was published in the *New York Times*, calling on military personnel to support the protest. A month after the D.C. protest, 1,000 Marines in Oceanside, California, staged their own military moratorium (Lewis, 2013).

On April 30, 1970, Nixon took to television to announce an "incursion" into Cambodia, really an invasion by tens of thousands of U.S. and South Vietnamese troops, in order to attack enemy sanctuaries, destroy the revolutionary forces' high command, and demonstrate support for Cambodia's new military ruler, Lon Nol, who had overthrown neutralist Prince Norodom Sihanouk in March. "The speech was dis-ingenuous and artful," historian Jeffrey Kimball noted. "Although making reference to the defenseless, neutral government in Phnom Penh, Nixon failed to mention the coup against Sihanouk, the American role in it, or the steps Lon Nol had taken in over-turning Sihanouk's policies." Nixon also lied to the American public, claiming that the United States had previously respected the neutrality of Cambodia, making no mention of long-running South Vietnamese and American cross-border raids and his own secret bombing campaign. "If, when the chips are down," he said, "the world's most powerful nation . . . acts like a pitiful, helpless giant, the forces of totalitarianism and anarchy will threaten free nations and free institutions throughout the world" (Appy 1993; Appy, 2003; Kimball, 1998, p. 212).

Again, Nixon's gamble of widening the war failed to force the Vietnamese revolutionaries to end their efforts to reunify their country. What the Cambodian incur-sion did instead was unleash a firestorm back home. Hundreds of thousands of students on more than 700 campuses went on strike, and about 30 Reserve Officers' Training Corps (ROTC) buildings were burned or bombed. The president of the United Auto Workers (UAW) criticized the invasion, former Peace Corps volunteers took over Peace Corps headquarters in Washington, D.C., in protest, GIs demonstrated at military bases across the U.S., 250 State Department employees signed a letter of protest, and two of Henry Kissinger's top aides resigned in opposition to the policy (Appy, 2003; Isserman & Kazin, 1999; Morgan, 1991; Young, 1991).

At Ohio's Kent State University, on May 4, 1970, National Guardsmen opened fire on student protesters, killing four. For the next four days, campus demonstrations erupted at the rate of more than 100 per day across the country; 1.5 million students went on strike; 536 schools shut down and 51 never reopened during the rest of the academic year. Ten days after the Kent State shootings, two more students were shot dead by state police and another 12 were left wounded at Jackson State College in Mississippi (Appy, 2003; Farber & Foner, 1994; Isserman & Kazin, 1999; Morgan, 1991; Young, 1991).

Four months after the killings at Kent State, a presidential Commission on Campus Unrest found that the use of lethal force by the National Guard was "unnecessary, inexcusable, and completely unwarranted." The public at large, however, followed the lead of the president, who seemed to blame the students for the violence. A Gallup poll shortly after the Kent State shootings found that 58% of Americans blamed the protesters for the shootings (Appy, 2015). In the wake of the Cambodia and Kent State protests, Nixon unleashed the CIA, FBI, and other operatives to sabotage the antiwar movement (Farber & Foner, 1994). This was just one facet of a concerted campaign of wiretaps, tax audits, spying, infiltration, provocation, intimidation, and various dirty tricks employed by the White House that would eventually end Nixon's presidency in a massive abuse-of-power scandal a few years later (Appy, 2015).

Despite the government's efforts, antiwar sentiment continued to spread. On August 29, 1970, for example, the National Chicano Moratorium Against the Vietnam War held a march and rally in East Los Angeles attended by as many as 30,000 protesters. One held a sign that read: "Traiga a mis carnales ahora" [Bring my homeboys home now]. Another read: "A mi me dieron una medulla y $10,000 por mi unico hijo" [They gave me a medal and $10,000 for my only son]. Still another seemed to reference the murder of civil rights leaders, the killings of Black Panthers, the gunning down of the antiwar protesters at Kent State, the shooting of the students at Jackson State, and the plight of the ghetto, in general: "Murdered in Vietnam, Murdered at Home. Ya Basta!" [Enough Is Enough!]. It would also, before the day was over, seem prophetic (Appy, 2015, pp. 204–205).

One of the journalists covering the protest was Ruben Salazar, a distinguished reporter for the *Los Angeles Times* and news director of a local Spanish-language television station. Salazar had covered the war in Vietnam and been the Mexico City bureau chief for the *Times* before returning to Los Angeles, where he covered the emerging Chicano rights and antiwar movements. He had just published several articles on police brutality and drawn the ire of the city police chief who dispatched officers to warn Salazar of the effects of his work on "the minds of barrio people" (Vigil, 1999, pp. 144–146).

The night before the protest, Salazar told organizers that his sources said the police and FBI were planning to incite violence during the demonstration. Indeed, participants recall what began as a peaceful and celebratory day turned into a "police riot" in which march organizers were clubbed by the police and protesters were attacked with tear gas. The crowd fought back. Hundreds were arrested, dozens injured, and two Chicanos died in the violence.

In the wake of the protests, Salazar headed to a bar many blocks away to relax and have a beer. Sherriff's deputies soon arrived, claiming they received a report of an armed man inside. Without attempting to clear the bar of patrons, a deputy fired a tear gas canister through the open door. It wasn't a standard cardboard-encased round but a metal projectile designed to be fired through doors or walls, and it struck Salazar in the temple and penetrated his skull. Police then cleared the bar and sealed it. It would be three hours before Salazar's corpse was found. The deputy claimed shooting the journalist was an accident, and no criminal charges were ever filed. Many in the community called it an assassination (Appy, 2015; Vigil, 1999).

The Final Years

As the United States increasingly seemed at be at war at home, the war in Vietnam was becoming more and more unpopular. In 1960, 63% of Americans said they wanted to see U.S. troops fighting "the Communist tide" abroad. By 1971, public opinion had dramatically shifted, with 71% of Americans reporting that the United States had made a "mistake" in ever sending troops to Vietnam, while 58% called the war "immoral" (Appy, 2003). Still, the conflict, which then had become Nixon's war, ground on with more than 400,000 personnel still serving in Vietnam as of July 1970—a month in which the United States carried out 64 large-scale (battalion-sized or bigger) operations (Lewy, 1981).

In February 1971, 15,000 South Vietnamese troops, supported by U.S. artillery, helicopters, fighter-bombers, and B-52s, invaded Laos in an effort to sever the Ho Chi Minh Trail. The operation, code-named Lam Son 719, was a disaster for the United States and South Vietnam. An operation slated to last three months was over in weeks. After running headlong into five North Vietnamese divisions and suffering 9,000 casualties, the ARVN retreated in a panic, abandoning 150 tanks as they fled back to South Vietnam. Television reports broadcast the devastating images of South Vietnamese soldiers clinging to the skids of helicopters as they fled pursuing North Vietnamese troops. And though they were officially serving only in a "support" role, hundreds of Americans were killed or wounded in the rout (Gettleman, 1985; Shkurti, 2011).

In spite of the failure of Lam Son 719, Nixon soon proclaimed that, "Vietnamization has succeeded" (Appy, 2003, p. 394). A March 1971 Gallup poll suggested that Americans thought otherwise. Only 19% of those who knew about the invasion of Laos believed it would shorten the war, and only 41% said they approved of the president's handling of the war. Distrust of the White House was also running high, with 65% of the public believing that the Nixon administration was not telling the public "all they should know about the Vietnam War" (Gallup, 1972).

At home, the invasion of Laos sparked a flurry of protests during the spring of 1971. In April, in an unprecedented act, highly decorated veterans descended on Washington, D.C., to return their medals and ribbons—honors that previous generations of American fighting men had treasured. Gloria Emerson, who had covered the war as a correspondent for the *New York Times*, described the emotional scene:

> They started to come on a Friday, an eccentric, a strange-looking army, wearing fatigues and field jackets, helmets and their old boonie hats, the same boots they had worn in Vietnam. Some brought bedrolls and all slept outdoors on a camping site on a small quadrangle on the Mall. . . . All came with their discharge papers so their bitterest critics could not accuse them of being imposters, although some did anyway. There were a few men who did not have two legs, a few who could not rise from wheelchairs, but they were in good spirits and among their own. (Emerson, 1976, p. 330)

When the authorities erected a barricade to stop the protestors from reaching Congress, they hurled their Purple Hearts and Bronze Stars over the wood and wire wall onto the steps of the Capitol, in perhaps the single most iconic antiwar act in American history. A few dozen tried to get someone to arrest them as war criminals, but no one would. When 110 of the veterans sat down on the steps of the Supreme Court to protest its failure to rule on the constitutionality of the war, however, the police moved in. Offering no resistance, the men placed their hands on their heads, as prisoners were made to do in Vietnam, and were taken away (Emerson, 1976).

Meanwhile, John Kerry—a spokesman for the largest antiwar veterans organization, Vietnam Veterans Against the War (VVAW) (and a future senator and secretary of state)—appeared before the Senate Foreign Relations Committee and demanded to know, "How do you ask a man to be the last man to die in Vietnam? How do you ask a man to be the last man to die for a mistake?" (Isserman & Kazin, 1999, p. 271; Prados, 2009). It wasn't an abstract question. A month before, the Vietnamese revolutionary forces carried out a devastating attack on a firebase named Mary Ann, located about 50 miles south of Da Nang.

On March 28, 1971, following a mortar barrage of hundreds of rounds, 60 enemy sappers attacked the base, which was in the process of being shut down. When it was over, 30 Americans lay dead and another 82 were wounded. The reasons for the carnage weren't hard to fathom. Officers had failed to send out reconnaissance patrols on the night of the attack or even post guards at each perimeter bunker or the entrances of the base's tactical operations center. Searchlights that should have lit up the base's perimeter were not working, and it was unlikely that mines, tear gas, napalm, and explosive charges were in place to repel an attack or that adequate lines of fire had been laid out for the soldiers defending the base. Of the 50 troops assigned to guard duty that night, not one noticed any sign of the massing enemy force. This last fact was hardly surprising, given that neither officers nor non-commissioned officers had bothered to check the bunker line even once that night.

An official inquiry revealed not just a field unit whose discipline had gone slack, but a systemic breakdown in authority extending to top commanders. High-ranking officers, including the division's commanding general, had failed to ensure that the troops on Firebase Mary Ann followed regulations, and the report's authors worried that as the war lurched to an end, an even greater disaster might lie on the horizon (Hammond, 1998).

Disaster was exactly what Colonel Robert Heinl, a distinguished combat veteran as well as a military historian and analyst, saw when he took stock of the entire U.S. military just a few months later. Examining the situation in the pages of *Armed Forces Journal*, his evaluation was dire:

> The morale, discipline and battleworthiness of the U.S. Armed Forces are, with a few salient exceptions, lower and worse than at anytime in this century and possibly in the history of the United States. By every conceivable indicator, our army that now remains in Vietnam is in a state approaching collapse, with individual units avoiding or having refused combat, murdering their officers and noncommissioned officers, drug-ridden, and dispirited where not near mutinous. (Heinl, 1971, p. 1).

The state of revolt in the armed forces, Heinl concluded, was just shy of "the French Army's Nivelle mutinies of 1917 and the collapse of the Tsarist armies in 1916 and 1917" (Heinl, 1971). A more dire description was hardly possible.

While only 5,000 U.S. troops were hospitalized for battle injuries in Vietnam in 1971, some 20,000 received treatment for drug abuse (Clodfelter, 1995). That same year, Army AWOL rates reached their highest levels in modern history, while desertions had skyrocketed nearly 400% since 1966. Antiwar GIs were also producing hundreds of underground newspapers that encouraged disobedience and rebellion (Cortright, 2005). While only three such papers had existed in 1967, some 245 had been or were being published by 1972. On top of this, Heinl counted no fewer than 14 "GI dissent organizations (including two made up exclusively of officers)" that were operating more or less openly and "at least six antiwar veterans' groups which strive to influence GIs" (Heinl, 1971). The best known of these groups, VVAW, began as a six-member speakers bureau in 1967. By 1972, its membership rolls exceeded 20,000 (Hunt, 1999).

Most veterans didn't belong to such organizations, but they found themselves no less affected—and changed—by the conflict. As the 1970s began, more men returned home with disturbing memories and uncertain futures. Specialist-4 Chris Mead saw a lot of hostile fire in Vietnam and several times thought he would be killed. But he wasn't. He did, however, see "trucks blown up, kids maimed, women killed, buddies bleeding and dying. Once he saw a Viet Cong running away on the stumps of his shot-away legs," wrote *Newsweek* reporter Karl Fleming (Fleming, 1971, p. 212). In 1971, Mead returned home to his boyhood bedroom, still adorned with rock band album covers and a flower he had drawn as a child, but now faced adult problems. His family's small dairy farm ceased to turn a profit, so they had sold off the cows. His friend didn't think the local seed company was hiring. His father thought the prospects of finding a job in nearby Flint, Michigan, were poor (Fleming, 1971).

Men like Chris Mead, who had grown up during the post–World War II economic boom, came home to a changing America. Not only were protests, rights' movements, and cultural shifts remaking the nation in profound ways, the economy was increasingly inhospitable. Between 1966 and 1971, the United States hemorrhaged nearly 1 million blue-collar jobs in key sectors like the automotive industry and steel manufacturing. In 1969, the average factory worker earned 82 cents per week less, in real terms, than he did in 1965. Inflation, under 2% in 1965, had climbed to 4.5% by 1971. Unemployment, at just 4% when Nixon took office, crept higher over the next two years, rising to 6%, as the nation slipped into recession. By the summer of 1971, 73% of Americans disapproved of the President's handling of the economy (Isserman & Kazin, 1999; Perlstein, 2008).

As the economy faltered and the American war effort limped toward an end, Daniel Ellsberg, a military analyst who had helped to write a secret history of the conflict while working in the government, had become disillusioned with the war and felt an imperative to expose the truth of it to the American people. An official cover-up of an atrocity scandal, involving the execution of a supposed spy by Green Berets, pushed Ellsberg over the edge, causing him to leak Robert McNamara's secret study of U.S. policy in Vietnam from the 1940s to 1968, which would soon become famous as the Pentagon Papers. He gave the documents to Neil Sheehan of the *New York Times*, Ellsberg later said, to expose "a system that lies automatically, at every level from bottom to top—from sergeant to commander in chief—to conceal murder" (Ellsberg, 2002, p. 289).

The Pentagon Papers contained candid analyses and secret documents outlining official lies that had misled the American public about the war through four presidential administrations. Chief among the revelations was the fact that, despite high-minded public rhetoric, U.S. war managers had little concern for the Vietnamese people, regarding South Vietnam as nothing more than a strategic site in the Cold War power struggle. Sheehan's first articles about the secret study ran in the *New York Times* in June 1971, and the airing of decades' worth of deceptions—along with the government's strenuous efforts to prevent newspapers from publishing more of the material—added to the growing public perception that Washington could not be trusted (Ellsberg, 2002).

In 1972, after repeated failures to turn around U.S. fortunes in Southeast Asia, Nixon embarked on a heralded trip to the People's Republic of China in an effort to drive a wedge between Beijing and Moscow and persuade both to pressure Hanoi to come to a settlement with the United States. Nixon's showy diplomatic effort, however, prompted China to sign a new agreement to increase military aid to North Vietnam, further undermining U.S. aims. In 1972, for instance, Beijing sent North Vietnam 220 tanks compared to the 80 they supplied the previous year. And just a month after the historic summit, Hanoi launched a major offensive (Appy, 2003; Prados, 2009).

On March 30, 1972, 30,000 North Vietnamese troops, equipped with 200 tanks, streamed through the DMZ into the South Vietnam's Quang Tri Province, capturing, in just two days, 12 bases that the United States had turned over to the ARVN, while winning control of most of the province, including its capital, Quang Tri City. At the same time, another 70,000 North Vietnamese troops attacked Dak To in South Vietnam's Central Highlands, and An Loc, an area just northwest of Saigon. While U.S. ground troops were now fewer in number (133,200 total U.S. military personnel remained in January, and just 45,600 by mid-year) and operating primarily in a non-combat role, American airpower was still formidable. U.S. aircraft relentlessly pounded North Vietnamese positions and halted the offensive before it toppled the Saigon government.

Nixon also launched the retaliatory Linebacker Raids, the first large-scale, sustained bombing of North Vietnam since 1968. That April alone, North Vietnam would be slammed by 700 B-52 raids, including a 48-hour sustained air assault on Hanoi and Haiphong (Appy, 2003; Lewy, 1981; Young, 1991). The massive U.S. bombing campaigns that followed the Easter Offensive were not, however, confined to north of the demilitarized zone. Forty specially designed B-52 bombers, each carrying almost 30 tons of ordnance, blasted Quang Tri on a daily basis, destroying up to 99% of all buildings in the southeastern quadrant of the province and all but obliterating Quang Tri City (Turley, 2009). One reporter on the scene described Quang Tri's capital as "no longer a city but a lake of masonry" (Isaacs, 1983, p. 26). Other areas of the province suffered a similar fate, with air strikes and artillery fire wiping out homes and killing thousands of civilians (Leslie, 1995).

American firepower saved South Vietnam from collapse, but, as historian Marilyn Young observed, "Hanoi's minimal goals had been achieved: the series of highly visible victories would convince any observer that the policy of Vietnamization was, if not completely forfeit, certainly very vulnerable" (Young, 1991, p. 271). That fall, after years of fruitless talks in Paris, the revolutionary forces and the United States reached an agreement on terms for an American withdrawal from Vietnam. The Saigon government, panicked by the thought of U.S. detachment from the war effort, raised a storm of protest and pressured the United States to renegotiate already settled terms. As a result, the United States reneged on the agreement and presented North Vietnam with new demands. Hanoi then issued counter-demands, and the diplomatic talks broke down. Following this, Nixon ordered a massive bombing raid on Hanoi and the port city of Haiphong. The "Christmas bombing," which began on December 17, 1972, and lasted for 11 days, saw more than 20,000 tons of munitions unleashed on targets throughout the North Vietnam. Military targets, warehouses, factories, railroad yards, bus stations, and even Hanoi's largest hospital, Bac Mai, were hit. The civilian death toll was kept low only because North Vietnamese authorities had ordered a mass evacuation of their capital. Following the bombing, the United States and North Vietnam returned to the negotiating table and agreed to cease-fire terms that were nearly identical to those that had been reached in October (Appy, 2003).

The End of American military Involvement in Vietnam

When the Paris Peace Accords were signed in January 1973, fewer than 20,000 U.S. troops were left in Vietnam. Under terms of the agreement, U.S. prisoners held by North Vietnam were returned, and American combat troops departed from Vietnam. Still, 9,000 American "civilians," many of them former U.S. military personnel, continued to play an important support role for the South Vietnamese armed forces; $5 billion in U.S. arms and equipment, including 500 fighter-bombers and 625 helicopters, were left for the South Vietnam's military forces (giving them the fourth largest air force in the world); and U.S. economic aid continued to flow into the country. The Saigon regime stayed in power in the South, however the Provisional Revolutionary Government—formed by the NLF—was also recognized as a legitimate government, and North Vietnam was allowed to leave its troops in South Vietnam as part of a stand-still cease-fire (Appy, 2003; Clodfelter, 1995; Farber & Foner).

Almost immediately, both North Vietnam and South Vietnam broke the terms of the accord, and two years later, the last remaining U.S. personnel were driven out of the country as North Vietnamese forces entered the southern capital. "As communist soldiers marched and rode atop Soviet tanks into the heart of [South Vietnam's] power," wrote historian Lien-Hang Nguyen, "exuberant masses lined the streets of Saigon to welcome the troops as liberators." There was no need for the type of general uprising envisioned during the planning of the 1968 Tet Offensive. South Vietnam's leaders had already fled the country (Nguyen, 2012, p. 271).

Back in the United States, Americans watched televised scenes of South Vietnam's frantic final moments, as Vietnamese refugees attempted to scale the fence of the U.S. embassy compound; American troops pushed helicopters into the sea to make room on crowded aircraft carriers for more evacuations; and the last U.S. helicopter departed Saigon, emphasizing the final defeat of America in Vietnam (Appy, 2003).

AFTERMATH

Nixon's embrace and expansion of the Vietnam War had spelled doom for his presidency, which crumbled amidst a string of criminal activities known collectively as "Watergate"—named for the 1972 illegal break-in at the Democratic National Committee headquarters in the Watergate hotel. What is often forgotten is that the Watergate crimes began with wiretaps of those suspected of leaking information on clandestine bombing of Cambodia in 1969 and also included the break-in, at the office of the psychiatrist treating Daniel Ellsberg, by a team of covert White House operatives, known as "the Plumbers" (Appy, 2003). With the House Judiciary Committee moving toward a vote to impeach the president for abuse of power and obstruction of justice and a Senate trial due to follow, Nixon resigned the presidency on August 9, 1974 (Appy, 2015).

The Human Cost

While Americans who served in Vietnam paid a heavy price, an extremely conservative estimate of Vietnamese deaths found them to be "proportionally 100 times greater than those suffered by the United States" (Hirschman, et al., pp. 793–797, 809). The military forces of the U.S.-allied Republic of Vietnam reportedly lost more than 254,000 killed and more than 783,000 wounded, while the casualties of the revolutionary forces were evidently far graver—perhaps 1.7 million, including 1 million killed in battle, plus some 300,000 personnel still "missing" according to the official but incomplete Vietnamese government statistics (Appy, 2003, p. 164).

Horrendous as these numbers may be, they pale in comparison to the estimated civilian death toll during the war years. At least 65,000 North Vietnamese civilians were killed, mainly by U.S. air raids (Clodfelter, 1995; Lewy, 1981). No one will ever know exactly how many South Vietnamese civilians were killed as a result of the conflict, but using fragmentary data and questionable extrapolations, one Department of Defense statistical analyst came up with a post-war estimate of 1.2 million civilian casualties, including 195,000 killed (Appy, 1993; Thayer, 1995). In 1975, a U.S. Senate subcommittee on refugees and war victims offered an estimate of 1.4 million civilian casualties in South Vietnam, including 415,000 killed (Appy, 1993, pp. 203–204).

In recent years, careful analyses, surveys, and official estimates have pointed toward a considerably higher number of civilian deaths. The most sophisticated analysis yet of wartime mortality in Vietnam, a 2008 study by researchers from Harvard Medical School and the Institute for Health Metrics and Evaluation at the University of Washington, indicates that a reasonable estimate might be 3.8 million violent war deaths, combatant and civilian (Obermeyer, et al.). Given the limitations of the study's methodology, there are good reasons to believe that even this figure may be a significant underestimate. Nonetheless, the findings lend credibility to an 1995 Vietnamese government estimate of more than 3 million deaths in total—including 2 million civilian deaths—for the years when the Americans were involved in the conflict (Turse, 2013).

From 1955 to 1975, the United States lost more than 58,000 military personnel in Southeast Asia—in excess of 47,000 in battle—33% of them draftees. Some 86% of the dead were enlisted men or warrant officers. Only 5,741 officers died in battle and just 72 men from National Guard units were among those killed. About 80% of Marines and 60% of Army soldiers killed were 21 years old or younger. U.S. troops were wounded around 304,000 times, with 153,000 cases serious enough to require hospitalization, and 75,000 veterans were left severely disabled (Appy, 2003, Clodfelter, 1995; Defense Manpower Data Center of the Office of the Secretary of Defense, 2008; Ebert, 2004; Kelley, 2002; Thayer, 1985).

After the war, films, books, and various commentators claimed that veterans were treated with opprobrium, even regularly spat upon by antiwar protesters upon their return to the United States (Appy, 2015; Lembcke, 1998). Jerry Lembcke, a sociologist and Vietnam veteran, investigated and found no persuasive evidence that veterans were commonly spat at by antiwar demonstrators. Instead, he chalks up this notion to a latter-day conservative backlash against protest movements of the 1960s and 1970s and an accompanying effort to restore honor to military service and blot out the fact that many veterans were actually prime participants in the antiwar movement (Appy, 2015; Lembcke, 1998).

Treatment of veterans by their government was another matter. After being gravely wounded in Vietnam, Ron Kovic began to lose faith in his country as he recovered in a VA hospital. "The wards are filthy," he wrote:

> The men in my room throw their breadcrumbs under the radiator to keep the rats from chewing on our numb limbs during the nights. . . . There are never enough aides to go around on the wards, and there is constant complaining by the men. The most severely injured are totally dependent on the aides to turn them. They suffer the most and break down with sores. These are the voices that can be heard screaming in the night for help that never comes. Urine bags are constantly overflowing onto the floors while the aides play poker on the toilet bowls in the enema room. The sheets are never changed enough and many of the men stink from not being properly bathed. It never makes any sense how the government can keep asking money for weapons and leave us lying in our own filth. (Kovic, 2005, pp. 51–52)

Even many of those who made it home without physical injuries were nonetheless affected in profound ways. A 1971 Louis Harris poll found, for example, that 58% of Vietnam veterans felt "people at home just don't understand" what they had experienced at war (Nicosia, 2001). Still, 95% of Vietnam veterans believed that their family and friends treated them warmly upon their return and 79% felt that "most people respect you." Such admiration was evident on March 31, 1973, for example, when 150,000 New Yorkers lined the streets for one of the largest parades in the city's history—a "Home With Honor" event, complete with 120 brass bands, celebrating Vietnam veterans (Napoli, 2013).

Recognition of Veteran Experiences

Even so, clinicians began to talk of a "Post-Vietnam Syndrome" affecting veterans. In a 1971 letter to the editor of the *New York Times* under that very title, Henry Rosett, a professor of psychiatry at New York's Mount Sinai School of Medicine, stated that while veterans of all wars suffered guilt over killing others and surviving their less fortunate comrades, veterans of previous conflicts were also "hailed by a grateful nation" and received "absolution for both the necessary homicide and any atrocities." Vietnam veterans, however, returned to "an ambivalent nation" and received no such social support, he claimed. As a remedy, he noted, the New York chapter of VVAW had developed "rap groups" in which veterans could "attain closeness, share outrage and grief and work through their depression" (Rosett, 1971).

In December 1969 and January 1970, psychiatrist and National Book Award winner Robert Jay Lifton testified before a Senate subcommittee that atrocities were endemic to the war in Vietnam and veterans were likely to experience mild to severe psychological fallout in the years ahead. Not long after, at the invitation of New York University psychoanalyst Chaim Shatan, Lifton spoke at a public forum in the wake of the Kent State killings that was also attended by members of VVAW. Impressed, the VVAW veterans invited Lifton to sit in on their rap sessions in New York City, and VVAW president Jan Barry asked him to participate in one of the organization's upcoming events—an effort to address "the severe psychological problems of many Vietnam veterans" (Hunt, 1999, p. 86; Nicosia, 2001).

In January 1971, Lifton joined more than 100 Vietnam vets who testified about atrocities they had witnessed or committed at the VVAW's "Winter Soldier Investigation" in Detroit, Michigan. (The name was taken from a pamphlet written by the revolutionary patriot Thomas Paine in 1776, which began: "These are the times that try men's souls. The summer soldier and the sunshine patriot will, in this crisis, shrink from the service of his country; but he that stands it now, deserves the love and thanks of man and woman.") The event included testimonies from every branch of the U.S. military and almost every major combat unit from all periods of the war. By their very act of speaking out, these veterans sought to put the lie to any notion of bad apples and isolated incidents. And many went beyond merely rattling off a list of individual war crimes. Instead, broadening their focus, the Winter Soldiers explicitly pointed to superior officers and command policies as the ultimate sources of the atrocities they had witnessed or committed.

Lifton, in turn, spoke about his experiences with the rap groups. This new generation of veterans, he said, was unique. "I think the first point I'd like to make, and make very strongly is the psychological difference of this war, for a veteran, as compared to other wars." He continued:

> There's a quality of atrocity in this war that goes beyond that of other wars in that the war itself is fought as a series of atrocities. There is no distinction between an enemy whom one can justifiably fire at and people whom one murders in less than military situations.

It's all thrown together so that every day the distinction between every day activities and atrocities is almost nil. Now if one carries this sense of atrocity with one, one carries the sense of descent into evil. This is very strong in Vietnam vets. It's also strong in the rest of society, and this is what we mean by the primitive or brutalized behavior that there has been so much talk about. I think that this brutalization and the patterns that occur in the war again have to do with the nature of the war we are fighting and the people we've chosen to make our enemies.

This has to do with the atrocities characterizing the war, as often happens in a counterinsurgency . . . we intervene in a civil war or in a revolution in a far-away alien place that you don't understand historically or psychologically, but also with the technological disparity. It's of great psychological significance that Americans go around with such enormous fire power in a technologically under-developed country and develop a kind of uneasy sense of power around their technological fire power, which they then use very loosely, and often with the spirit of a hunter, as we've again heard much about. In all this way, I would stress very strongly, the GI in Vietnam becomes both victim and executioner (Lifton, 1971).

Following the Winter Soldier investigation, members of the New York chapter of VVAW invited Lifton, Shatan and other therapists and counselors to join their rap groups not as authority figures but as equals (Hagopian, 2009). "The rap groups became known as the place where you could tell your story, even the most horrible parts and people would listen," recalled one veteran. Another remembered, "Here was the first opportunity that I really had to talk with guys who had gone through the same thing. They were having the same doubts about themselves . . . and digging inside themselves—and you didn't want to do that with just anybody" (Hunt, 1999, p. 87).

The psychiatrists began to create frameworks for understanding the trauma, anguish, alienation, and rage experienced and expressed by the veterans. "Post-Vietnam Syndrome confronts us with the unconsummated grief of soldiers—impacted grief, in which an encapsulated, never-ending past deprives the present of meaning," wrote Shatan.

Few in the military will admit—even to themselves—that counter-guerrilla training *and combat* are emotionally injurious. The injury is not so much the outgrowth of one or two traumatic incidents, but rather of a cumulative, chronic, recurring pattern of exposure— little by little—to unrecognized, depreciated, or unpublicized risk and peril. (Shatan, 1973, p. 645)

The syndrome, Shatan noted, often manifested itself between nine and 30 months after veterans returned from Vietnam (Hagopian, 2009; Shatan, 1973).

Lifton observed that, to avoid the painful feelings of guilt and anger, many veterans resorted to psychic numbing, which provided some psychological protections but forced them to live incomplete lives. Others were conversely crippled by "self-lacerating guilt." He proposed that veterans instead embrace "animating guilt"—a "survivor mission" of political action, speaking out in protest against the war that had dehumanized them and laying bare the atrocious nature of the conflict. In turn, the greater society owed it to veterans to listen to, as he put it, "the truths of American atrocities" that they were attempting to tell (Hagopian, 2009, pp. 54–55).

Soon, Lifton and Shatan were inundated with requests from veterans around the country to help organize their own rap groups. By the mid-1970s, hundreds of such groups had been set up. "The main reason for these approaches," writes historian Patrick Hagopian, "was the absence of effective treatment by the Veterans Administration (VA), the government-administered program of health and other benefits for veterans" (Hagopian, 2009, p. 56). Despite institutional resistance, some at the VA began setting up their own therapy groups. Floyd Meshad, a Vietnam veteran and former military psychiatrist working for the VA in California, encountered hundreds of homeless vets in and around Venice Beach. With assistance, he set up a Vietnam veterans–only clinic and persuaded some of the homeless vets to attend a rap group there (Hagopian, 2009).

While psychiatrists who worked with veterans were coming to understand the psychological effects of the war, their profession's "bible"—the *Diagnostic and Statistical Manual of Stress Disorders–II* (1968)—contained no reference to any type of war neurosis. As a result, veterans were commonly diagnosed with personality disorders, schizophrenia, or concurrent diseases like alcoholism, despite clinicians' understanding that the war had played a role in their psychological distress. When preparation of a third edition of the manual was announced in 1974, Lifton, Shatan, and others worked to have "post-combat syndrome" added to it. After much discussion, those involved in the preparation of the manual began to believe that "post-combat syndrome" might be part of a larger phenomenon not specifically linked to war and worked on creating a diagnosis that could cover both civilian and military experiences.

In 1978, the Committee on Reactive Disorders for the *Diagnostic and Statistical Manual of Stress Disorders–III* settled on Post-Traumatic Stress Disorder (PTSD)—a condition whose diagnosis involves a much broader set of conditions than war trauma—which appeared in the new manual when it was published two years later. The *DSM-III* PTSD included, for example, "recurrent painful, intrusive recollections" or "recurrent dreams or nightmares" due to a catastrophic stressor—a traumatic event far beyond the realm of normal human experience—like the atomic bombings, the Nazi Holocaust, war, or natural disasters like earthquakes and volcanic eruptions (Hagopian, 2009).

The official recognition of PTSD helped advocates in Congress win passage of a 1979 bill aimed at providing readjustment counseling to Vietnam veterans. Implemented under President Jimmy Carter and his VA chief Max Cleland, the law funded the Readjustment Counseling Service, which set up a nationwide network of 92 storefront "Vet Centers," which were separate from the existing VA medical center system (Hagopian, 2009; Kulka, 1990; Nicosia, 2001). The incoming administration of President Ronald Reagan sought to shut down the centers, but veterans began pouring into them, looking for help. By 1983, there were 135 centers—staffed by a mix of combat veteran counselors and mental health professionals—catering to the 4,000 new Vietnam veterans who came through their doors each month. By August, just three and a half years after they opened, 200,000 veterans had sought help at the Vet Centers (MacPherson, 2001; Nicosia, 2001).

Other evidence of difficulties in readjustment for Vietnam veterans also began to emerge (Kulka, 1990). A 1976 study by John Heltzer, Lee Robins, and Darlene Davis, for example, found that of a random sample of 470 enlisted Army veterans who returned from Vietnam in 1971, 26% reported some symptoms of depression, and 20% had either probable or full-blown depressive syndrome. Of those who saw combat, 29% had either probable or full-blown depressive syndrome, compared to 8% who didn't serve in combat (Helzer, Robins, & Davis, 1976). In 1977, John Wilson sampled 346 combat and noncombat Vietnam-era veterans in Cleveland for his Forgotten Warrior Project. He found 48% unemployment among black combat veterans, 39% among their white counterparts, and discovered that, among both races, 41% had alcohol problems (MacPherson, 2001).

A 1980 Louis Harris poll, conducted on behalf of the VA, found that about 36% of high combat veterans reported difficulties with memories of death and dying; 35% reported mental or emotional problems; and 30% reported issues with drugs and alcohol, compared to just 8%, 11%, and 10% among light combat veterans (Harris, 1980). Egendorf (1981) reported that military duty during the Vietnam war had a negative effect on post-military achievement . Numerous studies also indicated that Vietnam era veterans had lower incomes than those who didn't serve (Angrist & Chen, 2011; Berger & Hirsch, 1983; Martindale & Poston, 1979; Schwartz, 1986), except for African-Americans, who appeared to have done better than counterparts who avoided military service (Martindale & Poston, 1979; Xie, 1992).

The Vietnam Experience Study (VES), which followed 18,313 Army veterans from their date of discharge from active duty (1965–1977) through December 31, 1983, found that Vietnam veterans experienced excess all-cause mortality, primarily from external causes (such as motor vehicle accidents, suicides, and homicides) compared with veterans who served during the same period but not in Vietnam. The VES also found that drug-related deaths were higher among Vietnam veterans. (A 30-year follow-up of the VES indicated, however, that the excess mortality among Vietnam veterans was isolated to the first five years after discharge from active duty [Boehmer et al., 2004].)

At the same time that veterans and their allies were agitating for recognition of war neuroses due to service in Vietnam, others were doing the same for ailments they said were related to Agent Orange and other chemical defoliants used in Vietnam in order to deny food to civilians and guerrillas and jungle cover to enemy forces. The Pentagon and the manufacturers of the herbicides consistently denied they had harmed veterans, but a May 1978 VA memo drew attention to concerns that these chemicals might be "capable of producing adverse health effects" in exposed individuals (Wilcox, 2011). In the years after, studies began to suggest that exposure to the defoliants was associated with higher incidence of cancers among veterans as well as birth defects, such as anencephaly and spina bifida, among their children (Elliott, 2007; Kim et al., 2003; Kolko, 1985; Ngo et al., 2006; Tuyet & Johansson, 2001; Wilcox, 2011).

By the early to mid-1980s, the Department of Defense began accepting some liability for defoliant-related illnesses, and the VA began treating veteran victims (Westheider, 2007). In 1984, Congress passed legislation to provide compensation for soft-tissue carcinoma related to Agent Orange exposure, and that May, lawyers representing Vietnam veterans and their families agreed to a $180 million settlement with the manufacturers of Agent Orange (Westheider, 2007; Wilcox, 2011). Congress would also renew the VA's Vet Center program in 1983. At the time of the renewal, questions arose as to how many veterans who had not sought help might also be experiencing considerable post-war readjustment issues, since estimates of the number of those suffering from such problems varied widely—from 250,000 to more than 2 million (Kulka, 1990). In an effort to find answers, the 1983 legislation mandated a comprehensive study that would provide hard data on the incidence, prevalence, and effects of PTSD and related psychological problems affecting Vietnam veterans.

In September 1984, the VA awarded a contract to the Research Triangle Institute (RTI) to conduct the study that eventually became known as the National Vietnam Veterans Readjustment Study (NVVRS). More than four years later, having examined a sample population that was broader and more inclusive than previous studies, the researchers had completed what they described as "perhaps the most far-reaching and ambitious national mental health epidemiological study ever attempted with any population" (Kulka, 1990, p. 6, xxvi).

The findings of the NVVRS indicated that 15.2% of all male Vietnam veterans— 479,000 of 3.14 million who served in the theater of war—currently had PTSD. Among women who served with them, PTSD prevalence was estimated at 8.5% (or about 610 current cases out of a population of 7,200). The NVVRS also found that 30.6% of male theater veterans and 26.9% of their female counterparts had suffered from PTSD sometime during their lives (Kulka, 1990). In the years that followed, some conservative commentators would call the results of the NVVRS into question—claiming that veterans were fabricating aspects of their service or seeking undue compensation from the VA—but to many, the NVVRS helped to define the true costs of war for American veterans (Burkett & Whitley, 1998; Frueh, 2005; Kilpatrick, 2007; Satel, 2007). "The reasons for the dramatic psychological impact of fighting the Vietnam War on those who fought it remain a matter of controversy," Alan Cranston, the chairman of the Senate Committee on Veterans Affairs noted. "What can no longer be a controversy is our need to respond to these problems" (Kulka, 1990, pp. v–vi).

Just before work began on the NVVRS, another attempt by the country to come to grips with the Vietnam war came to fruition. On November 13, 1983, the Vietnam Veterans Memorial was dedicated in Washington, D.C. Designed by a 21-year-old Yale student named Maya Lin, the wall of polished black granite panels that form a 125-degree V, inscribed with the names of all the American military dead from the conflict, was a controversial choice among many veterans who felt that it was too abstract. Later, though, "the Wall," as it came to be known, was increasingly celebrated and was joined by more conventional nearby statues of soldiers (in 1984) and a women's memorial (in 1993) (Westheider, 2007).

The Wall was only the most visible manifestation of a 1980s movement that included the construction of hundreds of local and state Vietnam war memorials, retroactive "welcome home" parades, and other efforts to honor the service of Vietnam veterans (Appy, 2015). In May 1985, for example, the New York Times reported that amid a "blizzard of confetti," a "thunderously appreciative crowd" of 1 million gathered in New York to cheer a parade of 25,000 Vietnam veterans. "They are out there, welcoming us back home, and their enthusiasm should help the veterans realize what they did for their country. The war was bad, but the people who fought it were good," said John Behan, a Republican assemblyman from Long Island who lost both legs to a landmine in Vietnam in 1966 and led the march in a wheelchair pushed by New York Mayor Ed Koch (Gross, 1985, p. A1).

Political Controversies

These commemorations took place amidst a reevaluation and recasting of the war by conservatives. At about the same time that the notion of a "post-Vietnam syndrome" was giving way to the more expansive diagnosis of PTSD, right-wing commentators picked up the term "Vietnam Syndrome" and repurposed it as shorthand for a U.S. reluctance to employ military power abroad (Appy, 2015). Top officials with a stake in the memory of the war, including Henry Kissinger, Nixon's White House chief of staff Alexander Haig, and CIA director William Colby, as well as their supporters advanced the notion that the United States had won the conflict, but saw the victory squandered by various culprits such as the press, the antiwar movement, or weak-kneed members of Congress (Hogan, 1995). Speaking before the Veterans of Foreign Wars (VFW) convention in 1980, Ronald Reagan led this effort to rebrand the conflict in the eyes of Americans:

> For too long, we have lived with the "Vietnam Syndrome." . . . It is time we recognized that ours was, in truth, a noble cause. A small country newly free from colonial rule sought our help in establishing self-rule and the means of self-defense against a totalitarian neighbor bent on conquest. We dishonor the memory of 50,000 young Americans who died in that cause when we give way to feelings of guilt as if we were doing something shameful. . . . There is a lesson for all of us in Vietnam. If we are forced to fight, we must have the means and determination to prevail. . . . And while we are at it, let us tell those who fought in that war that we will never again ask young men to fight and possibly die in a war our government is afraid to let them win. (Appy, 2015, p. 286)

Reagan's history was deeply flawed and just how America was "forced to fight" was left unexplained, but it fed into popular reimaginings of the war that emerged during his presidency. A wave of movies, including *Uncommon Valor* (1983), *Missing in Action* (1984), and *Rambo: First Blood Part II* (1985), spun fictions about Americans still imprisoned in Vietnam and their rescue by former comrades. The movies attempted to redeem the memory of the war and championed the idea of Reagan and others that U.S. troops had been denied permission to win in Vietnam (Appy, 2015).

"Revisionist" historians provided a scholarly corollary to these cartoonish films with political scientist Guenter Lewy's *America in Vietnam* (1978) arguing that "the sense of guilt created by the Vietnam war in the minds of many Americans is not warranted" (p. vii), while Harry Summers, a Vietnam veteran and former member of the faculty of the Army War College, offered up the influential *On Strategy* (1982), which held that victory in Vietnam was squandered. In the years after, they were joined by others, most notably former Army officer and CIA analyst Lewis Sorley who, in 1999's *A Better War*, argued that by late 1970, "the fighting wasn't over, but the war was won" by the United States (Lewy, 1981; Prados, 2009; Sorley, 1999, p. 217; Summers, 1982). As a result, the meaning of the Vietnam war has been continuously contested in both academia and popular culture, while remaining a constant specter haunting U.S. foreign policy.

After Saddam Hussein's Iraq attacked Kuwait in 1990, President George H. W. Bush, Reagan's former Vice President, began a march to war. "It is not going to be another Vietnam," he announced of the impending conflict. The next year, basking in the apparent success of Operation Desert Storm, Bush boasted: "It's a proud day for America—and, by God, we've kicked the Vietnam syndrome once and for all" (Appy, 2015, p. 299). Twelve years later, however, Bush's son, George W. Bush, took the country to war against Saddam Hussein's Iraq over what turned out to be nonexistent weapons of mass destruction.

The ghosts of the Vietnam War reemerged as the United States found itself in an increasingly bloody and intractable conflict that caused many to draw attention to similarities between that war and the one in Iraq. After refusing to acknowledge parallels between the conflicts, president Bush finally—in 2007—invoked the history of the Vietnam war to insist on staying the course. Like Reagan, he spoke before the Veterans of Foreign Wars convention, and like Reagan, he offered a spurious history of the conflict while making his case. He argued that the United States should have remained in Vietnam and made a tenuous link to his own war in Iraq. "Here at home, some can argue our withdrawal from Vietnam carried no price to American credibility—but the terrorists see it differently," he told the highly receptive audience (G. W. Bush, 2007). Critics, in turn, pounced on Bush for badly misreading history (as well as Graham Greene's classic novel of the early U.S. efforts in Vietnam, *The Quiet American*) (Buckley, 2007).

The Vietnam War also featured prominently in the 2004 presidential campaign, which saw Massachusetts senator and former VVAW spokesman John Kerry, who had served on a Navy Swift Boat in Vietnam, run for president as the Democratic Party candidate against Bush. Bush had, like so many other sons of privilege, served stateside during the war—in his case, with the Texas Air National Guard. Kerry was attacked by a group called Swift Boat Veterans for Truth that impugned his record and claimed he exaggerated his exploits in Vietnam. While Navy documents contradicted their accusations, the group's book (O'Neill & Corsi, 2004), advertisements, and media appearances took a toll on Kerry's campaign and made the war a hot-button issue once again (Swift Boat Veterans for Truth, 2015; Zernike, 2008).

As a result, conservative, pro-military commentators found themselves defending a candidate who many saw as having dodged the war, while liberal supporters of Kerry—including those who had protested the Vietnam War—touted his military service in that conflict as a major strength of his campaign. In the end, Bush prevailed, "swift-boating" became shorthand for unfair and unfounded political attacks, and the Vietnam war continued to figure in debates on the war in Iraq and its companion conflict in Afghanistan. Almost a quarter century after George H. W. Bush announced the demise of the

Vietnam syndrome, the country was still at war in Afghanistan, for a third time militarily involved in Iraq, and the war in Vietnam continued to be evoked in foreign policy debates (Appy, 2015).

The conflicted nature of the Vietnam war in the American consciousness and how it was wielded for political gain in the nation's culture wars mirrors the contested assessments of the war in the minds of the men and women who served. According to Myths and Realities the comprehensive study conducted for the VA during 1979 and 1980, the war had a tremendous impact on Americans who served. Looking back, 48% of all Vietnam veterans, and 61% who were exposed to heavy combat, said "being in the Vietnam War was the biggest event of my life until now" (Harris, 1980, p. 15). Seventy-three percent of Vietnam veterans felt that their personal beliefs matched very closely with the phrase, "Looking back, I am glad I served my country," but a far fewer number, just 42%, said they enjoyed their military service to the same extent (Harris, 1980, pp. 28, 32).

Efforts to understand and explain various aspects of this war continue to the present. For example, in September 2017, a monumental documentary written by Geoffrey Ward and directed by Ken Burns and Lynn Novick, *The Vietnam War,* was aired on PBS, with a companion book being published the same month (Ward & Burns, 2017).

Against the historical background of the war presented in this chapter, the distinctive focus of all following chapters of this monograph is our investigation of psychological consequences, especially PTSD, of this war for U.S. veterans. We use data derived from military histories, military records, and not only the original NVVRS, conducted from 1986 to 1988, but also a follow-up Longitudinal Study, conducted from 2011 to 2013.

REFERENCES

Addington, L. (2000). *America's war in Vietnam: A short narrative history.* Bloomington, IN: Indiana University Press.

America takes charge: 1965-1967 [television series episode] (1983). In *Vietnam: A Television History.* PBS.

Anderson, D. (2007). *The war that never ends: New perspectives on the Vietnam war.* Lexington, KY: University Press of Kentucky.

Angrist, J., & Chen, S. (2011). Schooling and the Vietnam-era GI Bill: Evidence from the draft lottery. *American Economic Journal: Applied Economics,* 3, 96–119.

Anti-war group hears of "crimes." (1970, December 2). *New York Times,* p. A15.

Appy, C. (1993). *Working-class war: American combat soldiers and Vietnam.* Chapel Hill, NC: University of North Carolina Press.

Appy, C. (2003). *Patriots: The Vietnam war remembered from all sides.* New York: Viking.

Appy, C. (2015). *American reckoning: The Vietnam war and our national identity.* New York: Viking Penguin.

Bacevich, A. (2013). *Breach of trust: How Americans failed their soldiers and their country.* New York: Metropolitan Books, Henry Holt & Company.

Balaban, J. (2002). *Remembering heaven's face: A story of rescue in wartime Vietnam.* Athens, GA: University of Georgia Press.

Ball, P. (1998). *Ghosts and shadows: A marine in Vietnam, 1968-1969.* Jefferson, NC: McFarland.

Barnes, D. (2009, January 16). Dan Barnes, interview with Nick Turse [telephone interview].

Baskir, L., & Strauss, W. (1978). *Chance and circumstance: The draft, the war, and the Vietnam generation.* New York: Knopf.

Belknap, M. (2002). *The Vietnam War on trial: The My Lai massacre and the court-martial of Lieutenant Calley.* Lawrence, KA: University Press of Kansas.

Berger, M., & Hirsch, B. (1983). The civilian earnings experience of Vietnam-era veterans. *The Journal of Human Resources,18,* 455–479.

Bergerud, E. (1991). *The dynamics of defeat: The Vietnam war in Hau Nghia province.* Boulder, CO: Westview Press.

Betts, R., & Denton, F. (1967). *An evaluation of chemical crop destruction in Vietnam.* Santa Monica, CA: Rand.

Bibby, M. (1999). *The Vietnam war and postmodernity.* Amherst, MA: University of Massachusetts Press.

Bilton, M., & Sim, K. (1992). *Four hours in My Lai.* New York: Viking.

Boehmer, T., Flanders, W., McGeehin, M., Boyle, C., & Barrett, D. (2004). Postservice mortality in Vietnam veterans. *Archives of Internal Medicine, 164* (17), 1908–1916.

Borton, L. (1995). *After sorrow: An American among the Vietnamese.* New York: Viking.

Bourke, J. (1999). *An intimate history of killing: Face-to-face killing in twentieth-century warfare.* New York: Basic Books.

Bradley, M. (2009). *Vietnam at war.* Oxford: Oxford University Press.

Braestrup, P. (1977). *Big story: How the American press and television reported and interpreted the crisis of Tet 1968 in Vietnam and Washington.* Boulder, CO: Westview Press.

Bray, G. (2010). *After My Lai: My year commanding First Platoon, Charlie Company.* Norman, OK: University of Oklahoma Press.

Brenner, S. (Ed.). (2005). *Vietnam war crimes.* San Diego, CA: Greenhaven Press.

Buckley, G. (2001). *American patriots: The story of blacks in the military from the Revolution to Desert Storm.* New York: Random House.

Buckley, K. (1998). Firefight near Loc Ninh: October 1968, A small contribution. In M. J. Bates, L. Lichty, P. L. Miles, R. H. Spector, & M. Young, *Reporting Vietnam,* Part One (pp. 664–666). New York: Literary Classics of the United States, New York, NY.

Buckley, K. (1972, June 19). Pacification's deadly price, Newsweek, pp. 42–43.

Buckley, K. (2007). "The Graham Greene argument": A Vietnam parallel that escaped George W. Bush. *World Policy Journal, 24,* 89–98.

Burkett, B., & Whitley, G. (1998). *Stolen valor: How the Vietnam generation was robbed of its heroes and its history.* Dallas, TX: Verity Press.

Bush, G. W. (2007, August 22). Remarks made at the Veterans of Foreign Wars national convention, Kansas City, MO.

Caputo, P. (1996). *A rumor of war: With a twentieth anniversary postscript by the author.* New York: Henry Holt.

Chanoff, D., & Doan, V. (1986). *Portrait of the enemy.* New York, NY: Random House.

Clodfelter, M. (1995). *Vietnam in military statistics: A history of the Indochina wars, 1772–1991.* Jefferson, NC: McFarland & Co.

Colby, W. E. (1982). Oral History Interview II by Ted Gittinger, Internet Copy, 7, LBJ Library.

Cortright, D. (2005). *Soldiers in revolt: GI resistance during the Vietnam War.* Chicago, IL: Haymarket Books.

Cox, P. (2009, September 8). Paul Cox, interview with Nick Turse [telephone interview].

Daly, J., & Bergman, L. (2000). *Black prisoner of war: A conscientious objector's Vietnam memoir.* Lawrence, KA: University Press of Kansas.

Dellums, R. (1972). *The Dellums Committee hearings on war crimes in Vietnam: An inquiry into command responsibility in Southeast Asia.* New York: Vintage Books.

Department of Defense (1988). Vietnam war allied troop levels 1960–73. The American War Library.

Department of Defense (2008). Vietnam war U.S. Military fatal casualty statistics. Washington: National Archives.

Downs, F. (1978). *The killing zone: My life in the Vietnam war*. New York: Norton.

Duncan, D. (1967). *The new legions*. New York: Random House.

Durrance, D. (1988). *Where war lives: A photographic journal of Vietnam*. New York: Hill & Wang.

Ebert, J. (1993). *A life in a year: The American infantryman in Vietnam, 1965–1972*. Novato, CA: Presidio.

Ebert, J. (2004). *A life in a year: The American infantryman in Vietnam*. New York: Random House.

Edelman, B. (1985). *Dear America: Letters home from Vietnam*. New York: Norton.

Egendorf, A. (1981). *Legacies of Vietnam: Comparative adjustment of veterans and their peers: The final report to the Veterans Administration*. New York, NY: The Center for Policy Research, Inc.

Elliott, D. (2007). *The Vietnamese war: Revolution and social change in the Mekong Delta, 1930–1975* (Concise ed.). Armonk, NY: M. E. Sharpe.

Ellsberg, D. (2002). *Secrets: A memoir of Vietnam and the Pentagon Papers*. New York: Viking.

Emerson, G. (1976). *Winners and losers: Battles, retreats, gains, losses, and ruins from a long war*. New York: Random House.

Engelhardt, T. (1995). *The end of victory culture: Cold War America and the disillusioning of a generation*. New York: Basic Books.

Ewell, J. (1969). *Senior officer debriefing report: LTG Julian Ewell*. Department of the Army. Arlington, VA.

Ewell, J. (1979). *Senior officers debriefing program*. U.S. Army Military Institute. West Point, NY.

Ewell, J., & Hunt, I. (1974). *Sharpening the combat edge: The use of analysis to reinforce military judgment*. Washington, DC: Dept. of the Army [Supt. of Docs., U.S. Government Printing Office].

Falk, R., & Kolko, G. (1971). *Crimes of war: A legal, political-documentary, and psychological inquiry into the responsibility of leaders, citizens, and soldiers for criminal acts in wars*. New York: Random House.

Farber, D., & Foner, E. (1994). *The age of great dreams: America in the 1960s*. New York: Hill and Wang.

Farber, D. (2001). *The Columbia guide to America in the 1960s*. New York: Columbia University Press.

Ferrari, M., & Jobin, J. (Eds.). (2004). *Reporting America at war: An oral history*. New York: Hyperion Books.

Fit to Kill [television series episode] (2003). In CNN Presents. CNN.

FitzGerald, F. (1972). *Fire in the lake: The Vietnamese and the Americans in Vietnam*. Boston, MA: Little, Brown.

Fleming, K. (1998). A veteran returns: March 1971, The homecoming of Chris Mead. In M. J. Bates, L. Lichty, P. L. Miles, R. H. Spector, & M. Young, *Reporting Vietnam*, Part Two (pp. 212–216). New York: Literary Classics of the United States, New York, NY.

Frueh, B. (2005). Documented combat exposure of U.S. veterans seeking treatment for combat-related post-traumatic stress disorder. *The British Journal of Psychiatry, 186*, 467–472.

Gallup, G. (1972). *The Gallup poll: Public opinion, 1935–1971*. New York: Random House.

Gallup, G. (1978). *The Gallup poll: Public opinion, 1972–1977*. Wilmington, DE: Scholarly Resources.

Gartner, S., & Myers, M. (1995). Body counts and "success" in the Vietnam and Korean wars. *Journal of Interdisciplinary History, 25*, 377–395.

Gault, W. (1971). Some remarks on slaughter. *AJP American Journal of Psychiatry, 128*, 450–454.

Gettleman, M. (1985). *Vietnam and America: A documented history.* New York: Grove Press.

Gibson, J. (2000). *The perfect war: Technowar in Vietnam.* Boston, MA: Atlantic Monthly Press.

Gilje, P. (1996). *Rioting in America.* Bloomington, IN: Indiana University Press.

Graham, H. (2003). *The brothers' Vietnam war: Black power, manhood, and the military experience.* Gainesville, FL: University Press of Florida.

Gravel, M. (1971). *The Pentagon papers: The Senator Gravel edition.* Boston, MA: Beacon Press.

Gross, J. (1985, May 8). New Yorkers roar thanks to veterans. *New York Times, National edition,* p. A1.

Grossman, D. (1995, 1996). *On killing: The psychological cost of learning to kill in war and society.* New York; Boston: Little, Brown & Company.

Hackworth, D., & Sherman, J. (1989). *About face: Odyssey of an American warrior.* South Melbourne, Australia: Macmillan.

Hackworth, D., & England, E. (2002). *Steel my soldiers' hearts: The hopeless to hardcore transformation of 4th Battalion, 39th Infantry, United States Army, Vietnam.* New York: Rugged Land.

Hagopian, P. (2009). *The Vietnam War in American memory: Veterans, memorials, and the politics of healing.* Amherst, MA: University of Massachusetts Press.

Halberstam, D. (1972). *The best and the brightest.* New York: Random House.

Hammond, W. (1998). *Reporting Vietnam: Media and military at war.* Lawrence, KA: University Press of Kansas.

Harris, L. (1980). *Myths and realities: A study of attitudes toward Vietnam era veterans, submitted by the Veterans' Administration to the Committee on Veterans' Affairs, United States Senate. Print No. 29.* Washington, DC: U.S. Government Printing Office.

Hearts and minds [documentary film] (1974). Warner Bros. Entertainment Inc.

Heinl, R. (1971). The collapse of the armed forces. *Armed Forces Journal, 108,* 1–14.

Helzer, J., Robins, L., & Davis, D. (1976). Depressive disorders in Vietnam returnees. *The Journal of Nervous and Mental Disease, 163,* 177–185.

Hemphill, R. (1999). *Platoon: Bravo Company.* Fredericksburg, VA: Sergeant Kirkland's Museum and Historical Society, Inc.

Henry, J. (2005, October 1). James Henry, interview with Nick Turse [personal interview].

Herr, M. (1977). *Dispatches.* New York: Knopf.

Herring, G. (1986). *America's longest war: The United States and Vietnam, 1950–1975* (2nd ed.). New York: Knopf.

Hersh, S. (1970). *My Lai 4: A report on the massacre and its aftermath.* New York: Random House.

Hersh, S. (1972). *Cover-up: The Army's secret investigation of the massacre at My Lai 4.* New York: Random House.

Hirschman, Charles, et al. (Dec. 1995). Vietnamese casualties during the American war: A new estimate. *Population and Development Review, 21,* 793–797, 809.

Hogan, M. (1995). *America in the world: The historiography of American foreign relations since 1941.* Cambridge, UK: Cambridge University Press.

Hunt, A. (1999). *The turning: A history of Vietnam veterans against the war.* New York: New York University Press.

Hunt, I. (2010). *The 9th infantry division in Vietnam: Unparalleled and unequaled.* Lexington, KY: University Press of Kentucky.

Indochina Peace Campaign. (1973). *Women under torture.* Santa Monica, CA: Indochina Peace Campaign.

Isaacs, A. (1983). *Without honor: Defeat in Vietnam and Cambodia.* Baltimore, MD: Johns Hopkins University Press.

Isserman, M., & Kazin, M. (1999). *America divided: The civil war of the 1960s.* New York: Oxford University Press.

Johnson Library, Recordings and Transcripts. Recording of a May 27, 1964, telephone conversation between President Lyndon Johnson and McGeorge Bundy [radio series episode]. In *Tape 64.28 PNO 111*. U.S. Department of State, Foreign Relations of the United States, 1964–68, Volume XXVII.

Kaufman, F. (1968, March). Roll out the leaders: New model NCOs take to the field. *Army Digest, 23*, 17–19.

Kelley, M. (2002). *Where we were in Vietnam: A comprehensive guide to the firebases, military installations, and naval vessels of the Vietnam War, 1945–1975*. Central Point, OR: Hellgate Press.

Kilpatrick, D. (2007). Confounding the critics: The Dohrenwend and colleagues reexamination of the National Vietnam Veteran Readjustment Study. *Journal of Traumatic Stress, 20*, 487–493.

Kim, H., Kim, E., Park, Y., Yu, J., Hong, S., Jeon, S., et al. (2003). Immunotoxicological effects of Agent Orange exposure to the Vietnam War Korean veterans. *Industrial Health, 41*, 158–166.

Kimball, J. (1998). *Nixon's Vietnam war*. Lawrence, KA: University Press of Kansas.

King Jr., M. (1963). I have a dream. Speech given at the Lincoln Memorial, August 28, Washington, DC.

Kinnard, D. (1991). *The war managers: American generals reflect on Vietnam*. New York: Da Capo Press.

Knightley, P. (1975). *The first casualty: From the Crimea to Vietnam: The war correspondent as hero, propagandist, and myth maker*. New York: Harcourt Brace Jovanovich.

Kolko, G. (1985). *Anatomy of a war: Vietnam, the United States, and the modern historical experience*. New York: Pantheon Books.

Kovic, R. (2005). *Born on the Fourth of July*. New York: Akashic Books.

Krepinevich, A., Jr. (1986). *The army and Vietnam*. Baltimore, MD: The Johns Hopkins University Press.

Kulka, R. A., Schlenger, W. E., Fairbank, J. A., Hough, R. L., Jordan, B. K., Marmar, C. R., et al. (1990). *Trauma and the Vietnam war generation: Report of findings from the National Vietnam Veterans Readjustment Study*. New York: Brunner/Mazel.

Kunen, J. (1971). *Standard operating procedure: Notes of a draft-age American*. New York: Avon.

Laurence, J., & Ramsberger, P. (1991). *Low-aptitude men in the military: Who profits, who pays?* New York: Praeger.

Laurence, J. (2002). *The cat from Hué: A Vietnam war story*. New York: PublicAffairs.

Lembcke, J. (1998). *The spitting image: Myth, memory, and the legacy of Vietnam*. New York: New York University Press.

Lepre, G. (2011). *Fragging: Why U.S. soldiers assaulted their officers in Vietnam*. Lubbock, TX: Texas Tech University Press.

Leslie, J. (1995). *The mark: A war correspondent's memoir of Vietnam and Cambodia*. New York: Four Walls Eight Windows.

Lewis, P. (2013). *Hardhats, hippies, and hawks: The Vietnam antiwar movement as myth and memory*. Ithaca, NY: ILR Press.

Lewy, G. (1981). *America in Vietnam* (reprint ed.). New York: Oxford University Press.

Li, X. (2010). *Voices from the Vietnam war: Stories from American, Asian, and Russian veterans*. Lexington, KY: University Press of Kentucky.

Lifton, R. (1971). What Are We Doing to Ourselves? Part III. In *Vietnam Veterans Against the War, Winter Soldier Investigation*. University of Virginia, Charlottesville, VA: The Sixties Project.

Lifton, R. (1973). *Home from the war: Vietnam veterans neither victims nor executioners*. New York: Simon & Schuster.

MacPherson, M. (2001). *Long time passing: Vietnam and the haunted generation*. Bloomington, IN: Indiana University Press.

Mackenzie, A. (1997). *Secrets: The CIA's war at home*. Berkeley, CA: University of California Press.

Mangold, T., & Penycate, J. (1985). *The tunnels of Cu Chi*. New York: Random House.

Martindale, M., & Poston, D. (1979). Variations in veteran/nonveteran earnings patterns among World War II, Korea, and Vietnam war cohorts. *Armed Forces & Society, 5*, 219–243.

McCoy, A. (2006). *A question of torture: CIA interrogation, from the Cold War to the War on Terror*. New York: Metropolitan Books/Henry Holt.

McFann, H., Hammes, J., & Taylor, J. (1955). *TRAINFIRE I: A new course in basic rifle marksmanship*. Washington, DC: George Washington University, Human Resources Research Office.

McNamara, R., & VanDeMark, B. (1995). *In retrospect: The tragedy and lessons of Vietnam*. New York: Random House.

Morgan, E. (1991). *The 60s experience: Hard lessons about modern America*. Philadelphia, PA: Temple University Press.

Morris, C., & West, F. (1970). *U.S. fatalities during Vietnamization: Part II, Marine fatalities in Quang Nam: A method for analysis*. Santa Monica, CA: Rand.

Murray, M. (1992). "White gold or white blood"? The rubber plantations of colonial Indochina, 1910–1940. In Daniel, E., Bernstein, H., & Brass, T. (Eds.), *Plantations, proletarians, and peasants in colonial Asia*, p. 60. London: F. Cass.

Napoli, P. (2013). *Bringing it all back home: An oral history of New York City's Vietnam veterans*. New York: Hill & Wang.

Ngo, A., Taylor, R., Roberts, C., & Nguyen, T. (2006). Association between Agent Orange and birth defects: Systematic review and meta-analysis. *International Journal of Epidemiology, 35*, 1220–1230.

Nguyen, L. (2012). *Hanoi's war: An international history of the war for peace in Vietnam*. Chapel Hill, NC: University of North Carolina Press.

Nicosia, G. (2001). *Home to war: A history of the Vietnam veterans' movement*. New York: Crown.

Nolan, K. (2006). *House to house: Playing the enemy's game in Saigon, May 1968*. St. Paul, MN: Zenith Press.

Nordstrom, G. (2008, January 1). Gary Nordstrom, interview with Nick Turse [telephone interview].

Norman, E. (1990). *Women at war: The story of fifty military nurses who served in Vietnam*. Philadelphia, PA: University of Pennsylvania Press.

Obermeyer, Z., Murray, C., & Gakidou, E. (2008). Fifty years of violent war deaths from Vietnam to Bosnia: Analysis of data from the World Health Survey Programme. *British Medical Journal, 226*, 1482–1486.

Oberdorfer, D. (1985). *Tet!: The turning point in the Vietnam war*. New York: Da Capo Press.

O'Neill, J., & Corsi, J. (2004). *Unfit for command: Swift Boat veterans speak out against John Kerry*. Washington, DC: Regnery Publishing, Inc.

Ostertag, B. (2006). *People's movements, people's press: The journalism of social justice movements*. Boston, MA: Beacon Press.

Paine, T. (1776). *Common sense*. Published anonymously.

Peck, A. (1985). *Uncovering the sixties: The life and times of the underground press*. New York: Pantheon Books.

Peers, W. (1974). *Report of the Department of the Army review of the preliminary investigations into the My Lai incident 14 March 1970* (Book 19 ed., Vol. 2). Washington, DC: Government Printing Office.

Peers, W. (1976). *The My Lai massacre and its cover-up: Beyond the reach of law? The Peers Commission report*. New York: Free Press.

Perlstein, R. (2008). *Nixonland: America's second civil war and the divisive legacy of Richard Nixon, 1965–1972*. London: Simon & Schuster.

Pickerell, J. (1966). *Vietnam in the mud*. Indianapolis, IN: Bobbs-Merrill.

Prados, J. (2009). *Vietnam: The history of an unwinnable war, 1945–1975*. Lawrence, KA: University Press of Kansas.

Prados, J. (2011). *In country: Remembering the Vietnam war*. Lanham, MD: Ivan R. Dee.

Prokosch, E. (1995). *The technology of killing: A military and political history of antipersonnel weapons*. London: Zed Books.

Prugh, G. (1975). *Law at war, Vietnam, 1964–1973*. Washington, DC: Dept. of the Army.

Puller, L. (1991). *Fortunate son: The autobiography of Lewis B. Puller, Jr.* New York: Grove Weidenfeld.

Record, J. (1998). *The wrong war: Why we lost in Vietnam*. Annapolis, MD: Naval Institute Press.

Rosett, H. (1971, June 12). Letters to the editor: Post-Vietnam syndrome. *New York Times*, p. A28.

Saar, J. (1970, October 23). You can't just hand out orders. *Life Magazine, 69*, 30–37.

Safer, M. (1990). *Flashbacks: On returning to Vietnam*. New York: Random House.

Sallah, M., & Weiss, M. (2006). *Tiger Force: A true story of men and war*. New York: Little, Brown.

Satel, S. (2007, February 19). The trouble with traumatology: Is it advocacy or is it science? *The Weekly Standard*, p. A15.

Schell, J. (2000). *The real war: The classic reporting on the Vietnam war with a new essay*. New York: Da Capo Press.

Schiffrin, A. (2014). *Global muckraking: 100 years of investigative journalism from around the world*. New York: The New Press.

Schultz, B. (1989). *It did happen here: Recollections of political repression in America*. Berkeley, CA: University of California Press.

Schwartz, Saul. (1986). The relative earnings of Vietnam and Korean-era veterans. *Industrial and Labor Relations Review, 39* (July), 564–572.

Shatan, C. (1973). *The grief of soldiers: Vietnam combat veterans' self-help movement. American Journal of Orthopsychiatry, 43*, 640–653.

Sheehan, N. (1988). *A bright shining lie: John Paul Vann and America in Vietnam*. New York: Random House.

Shkurti, W. (2011). *Soldiering on in a dying war: The true story of the Firebase Pace incidents and the Vietnam drawdown*. Lawrence, KA: University Press of Kansas.

Smith, J. (1998). "Men all around me were screaming": November 1965, Death in the Ia Drang Valley. In M. J. Bates, L. Lichty, P. L. Miles, R. H. Spector, & M. Young, *Reporting Vietnam*, Part One (pp. 208–222). New York: Literary Classics of the United States, New York, NY.

Smith, W. (2008, June 19). Wayne Smith, interview with Nick Turse [telephone interview].

Sorley, L. (1999). *A better war? The unexamined victories and final tragedy of America's last years in Vietnam*. New York: Harcourt Brace.

Stanton, S. (1987). *Vietnam order of battle*. New York: Galahad Books, by arrangement with Kraus Reprint & Periodicals.

Sterba, J. (1970, October 18). Scraps of paper from Vietnam. *New York Times Magazine*, p. SM15.

Summers, H. (1982). *On strategy: A critical analysis of the Vietnam war*. Novato, CA: Presidio Press.

Terry, W. (1984). *Bloods, an oral history of the Vietnam war*. New York: Random House.

Thayer, T. (1975). *A systems analysis view of the Vietnam war 1965–1972* (Vol. 3). Washington, DC: OASD(SA)RP Southeast Asia Intelligence Division, Pentagon.

Thayer, T. (1975). *A systems analysis view of the Vietnam war 1965–1972* (Vol. 4). Washington, DC: OASD(SA)RP Southeast Asia Intelligence Division, Pentagon.

Thayer, T. (1975). *A systems analysis view of the Vietnam war 1965–1972* (Vol. 9). Washington, DC: OASD(SA)RP Southeast Asia Intelligence Division, Pentagon.

Thayer, T. (1975). *A systems analysis view of the Vietnam war 1965–1972* (Vol. 10). Washington, DC: OASD(SA)RP Southeast Asia Intelligence Division, Pentagon.

Thayer, T. (1985). *War without fronts: The American experience in Vietnam.* Boulder, CO: Westview Press.

The fog of war [documentary motion picture] (2003). Sony Pictures Classics.

Thompson, L. (1990). *The US Army in Vietnam.* Newton Abbot, UK: David & Charles.

Tucker, S. (1998). *The encyclopedia of the Vietnam war: A political, social, and military history.* Santa Barbara, CA: ABC-CLIO.

Turley, W. (2009). *The second Indochina War: A concise political and military history* (2nd ed.). Lanham, MD: Rowman & Littlefield.

Turse, N. (2008, July 28). War crimes hunter. *In These Times.* www.inthesetimes.com.

Turse, N. (2013). *Kill anything that moves: The real American war in Vietnam.* New York: Metropolitan Books/Henry Holt.

Tuyet, L., & Johansson, A. (2001). Impact of chemical warfare with Agent Orange on women's reproductive lives in Vietnam: A pilot study. *Reproductive Health Matters, 9*:18, 156–164. Published online: 01 November 2001.

United States v. Frank C. Schultz, Lance Corporal. (1969, March 7). U.S. Marine Corps, Appellant No. 21,055, United States Court of Military Appeals, 18 U.S.C.M.A. 133; 1969 CMA LEXIS 563; 39 C.M.R. 133.

Valentine, D. (1990). *The Phoenix program.* New York: Morrow.

Vietcong village to be bulldozed. (1967, January 11). *New York Times*, p. A4.

Vietnam National Defense Ministry. (2008). *History of the united resistance against invasion of the United States of America (1954–1975)* (Vol. 8).

Vietnam Veterans Against the War. (1971). Winter soldier investigation, testimony given in Detroit, Michigan, on January 31, 1971; February 1 and 2, 1971. In *Winter soldier investigation testimony* (pp. 2825–2900, 2903–2936). Congressional Record.

Vigil, E. (1999). *The crusade for justice: Chicano militancy and the government's war on dissent.* Madison, WI: University of Wisconsin Press.

Wallace, M. (1969, November 25). Transcript of interview of Vietnam war veteran on his role in alleged massacre of civilians at Songmy. *New York Times*, p. A16.

Ward, G., & Burns, K. (2017). *The Vietnam war: An intimate history.* New York: Knopf.

Warr, N. (1997). *Phase line green: The battle for Hue, 1968.* Annapolis, MD: Naval Institute Press.

Webb, J. (1978). *Fields of fire: A novel.* Englewood Cliffs, NJ: Prentice-Hall.

Westheider, J. (2007). *The Vietnam war.* Westport, CN: Greenwood Press.

Westmoreland, W. (1976). *A soldier reports.* Garden City, NY: Doubleday.

Wheeler, J. (1998). Khe Sanh under siege: February 1968, Life in the V Ring. In M. J. Bates, L. Lichty, P. L. Miles, R. H. Spector, & M. Young, *Reporting Vietnam*, Part One (pp. 576–580). New York: Literary Classics of the United States, New York, NY.

Wilcox, F. (2011). *Waiting for an army to die: The tragedy of Agent Orange* (2nd ed.). New York: Seven Stories Press.

Wilkins, W. (2011). *Grab their belts to fight them: The Viet Cong's big-unit war against the U.S., 1965–1966.* Annapolis, MD: Naval Institute Press.

Wolff, T. (1994). *In Pharaoh's army: Memories of the lost war.* New York, NY: Knopf.

Xie, Y. (1992). The socioeconomic status of young male veterans, 1964–1984. *Social Science Research, 73*, 2.

Yergin, D. (1977). *Shattered peace: The origins of the cold war and the national security state.* Boston, MA: Houghton Mifflin.

Young, M. (1991). *The Vietnam wars, 1945–1990.* New York: Harper Collins.

Young, M. (2002). *A companion to the Vietnam war.* Malden, MA: Blackwell.

Zernike, K. (2008, June 30). Veterans long to reclaim the name "Swift Boat." *New York Times,* A1.

PART II

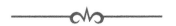

Veterans' War-Zone Experiences and Post-Traumatic Stress Disorder

CHAPTER 2

༚

Controversies About Rates of Post-Traumatic Stress Disorder in U.S. Vietnam Veterans

BRUCE P. DOHRENWEND, J. BLAKE TURNER, NICK
TURSE, BEN G. ADAMS, KARESTAN C. KOENEN, AND
RANDALL MARSHALL

PTSD is full of contradictions. Virtually every reaction that mental health professionals label a "symptom," and which indeed can cause havoc in your life after returning home from combat, is an essential survival skill in the war zone. The dilemma is that the reactions that are necessary for survival and success in combat are not easy to dial down and adapt after coming home.... (Hoge, 2010, pp. xii–xiii)

As historians have pointed out, all wars are different, and so have been the characterizations and understanding of their psychological effects on those who fought them. These differences are reflected in the terms used to describe war-related psychological problems. In World War I, the signature term was "shell shock"; in World War II, "battle fatigue"; and during and after the Vietnam war, "post-traumatic stress disorder" (PTSD) (Shephard, 2001, p. xix). Our concern here is with the Vietnam war and PTSD.

This was a very different kind of war than World War I or World War II, so-called industrial wars among nation states (e.g., Smith, 2007). In these inter-state wars, the fighting forces of the warring nations lined up against each other in fronts and fought for land. By contrast, Vietnam involved a U.S. intervention in a civil war between North and South Vietnam in which popular loyalties frequently departed from geographic lines. It was a "war amongst the people" in which the enemy was elusive and often difficult to distinguish from ordinary civilians. In this war, the "body count" of enemy combatants killed rather than the taking of territory was the gauge of military success. (See our Chapter 1, section War, *The American way of war, Fighting the war* and *Nixon's war*, for in-depth descriptions of how this war was fought.)

In the Vietnam war, the U.S. casualty rate was very low compared with the rates of U.S. fighting men killed in World Wars I and II, and military observers were impressed early in the war at how infrequently combat stress reactions involving inability to function in combat situations occurred (Bourne, 1970; Tiffany & Allerton, 1967). The relative rarity of combat breakdowns was considered an indicator of success in lessons learned from World War II. It was something of a surprise, therefore, when men who served in Vietnam returned home in seemingly large numbers with psychiatric problems. The formulation of PTSD in the third edition of the American Psychiatric Association (APA) *Diagnostic and Statistical Manual of Mental Disorders* (DSM-III; APA, 1980), and in later editions, is designed to describe the main features of these psychiatric problems among war veterans and others exposed to potentially traumatic experiences.

DESCRIPTION OF PTSD IN DSM-III-R

The diagnosis of PTSD was introduced in DSM-III amidst debate about the psychiatric effects of the Vietnam war on U.S. veterans a few years after the end of that war. The diagnosis included a novel syndrome of intrusive, avoidance/numbing, and arousal symptoms that last at least one month as the distinctive psychopathology following traumatic exposures. DSM-III-R, which we used in the present research, describes these three symptom clusters as follows:

B. The traumatic event is persistently reexperienced in at least one of the following ways:
   (1) recurrent and intrusive disturbing recollections of the event . . .
   (2) recurrent distressing dreams of the event
   (3) sudden acting or feeling as if the traumatic event were recurring . . .
   (4) intense psychological distress at exposure to events that symbolize or resemble an aspect of the traumatic event . . .
C. Persistent avoidance of stimuli associated with the trauma or numbing of general responsiveness . . . as indicated by at least three of the following:
   (1) efforts to avoid thoughts or feelings associated with the trauma
   (2) efforts to avoid activities or situations that arouse recollections of the trauma
   (3) inability to recall an important aspect of the trauma (psychogenic amnesia)
   (4) markedly diminished interest in significant activities . . .
   (5) feeling of detachment or estrangement from others
   (6) restricted feeling of affect . . .
   (7) sense of a foreshortened future . . .

D. Persistent symptoms of increased arousal (not present before trauma), as indicated by at least two of the following:

(1) difficulty falling or staying asleep

(2) irritability or outbursts of anger

(3) difficulty concentrating

(4) hypervigilance

(5) exaggerated startle response

(6) physiologic reactivity upon exposure to events that symbolize or resemble an aspect of the traumatic event . . . (DSM-III-R, 1987, pp. 250–251)

While PTSD is a relatively new diagnosis, Shay has found parallels in the experiences of Achilles and Odysseus, described by Homer, in ancient Greek wars (Shay, 1994 and 2002). Both Shay and Hoge (2010), more recently, have noted that many PTSD symptoms are adaptive responses that commonly occur when fighters are exposed to life-threatening situations in the war zone. It is when they persist after the fighter has returned to safety that they become evidence of psychiatric disorder. It seems to us that "living nightmare" might be an apt brief description of this constellation of symptoms when they persist or recur after the veteran leaves the war zone.

As set forth in DSM-III, this new diagnosis requires the antecedent presence of a traumatic event as "Criterion A." In this formulation, the adjective "traumatic" was used to describe stressors "outside the range of usual human experience" that would "evoke significant symptoms of distress in almost everyone" (APA, DSM-III, 1980, p. 236). Providing more examples than DSM-III, DSM-III-R emphasizes events that threaten the life or physical integrity of the individual or someone close to him or her; the definition also includes witnessing death or serious injury to others (APA, 1987).

Our assessments of the psychiatric toll of such stressor experiences on U.S. veterans of the Vietnam war come from our research with data from the National Vietnam Veterans Readjustment Study (NVVRS) (Kulka et al., 1988, 1990) and military records. We start with some details of how PTSD was measured in the NVVRS, present the controversy over the NVVRS reports of results, and provide our resolution of the controversy.

MEASUREMENT OF PTSD IN THE NVVRS

The NVVRS was a congressionally mandated, nationally representative study of psychological consequences of the Vietnam war for the veterans of that war. The fieldwork in the NVVRS was conducted from November 1986 to February 1988. It is the most important source of epidemiological data on PTSD in U.S. Vietnam veterans and a major focus of controversy about war-related rates of the disorder.

Some Characteristics of the Full Sample of Male Theater Veterans

The main NVVRS sample consists of 1,200 male U.S. Theater veterans—that is, men who served in Vietnam, in surrounding waters, or on U.S. bases in Thailand and elsewhere (e.g., Guam), usually for a year, at some time between August 1964 and May 1975. This sample of Theater veterans was drawn on a full probability basis from military records, with provision for oversampling black and Hispanic males and women. The completion rate was 83% of the Theater veterans designated for inclusion.

A consequence of this design is that, to obtain accurate population estimates, weights reflecting the different probabilities of selection into the NVVRS samples must be incorporated into statistical analyses of NVVRS data. With appropriate sampling weights, results of analyses of NVVRS data can be generalized to the population of about 3.14 million male Theater veterans, excluding only those (under 10%) still on active duty when the study was conducted 11–12 years after the war (Kulka et al., 1988).

The veterans were young when they went to Vietnam; according to the NVVRS data, 80.8% were under 25. (See our Chapter 1, section War, *Who Served and Why*, for a contrast between the fighting forces in World War II and those sent to Vietnam.)

When the NVVRS data were collected, the estimated mean age of the veterans was 41.5 years (*standard error [s.e.]* 0.18). Although only 19.8% of the men had a post–high school education at the time they went to Vietnam, by the time they were interviewed in this study, 60.0% had at least some college education. Similarly, although 83.5% had never been married when they went to Vietnam, by the time of the interview, only 5.5% were single and had never married, an estimated 55.2% were currently married with no history of being divorced or, in a few cases (0.04%) were widowed, and the remaining 39.3% had been divorced or were currently separated (with 55.9% of the divorced men remarried at the time of the interview). An estimated 11.5% of the male Theater veterans were black, 5.5% were Hispanic, and most of the remainder were non-Hispanic whites. Black and Hispanic veterans were oversampled in the NVVRS to provide adequate numbers for statistical analyses; this oversampling contributed to the complexity of the NVVRS multi-stage sampling procedure. More details of sampling procedures are available in Kulka et al. (1988, 1990).

Comparison Sample of Male Era Veterans

A comparison sample of 412 male Era veterans—i.e., those who served in the military during the same period of time but not in Vietnam—was also drawn by the same procedures, with a 76% completion rate.

An Intensively Studied Subsample of Male Theater Veterans

The NVVRS included a more intensively studied subsample of male Theater veterans consisting of 260 men from 28 standard metropolitan regions (SMRs), including the

15 largest SMRs. Veterans living in rural areas are unrepresented in the subsample (Dohrenwend et al., 2007).

Members of the subsample received diagnostic examinations by 28 experienced, doctoral-level clinicians (Kulka et al., 1988, Appendix D). The completion rate for male Theater veterans targeted for the subsample was 80% or more for each of the three main racial/ethnic groups (Kulka et al., 1990, p. 13). Veterans likely to have developed PTSD were oversampled; this included those with higher scores on the Mississippi Scale of Combat-Related PTSD (M-PTSD) (Keane, Caddell, & Taylor, 1998) and with higher levels of self-reported exposure to war-zone stress. Suitably weighted, the subsample results can be generalized to the population of male Theater veterans from the 28 SMRs.

Relevant data on PTSD status or information about sampling weights are missing for three members of the subsample. Racial/ethnic identity of 255 of the 260 veterans in the subsample was black, Hispanic, or white. Subtracting (a) the five subsample members who are neither black, Hispanic, nor white, (b) the three subsample members for whom relevant data on PTSD status or information about sampling weights are missing, and (c) four subsample members who had first onsets of PTSD that were prior to their service in Vietnam, the remaining 248 male veterans in the subsample included 70 who were black, 84 who were Hispanic, and 94 who were white.

All respondents in the NVVRS identified their racial background as American Indian, Alaskan Native, Asian, Pacific Islander, black, white, or other (asked to specify). They were then asked if they were of Hispanic (Spanish) origin and, if so, which of several groupings (e.g., Puerto Rican, Mexican) described their origin or ancestry. This information was used to cross-check the information in the military records on which the racial/ethnic stratification for sampling purposes was based (Hunt et al., 1994, pp. 21–23). The large majority of the 84 Hispanic respondents (63) were Mexican American; 15 were Puerto Rican; and the remaining six were from various other Latin American countries.

Suitably weighted, the demographic distribution of veterans from the three main racial/ethnic groups, and other demographic variables (rural location excluded), is very similar to that in the full 1,200-member sample of NVVRS Theater veterans (Dohrenwend et al., 2007). This is shown in Table 2.1.

Assessment of PTSD in the Full Sample

In the intensively studied subsample, PTSD was assessed with a rigorous semi-structured clinical interview administered by doctoral-level clinicians. To make their diagnoses, the clinicians used an instrument called the Structured Clinical Interview for Diagnosis (SCID) (Spitzer, Williams, & Gibbon, 1987). We describe this diagnosis in more detail later. But first, we focus on the assessment procedures used in the full sample.

Projected Current PTSD

In-person clinical diagnostic examinations were not conducted with most members of the full NVVRS sample of 1,200 male Theater veterans because it was deemed to be

Table 2.1 DEMOGRAPHIC AND MILITARY BACKGROUND CHARACTERISTICS
OF THE FULL NVVRS SAMPLE OF MALE VIETNAM THEATER VETERANS AND
OF THE DIAGNOSED SUBSAMPLE OF THOSE VETERANS

Background Characteristic	Full Sample %	Subsample %
Age at entry to Vietnam		
Under 20	24.9	27.7
20	22.1	20.5
21	14.7	13.4
22–24	18.9	19.1
25 and up	19.4	19.3
Total	100.0 ($n = 1180$)	100.0 ($n = 256$)
Race or ethnic group		
White	81.3	77.2
Black	11.2	13.2
Hispanic	5.4	6.5
Other	2.1	3.1
Total	100.0 ($n = 1200$)	100.0 ($n = 259$)
Educational attainment at follow-up		
Less than HS grad	6.4	8.1
HS grad	34.3	26.3
Some college	42.6	44.0
College grad	7.2	10.5
Grad/Prof Work	9.5	11.1
Total	100.0 ($n = 1200$)	100.0 ($n = 259$)
Marital status at follow-up		
Married	75.3	79.5
Separated	3.9	3.9
Divorced	13.5	9.2
Widowed	0.5	0.0
Never married	6.7	7.3
Total	99.9 ($n = 1200$)	99.9 ($n = 259$)
Grade at discharge		
Enlisted: E1–E4	51.3	46.8
E5–E6	33.2	38.7
E7–E9	8.6	8.3
Officer	6.9	6.2
Total	100.0 ($n = 1200$)	100.0 ($n = 259$)

Table 2.1 CONTINUED

Background Characteristic	Full Sample %	Subsample %
Branch of service		
Army	52.9	56.2
Air Force	16.0	15.4
Navy	21.1	19.9
Marines	9.8	8.3
Coast Guard	0.1	---
Total	99.9 ($n = 1197$)	99.8 ($n = 258$)

Record-based measure of probable severity of exposure to war-zone stress (Dohrenwend et al., 2006)		
Low	19.8	25.1
Moderate	68.4	64.0
High	8.5	7.6
Very High	3.2	3.4
Total	99.9 ($n = 1200$)	100.1 ($n = 259$)

Current PTSD according to the NVVRS algorithm (Kulka et al., 1990)		
Yes	15.2	15.4
No	84.8	84.6
Total	100.0 ($n = 1200$)	100.0 ($n = 259$)

Note. Percentages are weighted to the populations from which the samples were drawn.

Totals not equal to 100.0 are due to rounding error. Unweighted sample n's are in parentheses.

prohibitively expensive to hire experienced clinicians to conduct so many diagnostic assessments. Instead, PTSD in the full sample was measured by an algorithm applied to self-report symptom scales with the aim of creating a measure to approximate economically a diagnosis of current PTSD in the full sample. In brief, to develop this algorithm, data from the subsample were used to develop a criterion diagnosis. This criterion diagnosis consisted especially of the SCID diagnoses of current PTSD, but also of other measures such as the M-PTSD self-report scale of PTSD symptoms. These were combined into a composite diagnosis of current PTSD. Economical self-report measures, including M-PTSD in the full sample, were then calibrated against the composite diagnosis in the subsample to provide a measure of the projected probability of current PTSD (which we call the Projected Probability measure or algorithm) in the full sample. (More detail of the measurement procedure can be found in Kulka et al., 1988, Appendices D and E.)

The Projected Probability measure has been used in most of the NVVRS analyses to date, and its rate estimates are the focus of much of the controversy. The Projected Probability algorithm results in a 15.2% current prevalence of PTSD for Theater veterans, which is much higher than the 2.5% rate for Era veterans (Kulka et al., 1990).

For Theater veterans in the 28 SMRs, the rate of projected current PTSD according to the Projected Probability algorithm is 15.4%, almost identical to the rate in the Theater sample as a whole. Because the NVVRS Projected Probability algorithm focused solely on current PTSD symptoms, the often quoted but rarely analyzed lifetime rate, 30.9%, was extrapolated from the results of the SCID diagnoses in the subsample, which showed a roughly 2:1 ratio between lifetime and current PTSD (Kulka et al., 1988).

Meanwhile, two immediate limitations of the Projected Probability measure should be mentioned. First, the measure refers to current prevalence (i.e., course) of PTSD only. It does not include information about the onset (i.e., incidence) of the disorder; therefore, with this measure, we cannot distinguish between onset and adverse course of PTSD. Second, the Projected Probability measure does not fully specify whether or not PTSD was war-related; thus, PTSD assessed by this measure could have origins in any trauma experienced during the entire lifetime of the respondent. Nor are these the only problems with this measure, as we find and report more extensively in Chapter 4.

Mississippi scale of combat-Related PTSD (M-PTSD)

As noted previously, one of the main self-report measures of PTSD used in developing the NVVRS composite diagnosis (i.e., the criterion) in the subsample is the M-PTSD (Keane, Caddell, & Taylor, 1998). The M-PTSD was administered to the full Theater sample. It is a 35-item scale with a fixed alternative response format. On the M-PTSD scale, a score of 89 or higher is considered indicative of probable PTSD diagnosis (Hunt et al., 1994; Kulka et al., 1988). The M-PTSD was shown to have a high internal consistency of .94 in a reliability analysis of the scale items that was conducted as part of the NVVRS (Kulka et al., 1988). The M-PTSD scale was also shown to have a sensitivity of .77 and a specificity of .83 in relation to the diagnosis of current PTSD, which was assessed in the NVVRS subsample of 260 Vietnam Theater veterans referred to previously.

We, and others, have used the M-PTSD scale rather than the Projected Probability algorithm for assessing current PTSD in the full NVVRS sample. There are advantages and disadvantages to each approach. For example, the overall rate of current PTSD diagnosed by this algorithm, resulting in projected current PTSD in the full NVVRS sample (15.2%), is closer to the criterion rate assessed by the SCID in the subsample (13.4%) than the rate of PTSD diagnosed by the M-PTSD scale in the full sample (20.4%). Although the M-PTSD is likely to be more inclusive than the Projected Probability algorithm in relation to the SCID standard, in some cases (see, e.g., Dohrenwend et al., 2004) it seemed preferable to assess PTSD in the full NVVRS sample using the M-PTSD scale instead of the Projected Probability algorithm. One advantage of the M-PTSD scale is that it can be used in more types of statistical analyses.

Note, as pointed out before, the Projected Probability measure is actually a predicted probability of PTSD, computed by Kulka et al. (1988, 1990), for all veterans, and is based on the best-fitting model for predicting the composite diagnosis in the subsample receiving clinical assessment. This Projected Probability measure has been used to assess rates of the current prevalence of PTSD across subgroups of veterans (Hunt et al., 1994;

Kulka et al., 1988, 1990), but it cannot, like the M-PTSD, be used to identify current PTSD in individual veterans.

Diagnostic Histories of PTSD from the Subsample

Full, rigorous diagnostic assessments are available only in a diagnosed subsample of 260 Vietnam Theater veterans. As noted earlier, the diagnosed subsample was representative of the veterans who resided in 28 SMRs. As we showed in Table 2.1, it is demographically similar to the full sample, with the exception of under-representation of veterans from rural areas.

Examinations of individuals in the subsample were conducted by doctoral-level clinicians who, by design, were not employees of the Veterans Administration (VA). Examinations were tape-recorded, which permitted NVVRS clinicians to conduct a careful, independent reliability check of 30 of the taped clinical interviews. This check found inter-rater reliabilities (kappas) for the diagnoses of current and lifetime prevalence of PTSD of .87 and .94, respectively (Weiss et al., 1992).

PTSD and other psychiatric disorders were assessed in the subsample according to the then-current DSM-III-R criteria using the SCID. The SCID includes the Global Assessment of Functioning (GAF) scale to measure level of functioning using scores ranging from 9 (good functioning in all areas) to 1 (persistent danger of severely hurting self or others), with anchoring examples provided at each level of functioning.

The clinicians who conducted the evaluations in the subsample assessed the diagnostic history of PTSD and other disorders. The basic distinction called for in the SCID module for each PTSD symptom was between current and lifetime prevalence (i.e., whether or not the symptom occurred for a month or more at any time during the veteran's lifetime) and, if lifetime, whether the symptom was current (i.e., had a period prevalence of presence for a month or more during the six months prior to the examination). The clinician then ascertained whether the symptoms assessed as being present occurred together for at least a month in sufficient numbers and types to meet criteria for current prevalence, or for lifetime (but not current) prevalence, of PTSD (Schlenger, 1987).

Importantly, the clinicians assessed the times of occurrence of traumatic events and onsets of symptoms (Schlenger, 1987). This information made it possible for us to distinguish (in our 2006 reanalysis of the original NVVRS findings) war-related PTSD from PTSD with first onsets that were related to events that occurred prior to or after service in Vietnam (Dohrenwend et al., 2006).

During the interviews, the clinicians also hand-sketched graphs of variations in severity of PTSD symptoms across time, based on the reports of 84 respondents with first onsets of war-related PTSD. Analyzing these graphs, Villafranca-West (2010, pp. 135–136) found that onsets of PTSD symptoms generally occurred while serving in Vietnam or in the year after return to the United States. Consistent with Hoge's speculations about the problems of transition from service in the war zone to return to civilian life, she also found that the worst period of the symptoms usually occurred between one and two years after return.

For most present purposes, we focus on onsets of PTSD that were war-related. These consist of (a) first onsets of war-related PTSD that met full diagnostic criteria within the six months prior to SCID examination (current PTSD) and (b) first onsets that did not meet full diagnostic criteria within six months prior to the SCID diagnostic interview (past PTSD).

The subsample diagnostic examinations have received relatively little attention or analysis in the main reports of the NVVRS (Kulka et al., 1988, 1990) or in the wider literature, even though the diagnoses contain by far the most detailed data on PTSD and the only data on the history of this disorder. This is probably because of the loss of statistical power due to the much smaller size of the subsample (260) compared with the full sample of male Theater veterans (1,200). Nevertheless, most of the analyses that follow are based on the diagnostic data in the subsample. An example of the advantage of our subsample focus is evident when we confront, later in this chapter, controversies centered on results with projected current PTSD in the full sample.

RECORD-BASED MEASURE OF THE PROBABLE SEVERITY OF EXPOSURE TO WAR-ZONE STRESSORS

Also important in addressing these controversies is one of our measures of severity of exposure to war-zone stressors. This measure is based entirely on military records and cannot, therefore, be affected by possible recall biases in the veterans' self-reports. We call this the military/historical measure (MHM) of exposure.

We examined NVVRS data from military personnel files (201 files) together with military archival sources and historical accounts to construct the MHM. The first three components are the veteran's military occupational specialty, the monthly casualty rate during his Vietnam service, and the casualty rate in his larger military unit (e.g., division). Here are more details of each.

Military Occupational Specialty (MOS)

The MOS is a revision of a measure developed by Kulka et al. (1990) from military records of the respondent's MOS at time of discharge. Our revised measure, also based on military records, uses the more relevant MOS for each sample member at the time of his service in Vietnam. Discharge MOS is used only when the Vietnam MOS was missing from the military record, as was the case for 41 of the records. Like the original NVVRS measure, we grouped respondents into three levels of probable severity of exposure to war-zone stressors. We created the MOS exposure categories on the basis of information gleaned from military histories (e.g., Appy, 1993; Cash, Albright, & Sandstrum, 1985; Ebert, 1993; Thompson, 1990), U.S. military publications (e.g., Department of the Army, 1967; Department of the Army, Office of Personnel Operations, 1971; U.S. Army, Office of the Surgeon General, 1971), and judgments obtained from Vietnam veteran consultants.

The MOSs indicating the highest probable severity of exposure were those likely to be directly involved in combat operations and to receive enemy fire. An estimated 23.1% of male Theater veterans were in this category; examples include infantrymen, medics, combat engineers, cannon crewmen, and cannon-fire-direction specialists. The next, middle level of probable severity of exposure was composed of men in noncombat MOSs who were likely to be proximal to combat activity. An estimated 16.6% were in this category; examples include auto repair and motor transport operators, armored vehicle repairmen, and tactical wire specialists. Finally, MOSs indicating the lowest probable severity of exposure were service support occupations likely to be far away from heavy combat areas (e.g., finance specialists, storage specialists, and technical draftsmen). The large majority, 60.3% of male Theater veterans, were in this group.

Monthly Casualty Rate During Veteran's Vietnam Deployment

We also grouped respondents into three levels of probable severity of exposure to war-zone stressors on the basis of the average monthly rate of U.S. military personnel killed in action (KIA) during the period, usually about a year, that the veteran was in Vietnam. The monthly casualty rates from January 1966 through December 1971 have been published in various military histories (e.g., Clodfelter, 1995). The rates ranged from to 4.20 per 1,000 in February 1968 during the Tet Offensive to 0.11 per 1,000 in November 1971, shortly before the end of United States' fighting in Vietnam. The months of the respondent's tour(s) were included in the data extracted by Kulka et al. (1990) from military records. We classified veterans for whom the average monthly casualty rate during their tour of duty fell in the upper tertile of all of the monthly rates for the duration of the war as having the highest probable severity of exposure on this measure. Those whose average monthly casualty rate fell in the middle tertile were next. We classified the remaining veterans as having the lowest probable severity of exposure.

Casualty Rate of Veteran's Large Military Unit in Vietnam

Various military histories (Clodfelter, 1995; Palinkas & Coben, 1985) and National Archives and Records Administration electronic data files, retrieved in 2006 (Combat Area Casualties Current File and [U.S. Army] Casualty Information System), contain casualty figures for military divisions (usually about 20,000 men), separate brigades, and other larger units (e.g., 101st Airborne Division, 173rd Airborne Brigade) during the time period that the unit operated in Vietnam. The number of personnel in each unit was estimated from the nationally representative NVVRS sample, and a U.S. KIA rate for each unit was calculated. These ranged from a high of 78.3 U.S. KIA per 1,000 for the 1st Marine Division to a low of 0.6 U.S. KIA per 1,000 for Engineer Command. By use of these rates, military units were grouped into five levels of probable severity of exposure, from extremely high (1st Marines and 173rd Airborne Brigade, with rates of 78.3 and 70.3 per 1,000, respectively) to low (seven units with rates ranging from 7.5–0.6 per 1,000). The largest gap between adjacent rates in the rank order of units was 12.5 per 1,000 U.S. KIA (between 173rd Airborne Brigade and 101st Airborne Division). We used this to differentiate between extremely high casualties and very high casualties. The three additional points of division occurred when a gap of 6 per 1,000 U.S. KIA or more occurred between adjacent units in the rank order of rates.

Casualty data were often not available for smaller, unaffiliated units. Some of these units, although possessing their own name and designation, were attached to, and thus essentially part of, larger units for which casualty data were available. However, many combat support units (engineers, military police, and signal units) and service units (support commands and groups, adjutant general, composite service, maintenance, medical, ordinance, quartermaster, and transportation units) could not be assigned to any larger unit designation. For these units ($n = 25$), we used information contained in military histories (Clodfelter, 1995; Stanton, 1987), in conjunction with the casualty data that were available for similar units, to place these unaffiliated units within one of the five categories of probable severity of exposure. The resulting distribution of male Theater veterans in the five groups is as follows: 4.5%, extremely high; 19.2%, very high; 8.0%, high; 8.3%, moderate; and 60.1%, low.

Early (Three-Category) Composite Measure

In our first set of analyses (Dohrenwend et al., 2004), we combined the three measures described here into an overall measure of probable severity of exposure to war-zone stressors. This composite is a three-category variable: high, moderate, and low exposure probabilities. Information in historical accounts of the fighting during the course of the war provided the rationale for combining the measures. First, for units at the most extreme end of combat exposure, involvement in fighting was fairly constant, even during periods with low overall casualty rates (Casey et al., 1987; Sigler, 1992). Second, during periods with the highest casualty rates, as during the Tet Offensive in 1968, the level of exposure tended to be relatively high, regardless of the unit in question (Addington, 2000; Gibson, 2000; Stanton, 1985; Zabecki, 1998a, 1998b).

In view of these considerations, we constructed the composite measure according to the following scheme, which is also represented graphically in Figure 2.1.

We coded veterans in units with the highest levels of probable exposure on the basis of U.S. KIA (i.e., 173rd Airborne Brigade, 1st Marines) on the composite as having a high probability of severe exposure, and veterans in units in the next two combat levels (e.g., 101st Airborne Division, 1st Cavalry Division) as high on the composite if they served during the highest casualty rate period of the war. The only exceptions to this categorization were individuals in these high combat units with scores of 1 on the MOS variable—service support jobs with probable low combat exposure. Such MOSs are rare in the high-combat units, but they do exist.

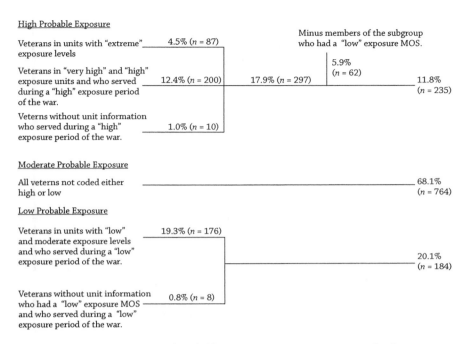

Figure 2.1 Composite MHM of probable war-zone stress exposure—weighted percentages (unweighted sample *n*'s are in parentheses). MOS = Military Occupational Specialty.

We coded veterans from military units that were in the bottom two of the five categories of probable severity of exposure (or who, if unit information was not available, had low combat MOSs) *and* who served during a low casualty period on the composite as having a probable low severity of war-zone exposure. We categorized all remaining veterans as having a probable moderate level of exposure.

Addition of Veteran's Company-Level Casualty Rates to (Four-Category) Measure

A few years later, we (Dohrenwend et al., 2006; 2007) validated and refined the first three components of the MHM just described with important new data from military records. These data consisted of information about the approximately 58,000 U.S servicemen killed in action in Vietnam (Coffelt, Arnold, & Argabright, 2002). It described the dates of these men's deaths and the KIA rates of the companies or other small units (about 200 men) in which they were serving when they died. This ranged from no KIA for 52.4% of veterans to 10 or more KIA for 9.4% of veterans.

We used this fourth measure to validate the first composite MHM measure (e.g., Dohrenwend et al., 2007).

As Table 2.2 shows, the company-level casualty rates vary directly with the Low, Moderate, and High probable severity of exposure groups defined by the first three indicators.

Table 2.2 RELATIONSHIP OF COMPANY RATES OF KIA DURING VETERAN'S
TOUR TO PREVIOUS COMPOSITE MHM OF PROBABLE SEVERITY OF EXPOSURE
TO WAR-ZONE STRESSORS IN MALE THEATER SAMPLE AS A WHOLE

Previous Composite MHM	Company KIA				
	None	1	2–9	10 or more	
Low combat exposure ($n = 151$)	71.4	9.8	16.0	2.9	100.0 %
Moderate combat exposure ($n = 641$)	53.5	14.3	24.9	7.3	100.0 %
High combat exposure ($n = 212$)	17.3	15.4	37.2	30.1	100.0 %
Total ($n = 1004$)	52.4	13.5	24.7	9.4	100.0 %

Note. Percentages are based on data weighted to reflect the complex sampling design; unweighted sample *n*'s are in parentheses. The number of KIA in the companies of 196 of the veterans could not be ascertained. These veterans were assigned to low, medium, or high probable severity of exposure based on the previous three-category MHM.

On the basis of the results given in Table 2.2, it was possible to refine the previous composite measure into a four-category variable that we summarize as follows. Veterans in the high and very high categories (11.7%) typically had high-exposure MOSs, were in large military units with high KIA rates, and served at times of high U.S. KIA rates; men in the very high category (3.2%) were further distinguished by having been in small units (e.g., companies) that suffered 10 or more KIAs during the veteran's service. In contrast, veterans in the low-exposure category (19.8%) typically had low-exposure MOSs, served in large units with low KIA rates, served at times of low KIA rates, and were in small units with no KIAs during the veteran's service. The remaining veterans in the moderate-exposure category (68.4%) differed from those in the low-exposure category mainly in that most served in Vietnam when KIA rates were moderate or high, rather than low. The distribution on MHM exposure in the psychiatrically assessed subsample is similar: 19.3% low; 65.3% moderate; 11.9% high; and 3.5% very high.

Figure 2.2 shows the relationship between the record-based MHM exposure variable we developed (Dohrenwend et al., 2007) and the NVVRS measure of war-zone stress based on retrospective reports by the veterans (see Kulka et al., 1988, Appendix C). The relationship is very strong. For example, only 8.5% of the veterans who had low MHM exposure reported high war-zone stress, compared with 72.1% of the veterans in the very high MHM exposure category.

CONTROVERSIES OVER THE ORIGINAL NVVRS FINDINGS ON RATES OF PTSD IN THE FULL THEATER SAMPLE AND STEPS TOWARD RESOLUTIONS

As we noted earlier, the findings from the NVVRS reported by Kulka and his colleagues (1990) that almost a third (31.9) of the Vietnam veterans developed PTSD and that PTSD was still current for 15.2% proved to be controversial. We now spell out the details of this controversy and what we have done to resolve it.

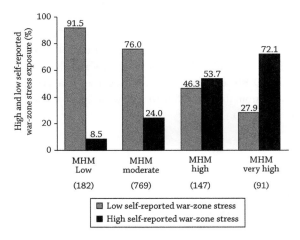

Figure 2.2 Percentages of veterans with Kulka et al. (1988) self-reported high and self-reported low war-zone stress exposure by military/historical measure (MHM) of probable severity of exposure to war-zone stressors (full sample *n* = 1,189, excluding 11 veterans with missing data on self-reported war-zone exposure). Percentages are based on data weighted to reflect the complex sampling design; unweighted sample *n*'s are in parentheses.

Differences in NVVRS and Centers for Disease Control (CDC) Reported Rates

As measured by rates of combat stress breakdowns (CSB), KIA, or wounded in action (WIA), Vietnam has been described as a "low intensity" war for U.S. forces (Jones & Wessely, 2001). Because CSB, KIA, and WIA rates have historically predicted adverse psychiatric outcomes (Bourne, 1970; Jones & Wessely, 2001; Pizarro, Silver, & Prause, 2006; Solomon & Mukulincer, 2006; Tiffany & Allerton, 1967), early expectations were that psychiatric casualty rates in Vietnam would be low (Wessely, 2005a). PTSD rates reported in 1988 by the CDC from a nationwide sample of U.S. Army veterans who served in Vietnam seemed consistent with these expectations: 14.7% lifetime PTSD and, especially, 2.2% still current 11–12 years after the war ended (CDC, 1988; Roberts, 1988). By contrast, the NVVRS findings of rates of 30.9% lifetime PTSD and 15.2% current at about the same time (Kulka et al., 1988, 1990) are inconsistent with these expectations.

There are problems, however, with the measure of PTSD used in the CDC research. The CDC used about half of the items (Thompson, Gottesman, & Zalewski, 2006) from a newly developed module from the Diagnostic Interview Schedule (DIS) (Robins, Helzer, Croughan, & Ratcliff, 1981) to diagnose lifetime and current PTSD on the basis of responses to closed questions asked by lay interviewers. This version of the DIS-PTSD module has been found to diagnose much lower rates of PTSD in the general population than the other diagnostic instrument that is most widely used by lay interviewers, the Composite International Diagnostic Interview (Kessler, Sonnega, Bromet, Hughes, & Nelson, 1995).

Against this background, it is not surprising that the abbreviated CDC adaptation of the DIS-PTSD module was found in the NVVRS to miss 78% of veterans who had diagnosable PTSD, according to the SCID clinicians (Kulka et al., 1988). These results suggest that PTSD is under-diagnosed in both military and civilian samples when this version of DIS-PTSD is used. However, this recognized weakness did not settle the controversies arising from the NVVRS reports of what were considered by many as unusually high rates of PTSD.

Questions About the Accuracy of Veterans' Reports

Critics, who argued that the NVVRS 30.9% lifetime rate is twice as high as the proportion of veterans (15%) who served in combat roles (Burkett & Whitley, 1998; Marlow, 2000; McNally, 2003; Satel, 2004; Shephard, 2001; Wessely, 2005b), raised questions about the accuracy of the retrospective reports of PTSD symptoms and war-zone stressors that qualify as traumatic.

As noted earlier, PTSD diagnoses require antecedent traumatic events, defined at the time of the NVVRS as events that are markedly distressing and "outside the range of usual human experience"—especially events that threaten the life or physical integrity of the individual or someone close to that person; the definition also includes witnessing death or serious injury to others (DSM-III-R; APA, 1987).

Anecdotes about fraudulent claims of military prowess in Vietnam by some individuals in the public eye (Burkett & Whitley, 1998), possible falsification of war-zone experiences by Vietnam veterans seeking compensation for psychiatric disability (Frueh et al., 2005), and evidence of recall biases in reports of combat experiences (e.g., Southwick, Morgan, Nicolau, & Charney, 1997) further fueled skepticism. Critics (Marlow, 2000; McNally, 2003; Satel, 2004) called for verification of veterans' retrospective reports using 201 files. Some suggested that the integrity of the PTSD database might be at stake (e.g., Frueh et al., 2005; McNally, 2003).

To address the full range of concerns expressed about the NVVRS findings, we (Dohrenwend et al., 2006) therefore studied military records, historical accounts, diagnostic histories of PTSD by experienced clinicians, Minnesota Multiphasic Personality Inverntory (MMPI) validity scales, and data on compensation-seeking.

Percentage of Theater Veterans Exposed to Combat

Dean (1997) was cited by McNally (2003) as the source of the figure of 15% involved in combat. This figure probably includes 10.5% who were infantrymen (Clodfelter, 1995, p. 238) and their combat counterparts in the Marines, Navy, and Air Force. However, the 15% clearly does not include 14% who were regularly exposed to combat hazards while serving in support roles, such as combat engineers and artillery personnel (Clodfelter, 1995, p. 256).

Estimates of the percentage exposed to combat dangers increase when Vietnam is recognized as a "war without fronts" rather than a conventional war (Thayer, 1985). For U.S. forces, 30.4% of combat engagements were "organized enemy attacks against U.S. static defense perimeter[s]" (Grave, 1971, pp. 461–462). From 1967 to 1972, U.S. fixed bases experienced an average of 15,000 such "stand-off attacks" per year by mortars, rockets, and recoilless rifles (Thayer, 1985, pp. 46–47). Against this background, Kolko (1985) estimates that, in all, 50% were considered "combat forces" (p. 361), and Baskir and Strauss (1978) conclude that about 1.6 million of the 2.5 million men assigned to tours in Vietnam itself "served in combat" (p. 53). The latter estimate is close to Kolko's when supporting troops on ships and bases in Laos and Cambodia are added, increasing the denominator to about 3.14 million.

Karnow (1997) has suggested that some degree of appreciable risk was nearly universal, noting that, "While infantrymen obviously faced greater risks, headquarters typists were also vulnerable" (p. 479). Michael Herr reached a similar conclusion and described it vividly as follows:

> You could be in the most protected space in Vietnam and still know that your safety was provisional, that early death, blindness, loss of legs, arms or balls, major and lasting disfigurement—the whole rotten deal—could come in on the freaky-fluky as easily as in the so-called expected ways, you heard so many of those stories it was a wonder anyone was left alive to die in firefights and mortar-rocket attacks. (1977, p. 13)

GAF Ratings of Impairment of Functioning in Veterans with War-Related First Onsets of PTSD

As we stated earlier, diagnostic examiners recorded the times of occurrence of traumatic events and onsets of symptoms (Schlenger, 1987). From this information, we (Dohrenwend et al., 2006) estimated that 1.3% of the veterans had first onsets of PTSD prior to Vietnam service, and that 0.1% had a first onset that could be attributed to a post-Vietnam traumatic event in the absence of prior Vietnam-related PTSD. There were too few veterans (4) with pre-Vietnam first onsets to analyze as a separate group. With these four removed, the rate of war-related first onsets of PTSD became 22.5% (*s.e.* 3.4%) and the rate of still current war-related first onsets, 12.2% (*s.e.* 2.3%).

Unlike DSM-IV (APA, 1994), DSM-III-R (APA, 1987) did not require impairment by either disability in social roles or elevated psychological distress. Fortunately, the SCID examiners assessed each veteran's present functioning on the GAF rating scale (Spitzer et al., 1987). It is possible, therefore, to check whether the high NVVRS rates included substantial numbers of veterans with only mild, un-impairing PTSD.

As noted earlier, the GAF used in the NVVRS ranges from 9 (good functioning in all areas) to 1 (persistent danger of severely hurting self or others), with anchoring examples of poor functioning or distress symptoms at each level.

Table 2.3 shows that the large majority, 84.8%, of the veterans with current war-related PTSD were rated as having more than slight impairment at the time of the examination.

The clinicians also made "severity" ratings of PTSD at its worst as well as of PTSD at the time of the examination. These severity ratings, which are strongly related to the GAF impairment ratings, suggest that the results in Table 2.3 underestimate impairment when the disorder was at its worst. For example, 36.1% with current war-related PTSD ("current group") were rated mild, 43.1% moderate, and 20.8% severe at the time of diagnosis. When PTSD was at its worst, 3.7% were rated mild, 31.8% moderate, and 66.5% severe.

Of those with past war-related PTSD ("past group"), only 7.2% were rated mild when the disorder was at its worst, 73.6% were rated moderate, and 19.2% severe. This suggests that the past group had disorders that were at least as severe at their peak as the disorders in the current group at the time of diagnosis. It follows that, like the current group (see Table 2.3), at least 85% in the past group had significantly impairing PTSD.

Table 2.3 ESTIMATED IMPAIRMENT ON GAF SCALE IN SUBSAMPLE VETERANS WITH NO WAR-RELATED FIRST ONSETS OF PTSD, PAST WAR-RELATED ONSETS, AND WAR-RELATED ONSETS THAT REMAINED CURRENT

War-Related First Onset

Functioning	None %	Past %	Current %
09 Good in all areas	46.6	43.6	0.0
08 No more than slight impairment	29.9	24.0	15.1
07 Some difficulty in social, occupational, or school functioning	18.3	23.9	40.5
06 Moderate difficulty	2.7	8.2	15.6
05 Any serious impairment	1.7	0.3	21.1
04 Major serious impairment in several areas	0.1	0.0	7.0
03 Inability to function	0.0	0.0	0.0
02 Some danger to self or others	0.0	0.0	0.0
01 Persistent danger to self or others	0.0	0.0	0.4
Subsample (*n*'s)	(158)	(30)	(59)

Note: Percentages are weighted to the populations from which the samples were drawn. Unweighted sample *n*'s are in parentheses.

A chi-square test shows that the overall difference in the percentages of male veterans with more than slight impairment is statistically significant at the 0.01 level. Individual tests show that the percentage impaired in veterans with current war-related PTSD is significantly greater at the 0.01 level than the percentage of impaired veterans with past PTSD and the percentage impaired with no PTSD ($N = 247$, omitting 4 with pre-war onsets, 2 missing onset information, 1 missing sampling weight, and 6 missing impairment scores).

Scrutiny of Veterans' Accounts

If some NVVRS veterans exaggerated their PTSD symptoms by outright lying or more subtle retrospective distortions (Young, 2004), these veterans should be over-represented among veterans who reported experiencing high war-zone stress, although record-based MHMs indicated low or moderate severity of exposure. Although interview and questionnaire methods for detecting dissembling are far from ideal (Rosen, 2004), data for constructing some of the more frequently used measures of dissembling were available for subsample veterans (i.e., three "fake bad" and "dissembling" validity scales from the MMPI) (Gough, 1947, 1950, 1957; Greene, 1988; Weiner, 1948). We (Dohrenwend et al., 2006) found that mean scores on each scale and percent above the usual cut-offs on all three scales were not elevated in the discordant exposure groups.

The one indication of possible exaggeration emerged in an analysis of projected current PTSD measured by the NVVRS Projected Probability algorithm in the full Theater sample. The PTSD rate among veterans reporting high war-zone stress was 46.9% in the context of low MHM exposure compared with 26.7% in the context of high MHM exposure and 37.4% in the context of very high MHM exposure. However, these differences were not statistically significant, and they did not replicate with SCID diagnoses in the subsample.

The possibility of receiving disability compensation might motivate falsification of symptoms and exposure reports (e.g., Frueh et al., 2005). Compensation-seeking for psychiatric disability was reported by 2.7% of the male Theater veterans in general and 5.7% of the subsample veterans who were diagnosed with current war-related PTSD. However, there was no elevation of compensation-seeking among veterans discordant on the exposure measures; for example, only 3.0% who reported high exposure in the context of low MHM exposure sought compensation, compared with 15.6% who were high on both exposure measures.

Veterans' 201 files do not systematically record information about specific war-zone experiences (U.S. National Archives & Records Administration, 2006). However, these files routinely contain, or make it possible to access from historical accounts, other valuable indicators of the likelihood of experiencing traumatic stressors, as we have shown in constructing the MHM of probable severity of exposure to war zone stressors. The indicators of interest here for present purposes are: High-exposure MOS; attachment to a high-casualty division; receipt of a Purple Heart, combat medal, or Combat Infantryman Badge; service in a company with one or more KIA during the veteran's tour; and service in Vietnam during the nationwide Tet Offensive. More than one of these indicators was present, of course, for all veterans in our high and very high MHM-exposure groups. One or more of these indicators was also present in the 201 files of 47 of the 60 subsample veterans diagnosed with war-related PTSD in the low and moderate MHM exposure groups.

To investigate the validity of the remaining 13 veterans' reports, we extracted verbatim descriptions of their war-zone experiences from their tape-recorded clinical

Table 2.4 SCID-DIAGNOSED WAR-RELATED PTSD
IN SUBSAMPLE (260) WITH AND WITHOUT ADJUSTMENTS
FOR IMPAIRMENT AND INDEPENDENT DOCUMENTATION
OF EXPOSURE

	Onsets (90)	Current (60)
Unadjusted SCID rate	22.5%	12.2%
Adjusted for impairment of functioning	21.0%	10.4%
Adjusted for documentation of exposure	20.3%	11.1%
Adjusted for both impairment and documentation	18.7%	9.1%

Note: Percentages are weighted to the population from which the subsample was drawn.
Unweighted subsample *n*'s are in parentheses.

interviews and responses to open-ended questions in the survey interviews (Kulka et al., 1988, 1990). We compared these narratives with information from military histories (e.g., Fox, 1979; Sigler, 1992) and from newspaper accounts of events in Vietnam published contemporaneously in *The New York Times* and *Los Angeles Times*. These independent sources confirmed the narratives of traumatic events of five veterans: Attacks on air bases reported by three veterans were reported in detail in a military history of Air Force actions (Fox, 1979); a harrowing rescue of U.S. personnel in a downed aircraft described by one veteran who served in a submarine was corroborated in a newspaper account, as was a typhoon that occurred during a series of attacks on another veteran's base.

This left eight veterans whose accounts could not be confirmed by any of these independent sources. However, record information was contradictory for only two of these veterans: One reported several combat medals, with no supporting evidence in his 201 file; the other's account of his exploits seemed out of proportion, and the diagnosing clinician noted that he may have been somewhat delusional.

Table 2.4 displays the rates of war-related PTSD onset and of current war-related PTSD after removal of cases without independent confirmation of exposure and cases with no more than slight impairment. Although these adjustments lower both rates, even the most conservative rates—18.7% for war-related onsets and, especially, 9.1% for current war-related PTSD—remain higher than the rates (14.7% and 2.2%, respectively) reported by the CDC.

Dose–Response Relationships

Figure 2.3 shows dose–response relationships between MHM exposure and war-related PTSD in the subsample.

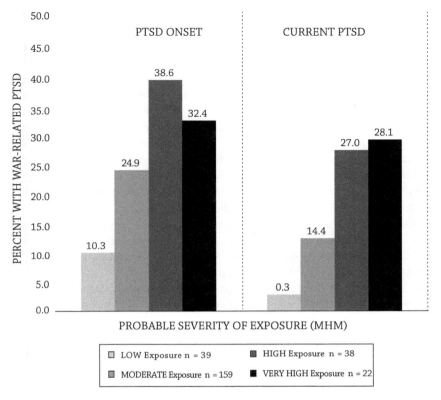

Figure 2.3 The percentages of veterans who had suffered from war-related PTSD during their lifetime (Onset of PTSD) and the percentages of those who still suffered from PTSD at the time of the NVVRS (Current PTSD) according to increases in MHM probable severity of exposure to war-zone stressors. Subsample n = 253, omitting 4 veterans with prewar onset, 2 missing onset information, and 1 missing sampling weight. Percentages are based on data weighted to reflect the complex sampling design. Unweighted subsample n's are provided for the various levels of combat exposure.

The relationship is especially strong for current PTSD, with less than 1% of the low-exposed receiving this diagnosis, compared to 28.1% in the very high exposure category. Omitting the veterans with unconfirmed traumatic exposure and/or those with no more than slight impairment has little effect; for example, with these veterans removed, current war-related PTSD in the very high-exposure group is reduced to 23.4% and in the low-exposure group to zero.

SUMMARY AND CONCLUSIONS

The conundrum posed by critics of the NVVRS involves the misleading juxtaposition of two questionable figures: a 30.9% lifetime prevalence of PTSD in Vietnam veterans and a 15% rate of Vietnam veteran exposure to combat. Our analyses show that neither figure represents the reality of the psychological risks and their consequences for U.S. forces in Vietnam.

First, consistent with estimates from military histories of this war without fronts, at least half the Theater veterans were involved in combat (Baskir & Strauss, 1978; Kolko, 1985), rather than 15%. Second, even the least conservative rates of SCID-diagnosed PTSD from Table 2.4 (22.5% war-related onsets, 12.2% war-related current) are lower than the previously published NVVRS rates (30.9% lifetime, 15.2% current). These latter rates are based on the Projected Probability algorithm that calibrates self-reports of symptoms to SCID-diagnoses and other criterion measures in the subsample (Kulka et al., 1988, Appendix E). As noted above, this algorithm does not distinguish between war-related PTSD and PTSD with other origins, and scores do not depend crucially on the presence of DSM-III-R (APA, 1987) traumatic events. These differences probably contribute to the higher rates found with the algorithm.

On the other hand, the SCID-based rates, even those fully adjusted for impairment and verification of exposure (18.7% onset, 9.1% current) are higher than the rates in the CDC study (CDC, 1988; Roberts, 1988). The CDC used a newly developed module from the DIS (Robins, Helzer, Croughan, & Ratcliff, 1981) to diagnose lifetime and current PTSD on the basis of responses to closed-ended questions asked by lay interviewers. This DIS-PTSD module was extensively tested and found to miss the large majority of veterans (78%) with diagnosable PTSD according to the NVVRS clinicians (Kulka et al., 1988, Appendix E). The DIS-PTSD module has also been found to diagnose much lower rates of PTSD in the general population than another widely used lay interview diagnostic instrument (Kessler et al, 1995). These results suggest that this version of DIS-PTSD under-diagnoses PTSD in both military and civilian samples.

In contrast, the SCID diagnostic results in the NVVRS have proven robust to record checks, investigation of compensation-seeking, and measures designed to detect outright falsification. In some cases, contemporary newspaper accounts or military histories confirmed the plausibility of the veterans' reports of war-zone experiences for which there was no confirmatory evidence in their personnel files. These results suggest that findings of a high rate of unverified trauma in some subgroups of compensation-seeking veterans (Frueh et al., 2005) must not be generalized to the population of Vietnam veterans as a whole.

The clear message is that the Vietnam war took a severe psychological toll on U.S. veterans. Our results, which focus on the subsample of veterans who received clinical examinations and independent measures of their combat exposure, provide compelling reasons to take this message seriously. The nature of this toll is suggested by substantial rates of war-related PTSD onset and current PTSD and the strong dose–response relationship of these rates with severity of exposure.

ACKNOWLEDGMENTS

This chapter expands on the following article:
Dohrenwend, B. P., Turner, J. B., Turse, N. A., Adams, B. G., Koenen, K. C., & Marshall, R. (2006), The psychological risks of Vietnam for U.S. veterans: A revisit with new

data and methods. *Science, 313,* 979–982. Publisher: American Association for the Advancement of Science.

Table 2.1 was originally published in the following article:
Dohrenwend, B. P., Turner, J. B., Turse, N. A., Adams, B. G., Koenen, K. C., & Marshall, R. (2007), Continuing controversy over the psychological risks of Vietnam for U.S. veterans. *Journal of Traumatic Stress, 20,* 449–465. Publisher: Wiley InterScience.

Figure 2.1 was originally published in the following article:
Dohrenwend, B. P., Neria, Y., Turner, J. B., Turse, N., Marshall, R., Lewis-Fernandez, R., et al. (2004), Positive tertiary appraisals and post-traumatic stress disorder in U.S. male veterans of the war in Vietnam: The roles of positive affirmation, positive reformulation, and defensive denial. *Journal of Consulting and Clinical Psychology, 72,* 417–433. Publisher: American Psychological Association.

REFERENCES

Addington, L. (2000). *America's war in Vietnam: A short narrative history.* Bloomington: University of Indiana Press.

American Psychiatric Association. (1980). *Diagnostic and statistical manual of mental disorders* (3rd ed.). Washington, DC: Author.

American Psychiatric Association. (1987). *Diagnostic and statistical manual of mental disorders* (3rd ed., rev.). Washington, DC: Author.

American Psychiatric Association. (1994). *Diagnostic and statistical manual of mental disorders* (4th ed.). Washington, DC: Author.

Appy, C. (1993). *Working class war: American combat soldiers and Vietnam.* Chapel Hill, NC: University of North Carolina.

Baskir, L., & Strauss, W. (1978). *Chance and circumstance: The draft, the war and the Vietnam generation.* New York: Knopf.

Bourne, P. G. (1970). Military psychiatry and the Viet Nam experience. *American Journal of Psychiatry, 127,* 481–488.

Burkett, B. G., & Whitley, G. (1998). *Stolen valor: How the Vietnam generation was robbed of its heroes and its history.* Dallas, TX: Verity.

Casey, M., Dougan, C., Lipsman, S., Sweetman, J., & Weiss, S. (1987). *Flags into battle.* Boston, MA: Boston Publishing.

Cash, J. A., Albright, J., & Sandstrum, A. W. (1985). *Seven firefights in Vietnam.* Washington, DC: U.S. Army, Office of the Chief Military History.

Centers for Disease Control. (1988). Health status for Vietnam veterans: 1. Psychosocial characteristics. *Journal of the American Medical Association, 259,* 2701–2707.

Clodfelter, M. (1995). *Vietnam in military statistics: A history of Indochina wars.* Jefferson, NC: McFarland & Company.

Coffelt, R. D., Arnold, R. J., & Argabright, D. (2002). *An electronic database of combat area casualties.* Washington, DC: National Archives and Records Administration.

Dean, E. T., Jr. (1997). *Shook over hell.* Cambridge, MA: Harvard University Press.

Department of the Army. (1967). *Enlisted military occupational specialties: Personnel selection and classification.* Washington, DC: U.S. Government Printing Office.

Department of the Army. (1970). *Office of Personnel Operations, Study of enlisted medical care and treatment, MOS Career Group (91).* Washington, DC: Department of the Army, Office of Personnel Operations.

Dohrenwend, B. P., Neria, Y., Turner, J. B., Turse, N., Marshall, R., Lewis-Fernandez, R. et al. (2004). Positive tertiary appraisals and posttraumatic stress disorder in U.S. male veterans of the war in Vietnam: The roles of positive affirmation, positive reformulation, and defensive denial. *Journal of Consulting and Clinical Psychology, 72,* 417–433.

Dohrenwend, B. P., Turner, J. B., Turse, N. A., Adams, B. G., Koenen, K. C., & Marshall, R. (2006). The psychological risks of Vietnam for U.S. veterans: A revisit with new data and methods. *Science, 313,* 979–982.

Dohrenwend, B. P., Turner, J. B., Turse, N. A., Adams, B. G., Koenen, K. C., & Marshall, R. (2007). PTSD and Vietnam veterans: Response to letters to the editor. *Science, 315,* 186–187.

Ebert, J. R. (1993). *A life in a year: The American infantryman in Vietnam, 1965–1972.* Novato, CA: Presidio.

Fox, R. P. (1979). Air base defense in the Republic of Vietnam, 1961–1973. Washington, DC: Office of Air Force History.

Frueh, C. B., Elhai, J. D., Grubaugh, A. L., Monnier, J., Todd, B., . . . Kashdan, J. A. (2005). Documented combat exposure of US veterans seeking treatment for combat-related posttraumatic stress disorder. *British Journal of Psychiatry 186,* 467–472.

Gibson, J. W. (2000). *The perfect war: Technowar in Vietnam.* Boston, MA: Atlantic Monthly Press.

Gough, H. G. (1947). Simulated patterns on the MMPI. *Journal of Abnormal and Social Psychology, 42,* 215–225.

Gough, H. G. (1950). The F Minus K Dissimulation Index for the MMPI. *Journal of Consulting Psychology, 14,* 408–413.

Gough, H. G. (1957). *California Psychological Inventory Manual.* Palo Alto, CA: Consulting Psychologists Press.

Gravel, M. (1971). *The Pentagon Papers, The Senator Gravel edition, Vol. 4, Type of engagements in combat narratives.* Boston, MA: Beacon Press.

Greene, R. L. (Ed.). (1988). *The MMPI: Use with specific populations.* New York: Grune & Stratton.

Herr, M. (1977). *Dispatches.* New York: Avon Books.

Hoge, C. W. (2010). *Once a warrior—always a warrior.* Guilford, CT: Globe Pequot Press.

Hunt, P. N., Schlenger, W. E., Jordan, B. K., Fairbank, J. A., LaVange, L. M., & Potter, F. J. (1994). *NVVRS public use analysis file documentation: Analysis variables from the National Vietnam Veterans Readjustment Study.* Research Triangle Park, NC: Research Triangle Institute.

Jones, E., & Wessely, S. (2001). Psychiatric battle casualties: An intra- and interwar comparison. *British Journal of Psychiatry, 178,* 242–247.

Karnow, S. (1997). *Vietnam: A history.* New York: Penguin Books.

Keane, T. M., Caddell, J. M., & Taylor, K. L. (1998). Mississippi scale for combat-related posttraumatic stress disorder: Three studies in reliability and validity. *Journal of Consulting and Clinical Psychology, 56,* 85–90.

Kessler, R. C., Sonnega, A., Bromet, E. Hughes, M., & Nelson, C. B. (1995). Posttraumatic stress disorder in the National Comorbidity Survey. *Archives of General Psychiatry, 52,* 1048–1060.

Kolko, G. (1985). *Anatomy of a war.* New York: Pantheon Books.

Kulka, R. A., Schlenger, W. E., Fairbank, J. A., Hough, R. L., Jordan, B. K., Marmar, C. R., et al. (1988). *National Vietnam Veterans Readjustment Study (NVVRS): Description, current status, and initial PTSD prevalence estimates.* Washington, DC: Veterans Administration.

Kulka, R. A., Schlenger, W. E., Fairbank, J. A., Hough, R. L., Jordan, B. K., Marmar, C. R., et al. (1990). *Trauma and the Vietnam War generation.* New York: Brunner/Mazel.

Marlowe, D. (2000). *Psychological and psychosocial consequences of combat and deployment.* Santa Monica, CA: Rand.

McNally, R. J. (2003). Progress and controversy in the study of posttraumatic stress disorder. *Annual Review of Psychology, 54,* 229–252.

Palinkas, L. A., & Coben, P. (1985). *Combat casualties among U.S. Marine Corps personnel in Vietnam: 1964–1972.* San Diego, CA: Naval Health Research Center.

Pizarro, J., Silver, R. C., & Prause, J. (2006). Physical and mental health costs of traumatic war experiences among Civil War veterans. *Archives of General Psychiatry, 63,* 193–200.

Roberts, L. (1988). Study raises estimate of Vietnam War stress. *Science, 241,* 788.

Robins, L. N., Helzer, J. E., Croughan, J., & Ratcliff, K. S. (1981). National Institute of Mental Health Diagnostic Interview Schedule: Its history, characteristics, and validity. *Archives of General Psychiatry, 38,* 381–389.

Rosen, G. M. (2004). Malingering and the PTSD data base. In G. M. Rosen (Ed.), *Posttraumatic stress disorder: Issues and controversies* (pp. 85–99). West Sussex, UK: Wiley.

Satel, S. (2004, March 5). Returning from Iraq, still fighting Vietnam. *The New York Times,* p. A23.

Shay, J. (1994). *Achilles in Vietnam: Combat trauma and the undoing of character.* New York: Scribner.

Shay, J. (2002). *Odysseus in America: Combat trauma and the trials of homecoming.* New York: Scribner.

Schlenger, W. E. (1987). *Supplemental user's guide for use of the Structured Clinical Interview for DSM-111-R in the National Vietnam Veterans Readjustment Study.* Research Triangle Park, NC: Research Triangle Institute.

Shephard, B. (2001). *A war of nerves.* Cambridge, MA: Harvard University Press.

Sigler, D. B. (1992). *Vietnam battle chronology: U.S. Army and Marine Corps combat operations, 1965–1973.* Jefferson, NC: McFarland & Co.

Smith, R. (2007). *The utility of force: The art of war in the modern world.* New York: Knopf.

Solomon, Z., & Mikulincer, M. (2006). Trajectories of PTSD: A 20-year longitudinal study. *American Journal of Psychiatry, 163,* 659–666.

Southwick, S. M., Morgan, C. A., & Nicolau, A. L. (1997). Consistency of memory for combat-related traumatic events in veterans of Operation Desert Storm. *American Journal of Psychiatry, 154,* 173–177.

Spitzer, R., Williams, J., & Gibbon, M. (1987). *Structured Clinical Interview for DSM-III-R, Version NP-V.* New York: New York State Psychiatric Institute, Biometrics Research Department.

Stanton, S. (1987). *Vietnam order of battle.* New York: Galahad Books.

Thayer, T. (1985). *War without fronts: The American experience in Vietnam.* Boulder, CO: Westview Press.

Thompson, L. (1990). *The U.S. Army in Vietnam.* New York: Sterling Publishing.

Thompson, W. W., Gottesman, I. I., & Zalewski, C. (2006). Reconciling disparate prevalence rates of PTSD in large samples of US male Vietnam veterans and their controls. *BMC Psychiatry, 6,* 19–28.

Tiffany, W. J., & Allerton, W. S. (1967). Army psychiatry in the mid-'60s. *American Journal of Psychiatry, 123,* 810–821.

U.S. Army, Office of the Surgeon General. (1971). *Enlisted medical occupational specialty training.* Washington, DC: Author.

U.S. National Archives & Records Administration. (2006). *Military service records and official military personnel files.* Retrieved February 8, 2006, through www.archives.gov

Villafranca-West, S. A. (2010). *Subtypes of disorder course in Vietnam veterans with war-related posttraumatic stress disorder.* Dissertation submitted to the graduate faculty in the doctoral subprogram of clinical psychology, Graduate Center of City University of New York.

Weiner, D. N. (1948). Subtle and obvious key for the MMPI. *Journal of Consulting Psychology, 12,* 164–470.

Weiss, D. S., Marmar, C. R., Schlenger, W. E., Fairbank, J. A., Jordan, B. K., Hough, R. L., & Kulka, R. A. (1992). The prevalence of lifetime and partial posttraumatic stress disorder in Vietnam veterans. *Journal of Traumatic Stress, 5,* 365–376. doi:10.1002/jts.249005030

Wessely, S. (2005a). Risk, psychiatry and the military. *British Journal of Psychiatry, 186,* 459–466.

Wessely, S. (2005b). War stories: Invited commentary on documented combat exposure of US veterans seeking treatment for combat-related post-traumatic stress disorder. *British Journal of Psychiatry, 186,* 473–475.

Young, A. (2004). When traumatic memory was a problem: On the historical antecedents of PTSD. In G. M. Rosen (Ed.), *Posttraumatic stress disorder: Issues and controversies* (pp. 127–146). West Sussex, UK: Wiley.

Zabecki, D. T. (1998a). Tet offensive: The Saigon circle (1968). In S. Tucker (Ed.), *The encyclopedia of the Vietnam war: A political, social and military history* (pp. 397–399). New York: Oxford University Press.

Zabecki, D. T. (1998b). Tet offensive: Overall strategy (1968). In S. Tucker (Ed.), *The encyclopedia of the Vietnam war: A political, social and military history* (pp. 396–397). New York: Oxford University Press.

CHAPTER 3

ॐ

Measurement of Severity of Combat, Involvement in Harming Civilians and Prisoners, and Personal Vulnerability Load

BRUCE P. DOHRENWEND, THOMAS J. YAGER,
MELANIE M. WALL, BEN G. ADAMS, AND NICK TURSE

The average age of the American soldier in Vietnam was nineteen, seven years younger than his father had been in World War II, which made him more vulnerable to the psychological strains of the struggle—strains that were aggravated by the special tension of Vietnam, where every peasant might be a Vietcong terrorist. (Karnow, 1997, p. 34)

For the common soldier, at least, war has the feel—the spiritual texture—of a great ghostly fog, thick and permanent. There is no clarity. Everything swirls. The old rules are no longer binding, the old truths no longer true. Right spills over into wrong. Order blends into chaos, love into hate, ugliness into beauty, law into anarchy, civility into savagery. The vapors suck you in. You can't tell where you are, or why you're there, and the only certainty is overwhelming ambiguity. (O'Brien, 1990, p. 88)

Here and throughout this monograph, we focus on the three main risk factors for the development of war-related PTSD. These are severity of exposure to combat, personal involvement in harming civilians and prisoners, and personal pre-Vietnam vulnerability. This chapter provides an account of how we measured each of these factors, focusing especially on the intensively studied subsample of veterans included in the National Vietnam Veterans Readjustment Survey (NVVRS).

SEVERITY OF COMBAT EXPOSURE

We developed a wide variety of measures of the combat situations and experiences of the men who served in Vietnam. Our measures are quantitative indicators of the severity of combat to which the veterans were exposed, both individually and collectively, while serving in Vietnam.

Record-Based Military/Historical Measure (MHM)

For use in much of our research with the NVVRS data, we constructed a measure of probable severity of combat exposure based on military records and historical accounts, a measure that is independent of the veterans' recall of their war-zone experiences. This military/historical measure (MHM) relies heavily on casualty rates of various kinds, as described in detail in Chapter 2. As we reported, the MHM shows a strong dose–response relationship with PTSD. We also ascertained from each veteran's military record whether or not he obtained a Purple Heart for being wounded.

Self-Report Measures

Though free of recall bias and indicating a general context of probable severity of combat exposure, the MHM does not provide information about the veteran's personal combat experiences. For example, the MHM does not describe his experiences with enemy mortar attacks, being caught in an ambush, involvement in injuring or killing enemy combatants, or being given dangerous assignments, any of which may have contributed to the development of PTSD symptoms (e.g., Grossman, 1995; Laufer, Gallops, & Frey-Wouters, 1984; Maguen et al., 2009; McNair, 2002; Yager, Laufer, & Gallops, 1984). It makes sense, therefore, to use measures carefully constructed on the basis of self-reports in combination with record-based measures to develop a comprehensive measure of stressful combat experiences.

The main NVVRS interview was called the National Survey of the Vietnam Generation (NSVG). The NSVG included items on traditional combat with the enemy and items on whether the veteran witnessed or participated in harm to prisoners and civilians (Kulka et al., 1988, Appendix C). We used NSVG items to develop four measures of combat exposure: a scale of life-threatening experiences; whether the veteran witnessed the death of a close friend in his unit; whether he killed enemy personnel; and whether he experienced betrayal involving life threat (usually in the form of friendly fire).

Our scale of intensity of exposure to life-threatening combat with the enemy is based on the veterans' reports of frequency of involvement in 11 types of war-zone situations, ranging from the most frequently reported experience of "received incoming fire from enemy artillery, rockets, or mortars" to the least frequently reported and far more dangerous situation of involvement in "hand-to-hand combat." Veterans were asked where they served, using Figure 3.1 as an aid to recall, and asked how often they had had each

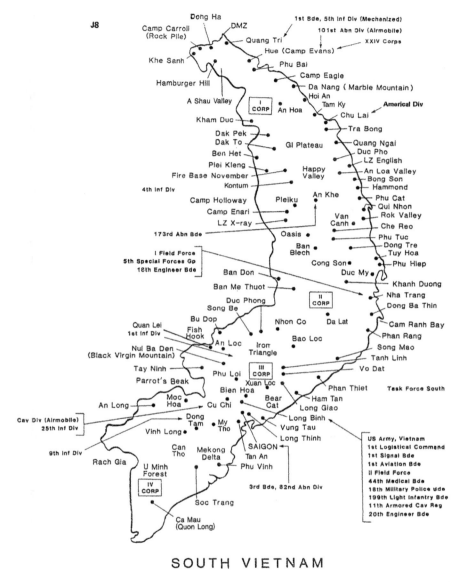

SOUTH VIETNAM

Figure 3.1 During the course of their NVVRS interviews, veterans were presented with this map of South Vietnam and instructed to mark the places on the map where they served.

of the 11 described experiences—*very often, often, sometimes, rarely,* or *never.* They were given concrete definitions of these terms, ranging from *Weekly or more* to *Experience did not occur.*

Following the questions about these 11 situations, the veterans were asked a general question:

In your opinion, how often were you in danger of being killed or wounded in (or around) Vietnam? Would you say *very often (more than 50 times), often (13–50 times), sometimes (3–12 times), rarely (1–2 times), or never?*

We examined the relationship of each of the 11 combat situations to the general life-threat item. Our aim was to dichotomize the items to lessen the potential for bias from extreme reporting, but to do it in a way that maximized each item's association with the general question of overall life threat. Usually, this resulted in dichotomizing the variable to indicate whether the veteran had ever had the experience. However, in two of the situations (identified later) we dichotomized the item to indicate whether the respondent had the experience *sometimes* or more frequently by contrast with *never* or *almost never*. The resulting frequencies for each of the 11 situations are set forth in Table 3.1, with percentages endorsing each dichotomized item weighted to represent the population.

The 11 dichotomized items were then summed to create a count of life-threatening experiences, which had an internal consistency reliability of .88 and exhibited properties of a Guttman (1950) scale, with a reproducibility of .93.

In addition, we reviewed veterans' responses to three questions relating to the deaths of individuals, as follows:

First, the veteran's response of more than *never* to the question, "How often did you see a close friend from your unit(s) killed or die?"

Second, the veteran's report about how often he knew that he had personally killed enemy combatants, indicated by a response other than *never* to the following query:

In the Vietnam arena, enemy personnel were often killed or wounded without any one American soldier being able to say definitely that he fired the shot that did it or was otherwise personally responsible for the casualty. But occasionally a soldier did know that

Table 3.1 PERCENTAGES OF VETERANS WHO EXPERIENCED SPECIFIC TYPES OF COMBAT SITUATIONS

81%	Received incoming fire from enemy artillery, rockets, and/or mortars
74%	Received sniper fire and/or sapper attacks
62%	Unit (patrol) engaged the Vietcong, guerrilla or unidentified troops in a firefight
60%	Received small arms fire from the enemy (*sometimes, often,* or *very often*)
54%	Unit (patrols) encountered anti-personnel weapons such as land mines, booby traps
54%	Unit (patrol) engaged the North Vietnamese Army or other organized . . . forces in a firefight
42%	Unit (patrol) ambushed
42%	Had to do . . . particularly dangerous tasks (e.g., walk point, check out bunkers or tunnels)
33%	Vehicle, aircraft, or boat in which you were traveling . . . was disabled by enemy fire
18%	Cut off/separated from your unit in hostile territory
4%	Experienced hand-to-hand combat (*sometimes, often,* or *very often*)

Note: Percentages are weighted to represent the population from which the subsample was drawn.

he was personally responsible for the death of an enemy. How often (if ever) were you in a combat situation where you were sure that you *personally* had killed enemy personnel?

Third, our research staff members rated betrayal involving life threat as having occurred (or not) from open-ended responses to various questions; it usually involved friendly-fire incidents.

The six individual combat exposure measures are substantially correlated with each other, with nine of the 15 correlations .50 or higher—for example, .59 between the record-based MHM and the self-report item on knowledge of personally killing enemy soldiers; .55 between having a record of receiving a Purple Heart for wounds and a self-report of having witnessed the death of a friend in his unit. Given the moderate to high correlations among the six combat exposure measures (i.e., MHM, Purple Heart, count of life-threatening experiences, witnessed death of a close friend in unit, betrayal involving life threat, killed enemy), we used a factor analytic method for ordered categorical items (Joreskog & Moustaki, 2001; Wirth & Edwards, 2007) to create a single score. This method combined the measures in such a way that the composite had the highest overall correlation with all of the original combat exposure measures. The resulting Combat Exposure Severity Scale (CESS) for each individual was calculated on the basis of the posterior predicted value from an ordered categorical item factor analysis fit using maximum likelihood in Mplus 6.1 (Muthen & Muthen, 1998). A simple sum score of the six combat exposure measures was also constructed. This score was highly correlated with the CESS, but the weighted scale was preferred because of its ability to capture additional variability in severity owing to different types of combat exposures.

Qualitative Examples of Combat Experiences Related to the Quantitative Measures of Combat Severity

In the responses to open-ended questions in the NSVG interview material and the tape-recorded clinical examinations of subsample veterans (previously described in Chapter 2), it was possible to obtain more detailed descriptions of the experiences related to some of the aforementioned quantitative indicators of the severity of combat exposure. This information was most frequently reported about being wounded and about losing close friends in combat situations. To analyze it, we grouped the veterans according to their percentile rank on the overall CESS and examined the described experiences of the veterans in each group, from those who fell above the 90th percentile on the CESS to those who fell below the 25th percentile. The percentiles were calculated using weights for members of the diagnosed subsample. The *n*'s in each resulting group are the unweighted subsample *n*'s, which, as described in the preceding section, overrepresent veterans in the larger sample who were likely to be exposed to severe combat situations.

Table 3.2 summarizes the main types of combat experiences that were described by veterans (i.e., being injured, seeing a close friend killed, or being subjected to friendly fire) in each group in response to open-ended questions about their experiences. More

Table 3.2 PROPORTIONS OF VETERANS GIVING OPEN-ENDED REPORTS
OF THREE KINDS OF TRAUMATIC EXPERIENCE GROUPED BY PERCENTILE
RANKING ON THE COMBAT EXPOSURE SEVERITY SCALE (CESS)

CESS Percentile Group	Injury	Seeing Close Friend Killed	Subjected to Friendly Fire	N
Above 90th	69.0%	45.2%	19.0%	42
Above 75th but at or below 90th	43.6%	25.5%	7.3%	55
Above 50th but at or below 75th	25.0%	25.0%	3.6%	56
At or below 50th but at or above 25th	18.9%	11.3%	1.9%	53
Below 25th	9.5%	4.8%	0.0%	42

Note: Percentile ranking is based on data weighted to represent the population. Unweighted subsample *n*'s are provided for the percentile groups.

detailed descriptions of severity of combat exposure based on the qualitative material follow.

Greater than 90th percentile

Over two-thirds (69%) of the most severely exposed men described experiences of being injured in combat situations. They describe injuries, sometimes multiple, variously to hands, arms, legs, hips, back, face, and head, coming most often as a result of shrapnel from enemy mortars, rockets, booby traps, land mines, or hand grenades. (These descriptions are consistent with official military records indicating that 65% of wounds and 36% of deaths resulted from explosive projectile fragments. Among hospitalized casualties, 36% received wounds to the lower extremities, 18% to the upper extremities, 14% to the head and neck, 7% to the thorax, and 5% to the abdomen, while 20% were wounded elsewhere or received multiple injuries [Neel, 1991]). These veterans frequently described gunshot wounds from sniper fire, being ambushed, exiting helicopters into landing zones near enemy camps, exiting landing zones in helicopters, and driving trucks. (Small arms, according to official records, accounted for 16% of wounds and 51% of deaths [Neel, 1991]). Veterans provided a couple of reports of injury by a knife and a machete in hand-to-hand combat.

Almost half (45.2%) of the men in this most severely exposed group described the death of at least one close friend in combat. The descriptions of the mortal wounds of comrades were often harrowing. Almost a fifth (19%) of the men in this group described being caught in fire from their own forces (so-called friendly fire). (Such incidents occurred, according to one expert, "with disconcerting frequency in Vietnam" (Garrett, 1993). A 1968 Pentagon study estimated that as many as 15–20% of U.S. casualties were caused by friendly fire [Appy, 1993]). Some veterans report these errant attacks coming from U.S. artillery, some from bombing by U.S. planes, and some from bullets fired by U.S. forces on the ground. In two cases, the veteran reported that, although friendly fire occurred, no U.S. personnel were hurt. More usually, however, they reported deaths and wounds.

Remarkably, there are no descriptions by these veterans or by the veterans in any of the other exposure groups of killing enemy fighters in battle, aside from descriptions of problems in distinguishing enemy forces from civilians. We report these latter results in Chapter 5, which focuses specifically on personal involvement in harm to civilians and prisoners.

Greater than 75th but less than or equal to 90th percentile

By and large, the differences between this group and the 90th percentile group of most severely exposed were in the lower rate rather than in the types of experiences described. For example, a substantial minority (43.6%) of the men in this group, rather than a substantial majority (69%) of the most severely exposed, described experiences of being injured. All but one veteran in this group referred to injuries received in combat situations. The sources of the injury again were mainly shrapnel from mortar attacks, as well as gunshot wounds. As was the case with the previous group, the injuries were to a variety of parts of the body, and the injuries occurred in a variety of situations, including ambushes and sniper fire.

About a quarter (25.5%) of the men in this group described deaths of close friends in combat. This is a lower rate than the 45.2% in the previous group. However, the types of situations reported do not differ from those described by the most severely exposed.

Only 7.3% of the men in this group, compared with almost a fifth of those in the most severely exposed, described experiences with friendly fire. One of the four descriptions specified the source as South Vietnamese allies. Another ascribed it to U.S. artillery units, who were said to have received incorrect coordinates.

Greater than 50th but less than or equal to 75th percentile

With this group of veterans, we found differences in both rate and type of experience reported. Only 25% (compared with 43.6% in the group between the 75th and 90th percentiles) described injuries that they experienced, and 29% of these wounds were from accidents that were not combat-related; for example, one veteran was burned as he tried to demonstrate to fellow soldiers how to disarm a grenade, another cut himself opening a can of food, while another broke a toe. This leaves only a fifth with combat-related injuries, usually from shrapnel.

A quarter of the veterans in this group reported one or more deaths of close friends. Usually, the cause of these deaths was stepping on mines. Only 4% of these veterans described experiences with friendly fire, and for one of them, the individual's unit was the source rather than the object of the fire.

Less than or equal to the 50th but more than or equal to the 25th percentile

Slightly less than a fifth (18.9%) of the veterans in this group described injuries that they received. Half of these were unrelated to combat situations. Examples are being injured by an attack from fellow soldiers (two veterans), shooting oneself in the leg by accident, hurting one's back in rear echelon work, and breaking ribs in a fall that took place outside Vietnam. Most of the other injuries were from mortar attacks on base camps.

A small minority (11.3%) of the veterans in this group described one or more deaths of close friends. Two of the six deaths were clearly not combat-related; one occurred in a fight with fellow soldiers, and the other in an accident servicing an aircraft. Most of the remaining deaths were from mortar attacks or sniper attacks. Only one veteran in this group described receiving friendly fire. This was related to guard duty, and it is unclear whether a combat situation was involved.

Less than the 25th percentile

Just under 10% (9.5%) of the veterans in this group described personal injuries. Most if not all of these injuries were not combat-related. There are reports of a leg injury in basic training, of cutting one's own hand, and of being hurt when a truck collided with another vehicle at an intersection. Between 1967 and 1970, in fact, an average of more than 361,000 days were lost to duty in Vietnam as a result of non-battle injuries (Neel, 1991, p. 34).

Two veterans (a weighted 6% of the group) described losing one or more close friends. For one veteran, the deaths were of friends whose planes were shot down. The other veteran does not describe the situation in which he saw a friend die. None of the veterans in this group reported experiencing friendly fire.

Satisfaction with the Excitement of Combat

Most of the qualitative descriptions of combat experiences are highly negative. We found few descriptions of positive experiences despite the fact that a number of anecdotal accounts were reported in the media and elsewhere of a welcome excitement in engaging in combat. Perhaps this is because such excitement is difficult to put into words, given the focus of so many of the NVSG questions that yielded the previously discussed accounts on negative aspects of combat. There was, however, in the NSVG the following closed question:

> Along with some of the unpleasant things and conflicts, many veterans found certain experiences they had in Vietnam satisfying in various ways. For each of these experiences, please describe how satisfying it was to you personally—*very satisfying, somewhat satisfying, not too satisfying, or not at all satisfying*? Or, if you never had this experience, please tell me.

The list of experiences included "camaraderie with friends," which was *satisfying* to almost all of the veterans: *very satisfying* to 69.2% and *somewhat satisfying* to an additional 24.2%. Substantial but lesser majorities expressed satisfaction with "the sense of doing something important" and "the opportunity to grow up quickly."

One item referred explicitly to combat and asked about satisfaction with "the excitement of combat." In response, 8% said they found the excitement of combat *very satisfying*, 17.4% *somewhat satisfying*, 23.6% *not too satisfying*, and 29.4% *not satisfying at all*. An additional 19.2% said they never had that experience. Those who never had that experience were concentrated in the bottom quartile with the least severe combat exposure.

Table 3.3 shows the distribution of satisfaction among the large majority of veterans who reported experiencing the excitement of combat. As can be seen in the Table 3.3 presentation of total rates of the various satisfaction responses, most (slightly over two-thirds) found the experience less than satisfying. In fact, only minorities of veterans at all levels of combat severity found the experience at least somewhat satisfying.

As noted earlier, most of the veterans (57.9%) in the quartile with the least severe combat exposure said they never experienced the excitement of combat. These and 24.4% in the second lowest exposure quartile giving the same response were excluded from Table 3.3. It is surprising that the remainder of the veterans in the bottom quartile had the highest proportion (27.7%) reporting that their experience with the excitement of combat was very satisfying. This is more than twice the 11.8% in the most severe exposure group who also said that their experience with the excitement of combat was very satisfying. The least exposed also had by far the lowest rate (1.3%) who said that their experience with the excitement of combat was not at all satisfying. In small doses,

Table 3.3 SATISFACTION WITH "THE EXCITEMENT OF COMBAT" BY QUARTILES OF COMBAT EXPOSURE, ELIMINATING THOSE VETERANS WHO "DID NOT EXPERIENCE" COMBAT

Combat Exposure Quartile	"The excitement of combat" was:				
	Very Satisfying	Somewhat Satisfying	Not Too Satisfying	Not At All Satisfying	TOTAL (*n*)
First (lowest)	27.7%	16.4%	54.6%	1.3%	100% (15)
Second	1.9%	24.6%	21.0%	52.6%	100% (42)
Third	7.7%	25.2%	35.9%	31.1%	100% (58)
Fourth (highest)	11.8%	19.5%	20.3%	48.6%	100% (99)
TOTAL	10.3%	22.1%	30.1%	37.5%	100% (214)

Combat exposure is measured by the Combat Exposure Severity Scale (CESS).

Percentages are weighted to reflect the population. *N*'s are unweighted sample *n*'s. Men more likely to have experienced high exposure were oversampled, hence the larger *n*'s in the higher quartiles of exposure.

Pearson's chi-square $p = .04$.

exposure to combat danger was, apparently, bracing for a substantial minority of veterans who experienced much less severe combat than the large majority of veterans who served in Vietnam.

INVOLVEMENT IN HARM TO CIVILIANS OR PRISONERS

In recent years, researchers have theorized that the types of guerrilla warfare encountered by U.S. forces in Vietnam, Iraq, and Afghanistan have led to the commission of "morally injurious events" involving "unnecessary cruel and abusive harm to others or lethal violence and killing violence in war zones"—actions commonly called "atrocities" or "war crimes" (see review by Litz et al., 2009, p. 695 and p. 697). Moreover, it has been speculated that involvement in such acts "may be deleterious in the long-term, emotionally, psychologically, behaviorally, spiritually, and socially" (Litz et al., 2009, p. 695).

Studying PTSD in relation to harm to noncombatants is difficult due to the nature of data dealing with such harm committed by U.S. military personnel. For example, allegations of incidents of harm that were identified as atrocities were rarely reported up the U.S. chain of command in Vietnam. Even in the few instances in which atrocities were reported, the evidence was often suppressed, inquiries were carried out with little rigor, and investigations were prematurely closed with no action taken (Turse, 2013). Beyond this, elements of the U.S. military, from the Pentagon down, took measures to ignore, bury, or cover up reports of such incidents during and after the war. Additionally, even micro-level harm incidents that were clearly atrocities—face-to-face crimes with no seeming military purpose, such as rape and mutilation—could be institutionalized in various ways (i.e., ears being cut off from corpses and turned in to commanders to prove a body count) and systemic acts of wanton violence, like home and village burning, were actually elements of official policy (Turse, 2013).

We, therefore, have relied on self-reports from veterans rather than military records. The questions used to identify involvement in harming civilians or prisoners followed a general introductory statement that was read to each veteran:

> In combat situations in (or around) Vietnam, Vietnamese prisoners or civilians were often injured because they were suspected of being enemy sympathizers, or to obtain information, or to avenge the deaths of American soldiers, or for other reasons.

This was followed by questions about the veteran's direct or indirect involvement in harming prisoners and civilians. For example, the veteran was asked whether he was ever in a situation in which a Vietnamese prisoner was injured or killed for any reason, and, if so, did he *only see this happen* or was he *directly involved*? Then, if directly involved, was he *personally responsible*? A similar series of questions was asked in a self-administered questionnaire about situations involving civilians and prisoners that inquired about the extent to which the veteran was involved in "terrorizing, wounding, or killing civilians" and "torturing, wounding, or killing hostages or prisoners of war." To define "extent," he was asked to choose among the following alternatives: *Not at all, Knew/heard about it, Saw it, Unit participated, I participated, I was responsible.* Admission of direct personal involvement (*I participated* or *I was responsible*) to the set of questions about harming prisoners or civilians was taken to indicate that the soldier had harmed prisoners or civilians, respectively.

On the basis of data from the full NVVRS sample of male Theater veterans from majority white, black, and Hispanic backgrounds ($n = 1183$), an estimated 11.8% personally harmed either civilians or prisoners. On the basis of the full, diagnosed subsample from these main racial/ethnic groups ($n = 254$), an estimated 13.3% harmed civilians or prisoners. Most of our analyses of involvement in harming civilians or prisoners focus on this subsample, minus the four veterans with pre-Vietnam PTSD first onsets and the two who were missing diagnostic information. In this remaining subsample ($n = 248$), an estimated 12.6% were identified as being personally involved in harming civilians or prisoners. In more detail, 5.9% reported harming civilians only; 3.4% prisoners only; and 3.3% both civilians and prisoners.

PRE-VIETNAM VULNERABILITY LOAD

There is now a considerable body of literature on vulnerability factors that are strongly associated with PTSD. This literature has been extensively reviewed (Brewin, Andrews, & Valentine, 2000; Dalgleish, 2004; Fontana & Rosenheck, 1994; Halligan & Yehuda, 2000; King, King, Foy, & Gudanowske, 1996; Macklin et al., 1998; Ozer et al., 2003; Schnurr, Lunney, & Sengupta, 2004). Here, we consider only vulnerability factors that either occurred prior to or were present at the start of the veteran's Vietnam service, thus ensuring that no vulnerability factor analyzed could have been caused by war-zone exposure.

In total, 15 possible indicators of pre-Vietnam vulnerability were extracted from the NVVRS data based on veterans' self-reports, military records, or both (Hunt et al., 1994; Kulka et al., 1990, p. 80). The self-report measures either were provided in the public use tapes (Hunt et al., 1994) or could be readily constructed from raw survey data provided by the Research Triangle Institute. The measures from the military records were based on data from the military records (201 files) that Kulka et al. (1990) extracted in relation to drawing the sample.

Total Vulnerability Load Score

Of the 15 vulnerability indicators, nine differentiated veterans with onsets of war-related PTSD or current war-related PTSD from other veterans with the lenient criteria of relative risks of 1.5 or more, or at least the .10 level of statistical significance. We subsequently used these nine indicators, shown in Box 3.1, to create a total vulnerability load score.

Box 3.1

PRE-VIETNAM VULNERABILITY LOAD: NINE INDICATORS SHOWN TO DIFFERENTIATE VETERANS WITH PTSD ONSETS OR CURRENT PTSD FROM OTHER VETERANS

- Reporting one or more family members having been arrested during the respondent's childhood (self-report)
- One or more family members with alcohol or drug abuse problems during the respondent's childhood (self-report)
- Childhood physical abuse involving being spanked or hit so hard by a parent or parent surrogate that the respondent had marks or bruises, had to stay in bed, or see a doctor more often than *hardly ever* (self-report)
- Childhood conduct disorder (subsample clinical interview)
- One or more other psychiatric disorders with pre-Vietnam onsets (subsample clinical interview)
- Low pre-Vietnam educational level (i.e., not beyond high school graduation) (military record)
- Average (category III) or worse on the Armed Forces Qualifications Test (military record) (see Dohrenwend et al., 2008, Table 3; and Sellman, 1990)
- Arriving in Vietnam younger than age 25 (military record)
- Having none of the following previous military experiences—exposure to enemy fire in the Korean War or other conflicts prior to Vietnam, attainment of rank of sergeant or equivalent, and military service at all (military record)

Measurement of Childhood Conduct Disorder and Other Psychiatric Disorders with Pre-Vietnam Onsets

These two risk factors are based on the clinical interview, so they are available only in the diagnosed subsample. Five of our colleagues—three psychiatrists and two doctoral-level clinical psychologists, blind to the original diagnoses—reviewed a random selection of 52 tapes of the SCIDs (described earlier in Chapter 2). We confirmed the good reliability of the PTSD diagnoses found by Weiss et al. (1992). In addition, our checks on diagnoses for psychiatric disorders other than PTSD showed that inter-rater reliabilities for most were satisfactory. For example, all but two of the kappas were over .80, as based on the weighted results for the current or lifetime presence of major depression, panic disorder, generalized anxiety disorder (current only), alcohol abuse or dependence, poly-substance abuse or dependence, and antisocial personality (lifetime only). The exceptions were .68 for current panic disorder and .56 for lifetime poly-substance abuse or dependence.

Because the clinicians probed for the dates of initial onsets of symptoms, it was possible to estimate whether the initial onsets of these disorders occurred prior to, during, or after service in Vietnam. Initial onsets prior to Vietnam, including those of childhood conduct disorder, are considered possible vulnerability factors. As noted earlier, only four subsample veterans had first onsets of PTSD prior to their service in Vietnam, and these veterans were eliminated from our investigation (i.e., too few to analyze).

With few exceptions, such as a correlation of .47 between pre-Vietnam educational level and AFQT score, the nine vulnerability factors shown in Box 3.1 are not highly inter-correlated. In contrast with the individual combat exposure measures, only one of the 36 correlations is .50 or higher (.93 between pre-Vietnam age and previous military experience); 18 of the correlations are below .20. Given these generally low correlations, our composite vulnerability load measure is a simple count of the nine vulnerability factors.

SUMMARY AND CONCLUSIONS

The three factors that we find most strongly affected the psychological impact of the Vietnam war on U.S. male veterans were their combat experiences, their involvement in harming civilians or prisoners, and their pre-Vietnam personal vulnerability load. We have developed and set forth in this chapter detailed measures of each of these factors. These descriptions are complete except for the even more detailed description in Chapter 2 of our use of military records to develop one of the most important measures of severity of combat experiences, the MHM. The detail on the MHM in the preceding chapter should be added to the summary description of the MHM set forth in the present chapter to get the full account.

Unlike the investigation of other variables we report later in other chapters of this monograph, we use these three in one way or another in most of the analyses. For this reason, we set forth in detail the procedures for measuring them here in one place. We describe the less central but perhaps no less important other variables and their measurement in subsequent chapters at the point where we first introduce them. Before proceeding to the remaining chapters, the reader should be thoroughly acquainted with the measures of war-related PTSD and other psychiatric disorders in Chapter 2, and these procedures for measuring severity of combat exposure, involvement in personally harming civilians and prisoners, and pre-Vietnam vulnerability load.

ACKNOWLEDGMENTS

This chapter expands on measures introduced in the following three articles:

Dohrenwend, B. P., Neria, Y., Turner, J. B., Turse, N. A., Marshall, R. D., Lewis-Fernandez, R., & Koenen, K. C. (2004), Positive tertiary appraisals and post-traumatic stress disorder in U.S. male veterans of the war in Vietnam: The roles of positive affirmation, positive reformulation, and defensive denial. *Journal of Consulting and Clinical Psychology*, 72, 417–433. Publisher: American Psychological Association.

Dohrenwend, B. P., Turner, J. B., Turse, N. A., Adams, B. G., Koenen, K. C., & Marshall, R. (2006), The psychological risks of Vietnam for U.S. veterans: A revisit with new data and methods. *Science, 313*, 979–982. Publisher: American Association for the Advancement of Science.

Dohrenwend, B. P., Yager, T. J., Wall, M. M., & Adams, B. G. (2013), The roles of combat exposure, personal vulnerability, and involvement in harm to civilians or prisoners in Vietnam war-related post-traumatic stress disorder. *Clinical Psychological Science, 1*, 223–238. Publisher: Sage Publications.

REFERENCES

Appy, C. G. (1993). *Working class war: American combat soldiers and Vietnam.* Chapel Hill, NC: University of North Carolina Press.

Brewin, C. R., Andrews, B., & Valentine, J. D. (2000). Meta-analysis of risk factors for posttraumatic stress disorder in trauma-exposed adults. *Journal of Consulting and Clinical Psychology, 68*, 748–766. doi:10.1037//0022-006X.68.5.748

Dalgleish, T. (2004). Cognitive approaches to posttraumatic stress disorder: The evolution of multirepresentational theorizing. *Psychological Bulletin, 130*, 228–260. doi:10.1037/0033-2909.130.2.228

Dohrenwend, B. P., Turner, J. B., Turse, N. A., Lewis-Fernandez, R., & Yager, T. J. (2008). War-related posttraumatic stress disorder in black, Hispanic, and majority white veterans: The roles of exposure and vulnerability. *Journal of Traumatic Stress, 21*, 133–141. doi:1002/jts.20327

Fontana, A., & Rosenheck, R. (1994). Posttraumatic stress disorder among Vietnam theater veterans: A causal model of etiology in a community sample. *Journal of Nervous and Mental Disease, 182*, 677–684. doi:10.1097/00005053-199412000-00001

Garrett, W. B., III (1993). *Fratricide: Doctrine's role in reducing friendly fire.* Fort Leavenworth, KS: U.S. Army Command and General Staff College.

Grossman, D. (1995). *On killing: The psychological costs of learning to kill in war and society.* Boston, MA: Little, Brown.

Guttman, L. (1950). The basis for scalogram analysis. In S. A. Stouffer et al. (Eds.), *Measurement and prediction* (pp. 60–90). Princeton, NJ: Princeton University Press.

Halligan, S. L., & Yehuda, R. (2000). Risk factors for PTSD. *PTSD Research Quarterly, 11*, 1–8.

Hunt, P. N., Schlenger, W. E., Jordan, B. K., Fairbank, J. A., LaVange, L. M., & Potter, F. J. (1994). *NVVRS public use analysis file documentation: Analysis variables from the National Vietnam Veterans Readjustment Study.* Research Triangle Park, NC: Research Triangle Institute.

Joreskog, K., & Moustaki, I. (2001). Factor analysis for ordinal variables: A comparison of three approaches. *Multivariate Behavioral Research, 36*, 347–387. doi:10.1207/S15327906347-387

Karnow, S. (1997). *Vietnam: A history.* New York: Penguin Books.

King, D. W., King, L. A., Foy, D. W., & Gudanowske, D. M. (1996). Prewar factors in combat related posttraumatic stress disorder: Structural equation modeling with national sample of female and male Vietnam veterans. *Journal of Consulting and Clinical Psychology, 64*, 520–531. doi:10.1037/0022-006X.64.3.520

Kulka, R. A., Schlenger, W. E., Fairbank, J. A., Hough, R. L., Jordan, B. K., Marmar, C. R., et al. (1990). *Trauma and the Vietnam war generation: Report on the findings from the National Vietnam Veterans Readjustment Study.* New York: Brunner/Mazel.

Kulka, R. A., Schlenger, W. E., Fairbank, J. A., Hough, R. L., Jordan, B. K., Marmar, C. R., et al. (1988). *National Vietnam Veterans Readjustment Study (NVVRS): Description, current status, and initial PTSD prevalence estimates.* Washington, DC: Veterans Administration.

Laufer, R. S., Gallops, M. S., & Frey-Wouters, E. (1984). War stress and trauma: The Vietnam veteran experience. *Journal of Health and Social Behavior, 25,* 68–72. doi:10.2307/2136705

Litz, B. T., Stein, N., Delaney, E., Lebowitz, L., Nash, W. P., Silva, C., et al. (2009). Moral injury and moral repair in war veterans: A preliminary model and intervention strategy. *Clinical Psychology Review, 29,* 695–706.

Macklin, M. L., Metzger, L. J., Litz, B. T., McNally, R. J., Lasko, N. B., Orr, S. P., et al. (1998). Lower precombat intelligence is a risk factor for posttraumatic stress disorder. *Journal of Consulting and Clinical Psychology, 66,* 323–326. doi:10.1037/0022-006X.66.2.323

Maguen, S., Metzler, T. J., Litz, B. T., Seal, K. H., Knight, S. J., & Marmar, C. R. (2009). The impact of killing in war on mental health symptoms and related functioning. *Journal of Traumatic Stress, 22,* 435. doi:10.1002/jts.20451

McNair, R. M. (2002). Preparation-induced traumatic stress in combat veterans. *Peace and Conflict: Journal of Peace Psychology, 8,* 63–72. doi:10.1207/S15327949PAC0801_6

Muthen, L. K., & Muthen, B. O. (1998). *Mplus user's guide* (6th ed.). Los Angeles, CA: Muthen and Muthen.

Neel, S. (1991). *Medical support of the U.S. Army in Vietnam 1965–1970.* Washington, DC: Department of the Army.

O'Brien, T. (1990). *The things they carried.* New York: Penguin Books.

Ozer, E. J., Best, S. R., Lipsey, T. L., & Weiss, D. S. (2003). Predictors of post-traumatic stress disorder and symptoms in adults: A meta-analysis. *Psychological Bulletin, 129,* 52–73. doi:10.1037/0033-2909.129.1.52

Schnurr, P. P., Lunney, C. A., & Sengupta, A. (2004). Risk factors for the development versus maintenance of posttraumatic stress disorder. *Journal of Traumatic Stress, 17,* 85–95. doi:10.1023/B:JOTS.0000022614.21794.f4

Sellman, W. S. (1990). *Project 100,000 testimony and report on the study of Vietnam war era low aptitude military recruits: Statement to the Subcommittee on Oversight and Investigations House Committee on Vets' Affairs 2-28-90.* Retrieved December 21, 2007, from http://members.aol.com/vetschoice/100-1.htm.

Turse, N. (2013). *Kill anything that moves: The real American war in Vietnam.* New York: Henry Holt & Company.

Weiss, D. S., Marmar, C. R., Schlenger, W. E., Fairbank, J. A., Jordan, B. K., Hough, R. L., et al. (1992). The prevalence of lifetime and partial posttraumatic stress disorder in Vietnam veterans. *Journal of Traumatic Stress, 5,* 365–376. doi:10.1002/jts.249005030

Wirth, R. J., & Edwards, M. C. (2007). Item factor analysis: Current approaches and future directions. *Psychological Methods, 12,* 58–79. doi:10.1037/1082-989X.12.1.58

Yager, T., Laufer, R., & Gallops, M. (1984). Some problems associated with war experience in men of the Vietnam generation. *Archives of General Psychiatry, 41,* 327–333. doi:10.1001/archpsyc.1984.01790150017003

CHAPTER 4

༗

A Puzzle About What the NVVRS "Projected Probability of Current PTSD" Measures

BRUCE P. DOHRENWEND, ELEANOR MURPHY,
THOMAS J. YAGER, MELANIE M. WALL,
AND STEPHANI L. HATCH

Somewhat surprisingly, the particular period in which male veterans served (for example, during the Tet offensive) is not related to variations in current rates of PTSD [as measured by the projected probability of current PTSD]. (Kulka et al., 1990, p. 66)

Throughout this monograph, we use clinical diagnoses made in the NVVRS subsample as our measure of PTSD. These diagnoses identify not only PTSD still current at the time of the interview, but also all onsets of PTSD, including the cases that had remitted before the interview. In addition to marking the course of the disorder in this way, the diagnoses offer the advantage that they are based on professional clinical assessments of the presence or absence of each symptom and trauma criterion specified in the DSM definition of PTSD itself. However, these diagnoses were conducted with only a minority of the NVVRS respondents. Use of the diagnoses comes, therefore, with the distinct disadvantage that the subsample's small size severely limits the statistical power of our analyses. What follows is an account of an additional reason that, nevertheless, it has proven so important to focus on the diagnostic histories despite the problem of sample size.

As explained in Chapter 2, the NVVRS devised a measure of current PTSD that could be used in the full sample. This projected probability of current PTSD measure was derived from a regression model fitted to the subsample on the basis of a variety of predictors of the NVVRS "composite diagnosis" of current PTSD, which in turn was largely based on the clinical diagnosis of current PTSD in the subsample and was highly correlated with it. The predictors include questionnaire responses to items about combat exposure and self-reported symptoms in the M-PTSD (Schlenger et al., 1992). We used this NVVRS variable (i.e., the Projected Probability measure) ourselves in some of our early, unpublished analyses as a way to overcome the size of the diagnosed subsample. One of these early analyses proved to be particularly important. It involved an examination of the possible effects of male veterans' attitudes toward the war on rates of PTSD for veterans who served in each of four distinct periods of the war. In the course of this earlier analysis, we discovered attributes of the Projected Probability measure that led us to question what it was in fact measuring, and, ultimately, to decide not to use it.

INVESTIGATION OF THE NVVRS MEASURE

Our starting point was the finding by Kulka et al. (1990) that rates of current PTSD did not vary with periods of the war. What made this finding surprising, of course, was that the intensity of combat exposure varied considerably over the course of the war, and that, as we and others have shown, there is a strong positive relationship between severity of combat exposure and PTSD. Neither Kulka et al. nor others, however, systematically investigated the factors that may have contributed to this puzzling finding.

Key Variables—Combat Intensity and Attitudes of The American Public

We set out to investigate the possible roles of two important variables that changed markedly with the passage of time. The intensity of ground combat was greatest in the middle years of the war and decreased as the American role in Vietnam was coming to an end, but unfavorable attitudes on the part of the American public increased steadily from year to year throughout the conflict. We thought it possible that the stress of combat itself might have been aggravated by the knowledge that the war was losing support back home—and, in fact, among the soldiers themselves while serving in Vietnam. We hypothesized that aggravating effects of these increasingly negative attitudes might have offset the declining risk of PTSD associated with combat intensity in Southeast Asia.

To address this possibility, we started out by using the Projected Probability measure to estimate rates of current PTSD among male theater veterans in the full sample who served during different periods of the war.

Four Distinct Periods of the Vietnam War

The NVVRS sample includes veterans who entered Vietnam as early as 1960 and as late as 1974. Times of their exits from the war range from 1964 to 1975, with dates of entry and exit for each veteran being ascertained through military records. We divided veterans' time of entry into four discrete periods, demarcated by specific cutoff dates. The first period of entry was on or before July 27, 1965, a time when relatively few U.S. troops were involved in combat operations (Bates et al., 1998). The second period started on July 28, 1965, when President Johnson's order to increase the number of U.S. troops prompted a massive upsurge in draft calls and large-scale U.S. involvement in ground operations for the first time. The third period of entry commenced on January 30, 1968, corresponding with the onset of the Tet offensive, during which the Vietnamese revolutionary forces launched coordinated attacks in five major cities, 35 of 44 provincial capitals, 64 district seats, and 50 other locations throughout South Vietnam. The fourth and final period of entry began on December 1, 1969, when a draft lottery was instituted in the United States, with the Selective Service taking steps to reduce the number of draft deferments. (See our Chapter 1 for a detailed chronology of the gradual commitment and eventual withdrawal of U.S. armed forces in Vietnam.)

Figure 4.1 shows levels of combat exposure experienced by the veterans in the subsample during each of these four periods of the war. Combat exposure is measured by five variables:

- The Military-Historical Measure (MHM) of probable combat exposure
- The Life-Threat Guttman scale of self-reported combat-exposure
- Having witnessed the killing of a close friend in the veteran's unit
- Having killed one or more enemy combatants
- Having received a Purple Heart medal (for having been wounded)

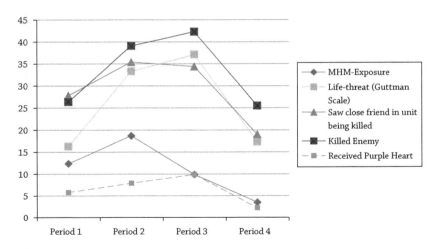

Figure 4.1 Distribution of combat exposure according to time of war entry.

Note: Figures represent weighted percentages of veterans in the subsample within each entry period that fell into the very high/high combat exposure categories on the MHM and life-threat (Guttman Scale), as well as the weighted percentage of those within each entry period who reported seeing a close friend in their unit killed, killing enemy combatants, or receiving Purple Hearts.

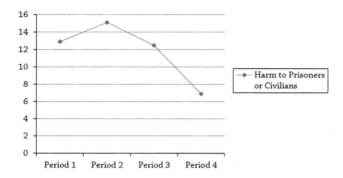

Figure 4.2 Distribution of involvement in harm to prisoners or civilians according to time of war entry.

Note: Figures represent weighted percentages of veterans in the subsample within each period of war entry who reported being involved in harm to prisoners or civilians.

These variables are described in Chapter 3. All five are components of the Combat Exposure Severity Scale (CESS), whose derivation we explain in that chapter. All five show combat exposure at its highest level during the middle two periods of the war.

As we later discuss in detail in Chapters 5 and 6, participation in harm to civilians and prisoners is also highly associated with PTSD as well as with severity of combat exposure.

Figure 4.2 shows that harm, too, was reported at higher levels during the middle periods of the war than in the final period. Note, in addition, that harm is much higher in the first period of the war than in the last period of the war, both of which were low combat periods. However, Figure 4.3 shows that rates of PTSD, as estimated in the full sample by the Projected Probability measure, are virtually constant across all four periods. This was Kulka et al.'s (1990) "surprising" finding.

As mentioned, it was in effect this very contrast between Figure 4.3's flat line and the curved lines in Figures 4.1 and 4.2 that first inspired us to investigate the relationship between PTSD and public attitudes toward the war. It is worth noting in this connection that the Projected Probability measure overestimates the rate of current PTSD in men with a low risk of combat exposure. Among men in the lowest category of the MHM—a measure of combat exposure based on the military record and therefore not subject to response bias—only 0.3% were diagnosed with current PTSD, but the Projected Probability measure estimates that rate as 3.1% in the diagnosed subsample and 12.0% in the full sample. Both differences are statistically significant at $p \leq .05$. (To compare the diagnosed rate of 0.3% in the subsample with the estimate of 12.0% based on the Projected Probability in the full sample, we simply determined that the two 95% confidence intervals do not overlap. In the subsample, the confidence interval of the difference between the diagnosed rate of 0.3% and the Projected Probability estimate of 3.1% does not include zero.)

For this low-combat-risk group, the fact that the Projected Probability measure overestimates the rate of current PTSD—even in the subsample where it was

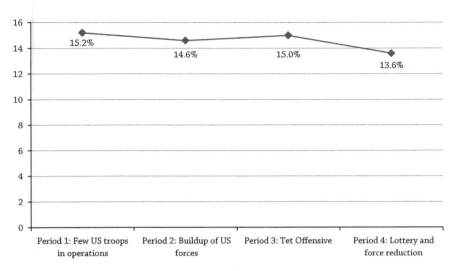

Figure 4.3 Rate of Projected Probability of current PTSD in the full sample by period of war entry.
Adjusted Wald F = .091, p = .964 (Wald F = .087, p = .967)

modeled—indicates that the estimate is problematic. The fact that the estimated rate is much higher still in the full sample strongly suggests that the Projected Probability measure is not doing the job it was meant to do—namely, to estimate the rate of current PTSD in the full sample. This overestimation in a group of men who had little combat exposure may help to account for the flat line, which represents an equally dramatic failure of the Predicted Probability measure to respond to variations in combat exposure in different periods of the war.

DIAGNOSED ONSETS AND DIAGNOSED CURRENT PTSD IN THE SUBSAMPLE

Because the attitude questions in the NVVRS (described later in detail in Chapter 10) inquire about the veteran's attitudes when he entered and when he left Vietnam, we decided to look at onsets of war-related PTSD—which would, of course, have occurred in reaction to traumatic experiences *during* his period of service in Vietnam, usually about one year. Information on PTSD onset was available only in the form of the clinical diagnoses made in the subsample. It was at this time that we learned, to our surprise, that diagnosed onsets of PTSD and diagnosed current PTSD both followed the same pattern as combat exposure and participation in harm to civilians and prisoners. All were highest in the two high-combat middle periods of the war. Furthermore, the Projected Probability measure for veterans in the subsample traced a curve whose shape was almost identical to that of *diagnosed* current PTSD, although the projected rates were higher in each period than those based on the diagnoses. In other words, the flat line we had seen in the full sample disappeared when we looked at the same variable in the subsample.

Figure 4.4 plots all three measures of PTSD across periods of the war in the subsample. We were surprised to see the Projected Probability measure in the subsample behave differently than this measure did in the full sample. Maybe we shouldn't have been surprised to see this Projected Probability measure in the subsample paralleling the diagnosis of current PTSD in the subsample, because it was fitted largely to the diagnoses in the subsample. The Projected Probability measure was not specifically modelled to predict the clinical diagnosis, but was instead modelled to predict the closely related "composite diagnosis," so the higher projected rates in comparison to the diagnosed rates are certainly within the realm of mathematical possibility. The mystery is why the Projected Probability measure in the full sample behaved so differently from the clinical diagnosis in the subsample.

We thought at first that the strikingly different results in the two samples might have been produced by differences in the composition of the subsample as compared to the full sample. However, the two samples have remarkably similar demographic characteristics and rates of projected current PTSD (see Chapter 2), differing only in the higher proportion of veterans from rural areas and small towns in the full sample. We compared these veterans with their urban peers and could find no differences in relevant risk factors such as severity of combat exposure and pre-Vietnam vulnerability load. We, therefore, considered the possibility that the Projected Probability measure in the full sample is tapping something different from the composite diagnosis of current PTSD. We next explored what that "something" might be.

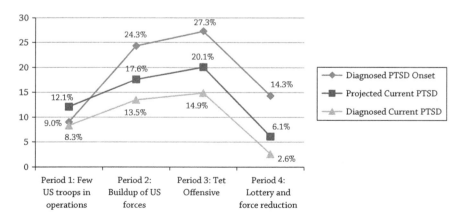

Figure 4.4 Weighted subsample rates of diagnosed onsets of PTSD, Projected Probability of current PTSD, and diagnosed current PTSD by period of the war.
Diagnosed PTSD onset: Adjusted Wald F = 1.349, p = .259 (Wald F = 1.632, p = .183)
Projected probability of current PTSD: Adjusted Wald F = 4.516, p = .003 (Wald F = 5.261, p = .002)
Diagnosed current PTSD: Adjusted Wald F = 3.765, p = .011 (Wald F = 4.341, p = .005)

THREE STUDIES POINTING TO NON-SPECIFIC, GENERAL DISTRESS

We found clues in the following studies.

Combat Veterans Returning from Iraq

In the first study, a non-patient sample of 345 U.S. National Guardsmen was given two widely used screening scales composed of self-report items two months after they returned from combat in Iraq. One, designed to screen for PTSD, was the military version of the PTSD Symptom Checklist (PCL-M), which asked the soldiers to rate each of 17 items "as a response to stressful military experiences" (Arbisi et al., 2012, p. 1035). The other was the Beck Depression Inventory (BDI-II) designed to screen for major depression. Three months later, the soldiers were examined using the Clinician Administered PTSD Scale (CAPS), the state-of-the-art instrument for diagnosing PTSD that the study used as a gold standard. The researchers found that both the PCL-M and the BDI-II had very high false-positive rates (e.g., between 65% and 76% for the PCL-M). Moreover, the PCL-M was not more accurate than the BDI-II in predicting CAPS diagnoses. The authors concluded that their findings "suggest that the PCL, along with the BDI-II, is primarily functioning by assessing general distress and demoralization rather than unique facets of PTSD" (Arbisi et al., 2012, p. 1038).

Civilians Exposed to Trauma

On the same problem, Marshall, Schell, and Miles (2010) studied two samples of trauma-exposed respondents. One sample consisted of 294 persons exposed to community violence; the other, of 234 persons evacuated from areas consumed by wildfires. The authors found that all 17 PCL items were highly correlated with a measure of "general distress" drawn from the SCL-90 depression and anxiety scales and the PHQ-8. Perhaps more surprisingly, the PCL items on intrusiveness and avoidance were as highly correlated with the measures of general distress as the PCL items apparently intended to tap dysphoric mood—items that, on their face, seemed more similar to general distress.

Civilian Version of the Mississippi PTSD Scale

A third study focused specifically on the Mississippi PTSD scale (M-PTSD), the forerunner of the PCL that was, uniquely, a major component of, and highly correlated with, both the composite diagnosis of current PTSD in the NVVRS subsample and its Projected Probability measure in the full sample. These authors found that the civilian version of the M-PTSD was more highly correlated with symptom scales of depression (the BDI) and anxiety (STAI-T) than with two scales of PTSD symptoms—namely, the IES and the

Purdue PTSD Questionnaire–Revised. The investigators concluded that the civilian version of the M-PTSD "may be more a general measure of psychological discomfort rather than a specific measure of PTSD symptomatology" (Lauterbach et al., 1997, p. 510).

Unlike the diagnosis of current PTSD in the NVVRS subsample, the Projected Probability measure relies heavily on self-reported symptom scale items—particularly the M-PTSD (Kulka et al., 1988, Appendix E). We, therefore, questioned whether, as in the three studies described, the Projected Probability measure might be similar to a measure of nonspecific distress or demoralization when used outside the sample on which it was calibrated.

Fortunately, we had a measure of nonspecific distress that, following Jerome Frank (1961), we think of as indicating demoralization in the NVVRS data set (Dohrenwend et al., 1980). The demoralization scale consists of 27 items on helplessness, hopelessness, depressed mood, dread and anxiety, low self-esteem, and psychophysiological disturbances. Its internal consistency reliability in the NVVRS male subsample is .94. The scale score is the mean of the item scores and ranges from zero to four. We dichotomized this scale for the present analysis. "High Demoralization" indicates a demoralization score above .9259, which is a level that detects the presence of any current psychiatric disorder with roughly equal sensitivity and specificity.

As we hypothesized on the basis of the studies just cited, High Demoralization is more highly correlated with the Projected Probability of current PTSD (.48) than with the diagnosis of current PTSD (.31) in the subsample. The same is true of the continuous demoralization scale, which produces correlations of .68 and .52, respectively.

Figure 4.5 shows that, unlike the diagnosis of current PTSD in the subsample, High Demoralization does not differ significantly in high and low combat periods of the war

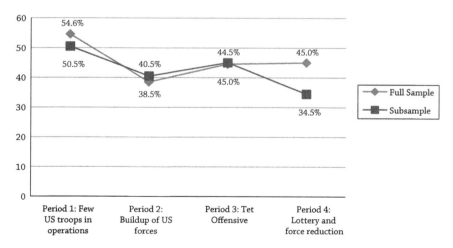

Figure 4.5 Weighted rates of high demoralization in the full sample and in the subsample by period of the war.
Note: Percentages are weighted to the populations from which the samples were drawn. Upper figures are for the full sample; lower figures for the subsample. Full sample: Adjusted Wald F = 1.755, p = .154 (Wald F = 1.882, p = .131) Subsample: Adjusted Wald F = .358, p = .776 (Wald F = .341, p = .795)

in either sample. In this regard, of course, demoralization behaves like the Projected Probability measure in the full sample. That Projected Probability of current PTSD behaves more like the diagnosis of current PTSD in the subsample we think is due to the fact that Projected Probability of current PTSD was calibrated in the subsample rather than in the full sample.

CONCLUSION

A likely explanation of why Kulka et al. (1990) found no difference in rates of projected probability of PTSD in high and low combat periods of the war is that the NVVRS Projected Probability measure reflects symptoms of general distress more than it reflects symptoms of PTSD. It is, therefore, a weak, if not misleading, measure of war-related PTSD. If Kulka et al. (1990) had been able to use diagnoses of PTSD in the full sample, they would probably have found differences in outcomes between high and low combat periods of the war, as is found in the subsample. This apparent problem with the NVVRS Projected Probability of PTSD as a measure of current war-related PTSD reinforced our decision to use the clinical diagnosis of war-related PTSD in most of the analyses in this monograph, despite the loss of statistical power that comes with being confined to the clinically examined subsample. With the need to focus on the diagnoses of PTSD in the subsample, we later return to consideration of the effects of changing public attitudes toward the war in Chapter 10.

REFERENCES

Arbisi, P. A., Kaler, M. E., Kehle-Forbes, S. M., Erbes, C. R., Polunsy, M. A., & Thuras, P. (2012). The predictive validity of the PTSD Checklist in a nonclinical sample of combat-exposed National Guard troops. *Psychological Assessment, 24*, 1034–1040.

Bates, M. J., Lichty, L., Miles, P., Spector, R. H., & Young, M. (1998). Chronology 1945–1995. In *Reporting Vietnam, Part 1: American journalism, 1959-1969* (pp. 775–803). New York: Library of America.

Dohrenwend, B. P., Shrout, P. E., Egri, G., & Mendelsohn, F. S. (1980). Measures of nonspecific psychological distress and other dimensions of psychopathology in the general population. *Archives of General Psychiatry, 37*, 1229–1236.

Frank, J. D. (Ed.). (1961). *Persuasion and healing: A comparative study of psychotherapy* (1st ed.). Baltimore, MD: The Johns Hopkins University Press.

Kulka, R. A., Schlenger, W. E., Fairbank, J. A., Hough, R. L., Jordan, B. K., Marmar, C. R., et al. (1988). *National Vietnam Veterans Readjustment Study (NVVRS): Description, current status, and initial PTSD prevalence estimates*. Washington, DC: Veterans Administration.

Kulka, R. A., Schlenger, W. E., Fairbank, J. A., Hough, R. L., Jordan, B. K., Marmar, C. R., et al. (1990). *Trauma and the Vietnam War generation: Report on the findings from the National Vietnam Veterans Readjustment Study*. New York: Brunner/Mazel.

Lauterbach, D., Vrana, S., King, D. W., & King, L. A. (1997). Psychometric properties of the civilian version of the Mississippi PTSD Scale. *Journal of Traumatic Stress, 10*, 499–513.

Marshall, G. N., Schell, T. N., & Miles, J. N. V. (2010). All PTSD symptoms are highly associated with general distress: Ramifications for the dysphoria symptom cluster. *Journal of Abnormal Psychology, 119,* 126–135.

Schlenger, W. E., Kulka, R. A., Fairbank, J. A., Hough, R. L., Jordan, B. K., Marmar, C. R., et al. (1992). The prevalence of post-traumatic stress disorder in the Vietnam generation: A multimethod, multisource assessment of psychiatric disorder. *Journal of Traumatic Stress, 5,* 333–363.

CHAPTER 5

ᔪᔭ

The Roles of Combat Exposure, Personal Vulnerability, and Involvement in Harm to Civilians or Prisoners in War-Related Post-Traumatic Stress Disorder

BRUCE P. DOHRENWEND, THOMAS J. YAGER,
MELANIE M. WALL, AND BEN G. ADAMS

The severity, duration, and proximity of an individual's exposure to the traumatic event are the most important factors affecting the likelihood of developing this disorder [PTSD]. (APA, 1994, p. 426)

As noted earlier, the diagnosis "post-traumatic stress disorder" (PTSD) was introduced in the third edition of the American Psychiatric Association's (APA; 1980) *Diagnostic and Statistical Manual of Mental Disorders* (DSM-III) amid debate about the psychiatric toll of the Vietnam war (e.g., Friedman, Resick, & Keane, 2007). The new diagnosis described a novel syndrome of intrusive, avoidance/numbing, and arousal symptoms as the distinctive psychopathology following exposure to traumatic stressors. (See our Chapter 1, section Aftermath, *Recognition of Veteran Experiences*, which summarizes the post-war political and scientific discussions that led to the official recognition of PTSD in DSM-III.)

PTSD is unusual among psychiatric diagnoses in that it requires a putative main-cause "Criterion A" stressor exposure, among its other indicators. The subsequent, revised edition (DSM-III-R; APA, 1987) was used by NVVRS clinicians to make the diagnoses in the present research. Its description of Criterion A emphasizes events that threaten the life or physical integrity of the individual, or of someone close to him or her, and includes witnessing death or serious injury to others.

The role of Criterion A stressors is spelled out in the fourth edition (DSM-IV) as follows:

> The severity, duration, and proximity of an individual's exposure to the traumatic event are the most important factors affecting the likelihood of developing this disorder. There is some evidence that social supports, family history, childhood experiences, personality variables, and preexisting mental disorders may influence the development of Post-traumatic Stress Disorder. This disorder can develop in individuals without any predisposing conditions, particularly if the stressor is especially extreme. (APA, 1994, pp. 426–427)

In DSM-III through DSM-IV, stressor exposure, in and of itself, was assumed to be capable of producing the underlying disturbance that resulted in persistent symptoms. As Friedman (2005) put it,

> armed with this diagnosis . . . , we have begun to appreciate the profound and sometimes irreversible changes produced by overwhelming stress. These include fundamental alterations in perception, cognition, behavior, emotional reactivity, brain function, personal identity, world view, and spiritual beliefs. (p. 1288)

The implication is that the Criterion A stressor exposure itself can produce the underlying disorder, which is manifested by symptoms that are far from transient. Such stressor exposure has been retained as a requirement for the diagnosis of PTSD in the latest manual, DSM-5 (APA, 2013).

This formulation of the role of the Criterion A stressors in PTSD differs from the treatment of exposure to life-threatening stressors and situations in previous American diagnostic manuals. In DSM-I, whose publication followed World War II, the diagnosis was called "gross stress reaction" and was grouped under a broader heading of "transient personality disorder" (APA, 1952, p. 40). This formulation was carried over to DSM-II (APA, 1968), which emphasized "reactions [that] differ from those of neurosis and psychosis chiefly with respect to clinical history, reversibility of the reaction" (APA, 1952, p. 40). The reactions were thought to be transient in persons with "good adaptive capacity"; if they persisted after the stressful exposure lessened, this was evidence of "a more severe underlying disturbance" (p. 48). The implication of these earlier formulations is that symptom responses to traumatic events will usually be transient unless the exposed individuals had prior vulnerabilities, such as a previous history of serious psychiatric disorders.

CONTROVERSY SURROUNDING CRITERION A STRESSORS

The assumption that Criterion A stressors are the primary causes of the disorder has become a center of controversy. There are arguments over whether Criterion

A should be broadened, narrowed, or done away with altogether (Brewin et al., 2009; Maier, 2007; McNally, 2003; Weathers & Keane, 2007). Some critics have argued that predisposing personal vulnerability factors contribute more to the development of the disorder than does exposure to traumatic events (e.g., Breslau, 2002; Yehuda & McFarlane, 1995). War-zone stressors in Vietnam, whose U.S. veterans' readjustment problems gave rise to the diagnosis, are included in this generalization by Yehuda and McFarlane (1995). They cite data on the prevalence of PTSD from the most important psychiatric investigation of U.S Vietnam veterans, the National Vietnam Veterans Readjustment Study (NVVRS), that suggest to them that many veterans exposed to war-zone stressors do not develop PTSD. However, their critique does not adequately consider the fact that there are often marked individual differences in "severity, duration, and proximity of an individual's exposure to the traumatic event" (APA, 1994, p. 426) and corresponding dose–response differences in rates of the disorder (Dohrenwend, 1998).

As noted earlier, the novel symptom criteria for the diagnosis of PTSD in DSM-III through DSM-IV, like the stressor Criterion A, have also been grouped into alphabetically designated types: Criterion B (intrusive symptoms), Criterion C (avoidance/numbing symptoms), and Criterion D (symptoms of arousal). We refer here to the required co-occurrence with Criterion A and duration (at least 1 month) of Criteria B, C, and D as the PTSD symptom syndrome (PSS).

Fortunately, the clinical examinations for the diagnosis of PTSD in a subsample of veterans from the NVVRS were conducted so that all PTSD symptoms were rated for all veterans regardless of whether the clinician judged that the veteran had experienced a Criterion A stressor in Vietnam. It is possible, therefore, to assess the presence or absence of PSS independently of the presence of Criterion A stressors that are needed for the full PTSD diagnosis.

PURPOSE

Our purpose is to use measures of PSS, personal vulnerability, and combat stressors—obtained from the NVVRS (Kulka et al., 1990) or constructed by us from the NVVRS interview data and military records—to investigate the primacy of the stressor assumption. In doing so, we take into account involvement in harm to civilians and prisoners in a type of war that was new for this generation of Americans. It has been described as a "war amongst the people" (Smith, 2007), in which it was often hard to distinguish civilians from enemy combatants, and as a "war without fronts" (Thayer, 1985), for which the body count of presumed enemy dead became a substitute for the taking of territory as an indicator of military success (Turse, 2013). (See our Chapter 1, section War, *America in Vietnam* and *Fighting the War*.)

We ask and seek to answer three main questions:

1. Were Criterion A combat stressors—that is, exposures that meet Criterion A specifications (e.g., life-threatening combat experiences)—necessary for the onset

of war-related PSS, defined as meeting Criteria B through D? Alternatively, was it possible for a veteran to experience PSS onset based on his general experience in Vietnam without having experienced one or more Criterion A war-zone stressors?

2. Are there specific types or severities of Criterion A war-zone stressors that were sufficient for the onset of war-related PSS?

3. What were the effects of (a) pre-Vietnam vulnerability factors, and (b) harming civilians or prisoners during service in Vietnam on the onset and adverse course of war-related PSS?

Part of the third and last question bears directly on the issue of the relative importance of exposure and personal vulnerability in the development of PTSD; that is, its onset and adverse course. To assess the claim of some investigators that pre-Vietnam vulnerability factors contribute more than does Criterion A exposure in the war zone to the development of the disorder, we must first define in operational terms what it might mean to "contribute more."

We address the question in three ways. First, exposure will contribute more if its effect on war-related PSS, with vulnerability controlled, is greater than the effect of vulnerability, with exposure controlled. Second, exposure will contribute more if the effect of vulnerability diminishes or disappears at very high levels of exposure—levels "that would evoke significant symptoms of distress in almost anyone" (DSM-III; APA, 1980, p. 236). In other words, we would expect a negative interaction between combat exposure and vulnerability. Finally, if, as suggested by previous research (e.g., Laufer, Gallops, & Frey-Wouters, 1984; a review in Lidz et al., 2009), personal involvement in harm to civilians or prisoners is found to be strongly related to PTSD, we can investigate whether such harm showed a stronger association with combat exposure than with vulnerability. If so, this would be another indication of the greater importance of exposure compared with vulnerability in the development of the disorder.

RESPONDENTS

The respondents consist of 248 of the 260 veterans in the diagnosed subsample of the NVVRS. Excluded as too few to analyze are five subsample members from ethnic minorities who are not either black or Hispanic, and four veterans in the subsample with pre-war first onsets of PTSD. In addition, we exclude three in the subsample for whom relevant data on PTSD status or information about sampling weights is missing.

MEASUREMENT OF RELEVANT VARIABLES

To investigate these questions, we needed measures of relevant variables, especially the onset of war-related PTSD and its adverse course, represented by current war-related

PTSD; the types and severities of combat exposure that the veterans experienced in Vietnam; indicators of the nature and extent of their pre-war vulnerabilities; and their involvement, if any, in harming civilians and prisoners. These measures are described in detail in Chapters 2 and 3.

DATA ANALYSIS PLAN

All analyses incorporated sampling weights so that estimates are representative of the entire population of Vietnam veterans from the 28 standard metropolitan regions.

Necessity of Criterion A stressors

To address the question of the necessity of Criterion A stressors for PSS, we examined the count (and proportion) of veterans with PSS who did not have Criterion A stressors, as identified by clinical diagnosticians. We conducted qualitative assessments of military records, news reports, and historical accounts to verify the clinicians' judgments about the presence or absence of Criterion A stressors for those with PSS.

Sufficiency of Combat Exposure

To address the question of sufficiency of combat exposure, we first examined veterans with a clinician-identified Criterion A stressor and calculated the proportion who met criteria for PSS as well as for other psychiatric disorders. Second, we elaborated rates and relative risks of PSS onset and current PSS across all of the record-based and self-reported combat exposure measures described earlier. Third, we used the single composite measure of the severity of combat exposure that combined the six specific combat exposure measures, as described in Chapter 3, into the Combat Exposure Severity Scale (CESS).

Vulnerability Factors

To address the role of vulnerability, we first examined the relative risk of PSS onset and current PSS with each vulnerability factor described in Chapter 3. Then we used the single measure of vulnerability load (or vulnerability) to examine rates of PSS onset and current PSS among veterans grouped by percentiles of the vulnerability measure, and performed logistic regression on the scale, treated as continuous and standardized, to test for dose-response relationships.

Harm to Civilians or Prisoners

To address the question of harm to civilians or prisoners, we used the measures described in our Chapter 3, especially the dichotomous variable, harm to civilians or prisoners (or harm), to indicate whether respondents reported having personally participated in such harm. We combined the two types of harm in order to insure an adequate number (n) for the analyses.

Assessment of Independent Contributions of Risk Factors

To assess the independent contributions of combat exposure and vulnerability, as well as harm to civilians or prisoners, to PSS onset and current PSS, we used a series of logistic regressions. We standardized both the CESS and the vulnerability measure to have mean 0 and variance 1 so that the magnitude of the associated odds ratios could be compared directly. The skew and kurtosis for the CESS were −0.5 and 1.6, and for the vulnerability load measure, −0.1 and 1.8, respectively, within ranges satisfying typical rules of thumb for normality assumptions, thus justifying direct comparison in standard-deviation (SD) units (Kline, 2010). Racial/ethnic background was included as a control variable in all models. For each outcome separately (i.e., PSS onset, current PSS), Model 1 was a logistic regression on combat exposure and vulnerability, both of which are continuous measures. Model 2 additionally included harm. Odds ratios for each predictor and associated 95% confidence intervals (CIs) were obtained from the fitted models.

Next, we considered tests for two-way interactions among combat exposure, vulnerability, and the harm indicator on the additive risk scale (Rothman, Greenland, & Lash, 2008). The test for interaction was conducted on the additive (risk difference) scale rather than the multiplicative (odds ratio) scale because the additive scale more closely represents synergy from a causal framework perspective (Rothman et al., 2008; Schwartz, 2006). Furthermore, because of the expected broad range from low to high risk for PSS onset and current PSS associated with the wide range of exposure and vulnerability, interpretation of the interaction is facilitated by examining risk directly (and risk differences) rather than focusing entirely on odds ratios, which can be more difficult to interpret when overall risk is not low. For tests of interactions on the additive scale, a logistic regression model was fitted with cross-product terms included between the variables of interest. Then, with use of a back transformation to the probability scale, an interaction risk difference contrast (Greenland, 2004; Rothman et al., 2008) was formed. This interaction risk difference contrast was associated with a one-standard-deviation increase from zero in each predictor while holding the other predictor in the interaction at zero and the other control variables at their marginal means. Tests for the significance of the interaction risk difference contrast were obtained using the SAS procedure PROC NLMIXED—code is available upon request.

After assessing interactions among the predictor variables, we then considered a more flexible Model 3, which allowed for the possibility of a breakpoint along the continuum of exposure, at which point the odds ratio (OR) of PSS onset (or current PSS) could increase or decrease. The optimal breakpoint was empirically chosen to minimize the Akaike information criterion obtained from a logistic regression of the outcome on a piecewise linear indicator for combat exposure (two slopes: one corresponding to continuous changes in combat exposure before the breakpoint, and one after), continuous vulnerability, racial/ethnic background, and harm. An exhaustive search along the combat exposure continuum was conducted to identify the optimal breakpoint. The Akaike information criterion for Model 3 was then compared to the Akaike information criterion for Models 1 and 2 and to the interaction models described earlier, to identify the best-fitting model for PSS onset and current PSS.

Finally, we present plots of predicted probabilities (i.e., estimated rates) from the best-fitting models to facilitate interpretation of results. Both exposure and vulnerability are continuous predictors in the models, but in plotting estimated rates of PSS, we present values of vulnerability load fixed at 2, 4, and 6, corresponding to low, moderate, and high values across the distribution of vulnerability—respectively, 5th–25th, 50th–75th, and 90th–99th percentiles. All regression analyses were performed in SAS 9.2.

RESULTS

Criterion A Combat Stressors as Necessary (Central Question 1)

Most symptoms of PTSD (e.g., flashbacks, nightmares, other intrusive thoughts, and avoidance of reminders) include memories of the exposure to stressful events in their definitions. The exposures are, in this sense of inclusion in symptom memory, always necessary for the diagnosis. Whether these exposures qualify as Criterion A stressors, however, remains a debatable issue. We can, therefore, still ask whether the exposures that meet specifications to type (e.g., life-threatening combat) and severity (e.g., long duration, frequent occurrence) are necessary for the symptom syndrome to develop.

Every PTSD symptom, as noted earlier, was evaluated for all subsample veterans, regardless of whether they reported experiences that the clinicians considered evidence of exposure to Criterion A stressors. This convention offers the opportunity to investigate whether Criterion A stressors were necessary for the occurrence of war-related PSS.

Only two veterans were classified as meeting the symptom criteria for first onsets of war-related PTSD but not the clinician-rated exposure criterion. Suitably weighted, these two veterans represent much less than 1% (0.15%) of the population of veterans from the 28 standard metropolitan regions (SMRs). Although, in the clinicians' judgment, neither provided evidence during the examination of exposure to Criterion A combat stressors, there was ample evidence of such exposure in these veterans' other NVVRS interviews and military records. For example, both veterans were infantrymen, according to their military records and self-reports. One of the veterans was scored in the second of the two most severe categories on the record-based MHM and reported that he was often (13–50 times) in danger of being killed or wounded. The other veteran was scored on the MHM in the intermediate category of *moderately severe* probable exposure and reported having been in danger of being killed or wounded "sometimes" (3–12 times).

We checked the plausibility of the clinicians' positive Criterion A ratings for veterans whom they diagnosed as meeting both the PSS and Criterion A requirements. Weighted back to the population from which the subsample was drawn, only 1.8% of these veterans diagnosed with war-related PTSD had a clinician-rated Criterion A stressor that we could not corroborate as being plausible with external sources, especially military records (Dohrenwend et al., 2006; Dohrenwend et al., 2007; and our Chapter 3). It seems, then, that at most 2% of the veterans' onsets of PSS occurred in the absence of one or more Criterion A stressors.

Combat Stressors as Sufficient (Central Question 2)

The results on the question of sufficiency are more complicated. Suitably weighted, only 31.6% of the veterans judged by the clinicians to have experienced Criterion A stressors had PSS onsets. However, PTSD is often comorbid with other psychiatric disorders (e.g., Kessler, Sonnega, Bromet, & Nelson, 1995), and this is the case here.

As Table 5.1 shows, over three quarters (78.3%) of the veterans with PTSD also had onsets of other Axis I disorders during or after their service in Vietnam. More important for our purposes, almost half (49.5%) of the veterans who did not develop war-related

Table 5.1 RATES OF PSYCHIATRIC DISORDERS OTHER THAN PTSD WITH ONSET DURING OR AFTER SERVICE IN VIETNAM BY PTSD CRITERIA MET

The Veteran Met:

Psychiatric Disorder	Trauma and Symptom Criteria (PTSD Onset)	Trauma Criterion Only	Neither Symptom Nor Trauma Criterion	Total
Alcoholism	48.0%	32.1%	19.7%	31.6%
Drug abuse	39.3	8.8	8.0	15.1
Major depression	43.0	9.5	9.2	16.7
Panic disorder, phobia or OCD	20.0	6.2	0.2	7.3
Any non-PTSD disorder rated	78.3	49.5	27.9	48.8
Sample *n*	(88)	(105)	(53)	(248)

Note: The two respondents who satisfied the symptom criteria but not the trauma criterion are included only in the Total column. Proportions are weighted to represent the population. Unweighted subsample *n*'s are in parentheses.

PSS following clinician-rated Criterion A stressors developed one or more other Axis 1 disorders, with alcoholism being the most prevalent, at 32.1%.

As noted, 31.6% of those exposed to Criterion A stressors had PSS onsets. All told, almost two-thirds (65.5%) developed either PSS or some other psychiatric disorder. The question arises as to how many of the non-PSS disorders were in fact consequences of Criterion A exposure; some of them could have developed long after the war ended and are probably not war related. To investigate this possibility, we calculated the rate of disorders other than PSS in veterans who did not experience a Criterion A stressor and did not develop PSS. We found that a substantial 27.9% of these veterans did develop disorders other than PTSD, with 19.7% developing alcoholism, during or after their service in Vietnam. If we consider their 27.9% rate of other disorders as non-war related, and subtract these 27.9% from the 65.5%, we have a rate of 37.6% who developed either war-related PSS or other psychiatric disorders, especially alcoholism, rather than PSS following clinician-rated Criterion A stressors. This 37.6% onset of disorder rate is substantial, but it is far from evidence that exposure to Criterion A stressors is sufficient.

Our findings thus far are based on the clinicians' judgments about the presence or absence of Criterion A stressors. However, these "either/or" clinical judgments do not differentiate among stressors of varying types and, even within a narrowed range, severities of experience in the war zone. Would any of these different types and severities of combat experience be sufficient for the onset of war-related PSS?

As Table 5.2 shows, all six combat exposure measures are strongly related to both PSS onset and current PSS. For example, 72.1% of the veterans reporting the highest number of life-threatening experiences had onsets of PSS, compared with only 7.5% in the lowest group. However, no measure, even at its most extreme exposure end, was close to being sufficient (i.e., risk was always much less than 100%). We therefore

Table 5.2 DISTRIBUTION OF COMBAT EXPOSURE MEASURES AND THEIR ASSOCIATIONS WITH RISK OF WAR-RELATED PSS ONSET AND CURRENT PSS

Variable	% (n)[a]	Onset		Current	
		Risk (%)	RR (95% CI)	Risk (%)	RR (95% CI)[b]
Sample	100 (248)	21.7		10.9	
Military historical measure					
Lowest severity	26.1 (38)	10.3	Ref	0.3	Ref
Moderate severity	63.1 (152)	23.4	2.28 (0.62, 8.39)	12.3	39.61 (8.47, 99)
High severity	7.8 (37)	40.1	3.91 (0.92, 16.58)	27.0	87.16 (16.90, 99)
Very high severity	3.0 (21)	38.7	3.77* (0.88, 16.14)	33.6	108.22* (21.4, 99)
Purple Heart					
No	90.9 (212)	19.8	Ref	9.1	Ref
Yes	9.1 (33)	45.9	2.32 (1.24, 4.32)	31.7	3.47 (1.57, 7.69)

(*continued*)

Table 5.2 CONTINUED

Variable	% (n)[a]	Onset Risk (%)	Onset RR (95% CI)	Current Risk (%)	Current RR (95% CI)[b]
Life-threatening experiences					
0-2	29.4 (44)	7.5	Ref	0.4	Ref
3-6	24.5 (62)	20.9	2.78 (0.64, 12.00)	8.5	19.27 (3.44, 99)
7-9	34.9 (89)	19.2	2.54 (0.60, 10.68)	7.6	17.17 (3.33, 88.6)
10-11	11.2 (50)	72.1	9.55 (2.49, 36.63)	56.3	127.97 (29.0, 99)
Witnessed death of a close friend in unit					
No	67.9 (125)	12.7	Ref	4.3	Ref
Yes	32.1 (119)	41.7	3.28 (1.68, 6.41)	25.3	5.94 (2.52, 13.99)
Betrayal involving life threat (friendly fire)					
No	90.3 (224)	19.4	Ref	8.2	Ref
Yes	9.7 (22)	46.7	2.40 (1.23, 4.71)	38.2	4.65 (2.12, 10.21)
Killed enemy					
No	66.4 (126)	15.1	Ref	4.6	Ref
Yes	33.6 (106)	34.9	2.31 (1.20, 4.45)	23.7	5.17 (2.21, 12.10)

Note: PSS = posttraumatic stress disorder symptom syndrome; RR = relative risk; CI = confidence interval; Ref = reference group.

[a]All percentages are weighted to represent population estimates. Unweighted subsample *n*'s and CI's are in parentheses. Total sample does not always equal 248, owing to missing values on exposure variables.

[b]A CI value of 99 represents extreme upper limit estimate, owing to small risk in reference group.

*Trend test for increasing risk by increasing severity of military historical measure score is significant: *p* = .016 for onset, *p* < .0001 for current.

examined the possibility that a composite measure would have a greater impact than any one of the six alone.

Table 5.3 shows a clear dose-response relationship between the CESS, our continuous scale of combat exposure based on all six individual measures, and the risk of both PSS onset and current PSS. In the most severe group on this scale (above the 99th percentile), the onset rate is 88.5%, which is nearer to sufficiency than exhibited by any of the individual combat exposure measures. The overall odds ratios for trend (not shown in the table) are both statistically significant—namely, 2.78 (95% CI 1.67–4.64) for PSS onset, and 5.64 (95% CI 2.53–12.57) for current PSS; each unit increase in either odds ratio indicates the effect of a one-standard-deviation increase in combat exposure.

Vulnerability Factors (Central Question 3a)

Like the combat exposure measures, the individual vulnerability measures were positively associated with increased risk of PSS onset and adverse course represented by current PSS—but generally less so than the combat exposure measures.

Table 5.3 RELATIONSHIP OF COMBAT EXPOSURE
SEVERITY SCALE WITH PSS: ONSET AND CURRENT

Percentile[c] of Predictor	n[b]	Predictor: Combat Exposure Severity[a]	
		Onset (%)	Current (%)
Below 10th	15	0.0	0.0
Below 25th	42	7.4	0.2
Below 50th	95	12.8	3.0
Above 50th	153	31.0	19.2
Above 75th	97	46.9	30.5
Above 90th	42	69.9	55.4
Above 99th	4	88.5	27.4

[a]Scale created from factor analysis using the six combat exposure variables as indicators.

[b]Samples (n) are unweighted sizes within each weighted percentile group for combat exposure severity or total vulnerability. Weighted sample percentages within each percentile category differ slightly from nominal (e.g., below 25th percentile for combat exposure severity has 28.6% of sample) owing to ties at percentile cut points.

[c]Categories are not mutually exclusive (e.g., veterans above 90th percentile on combat exposure severity are a subset of those above 75th percentile).

As Table 5.4 shows, the two pre-war vulnerability factors with the highest statistically significant risk of PSS onset (approximately 39%) were childhood experience of physical abuse and childhood conduct disorder. Almost as high were one or more other pre-Vietnam psychiatric disorders (34.3%) and having one or more family members with an arrest record (38.4%). Age was also a substantial factor; men who entered Vietnam at an age under 25 were nearly seven times as likely (25.8%) to have PSS onset as men aged 25 or older (3.7% PSS onset).

Table 5.5 shows that, like the CESS, the composite continuous measure of vulnerability load has a strong dose-response relationship with PSS onset and current PSS. The overall odds ratios for trend are statistically significant, with a one-standard-deviation increase in the total vulnerability load being associated with 2.85 (95% CI 1.89–4.31) odds of PSS onset and 3.56 (95% CI 2.28–5.57) odds of current PSS. The combat exposure severity and vulnerability load measures are only moderately correlated ($r = .28$, $p < .001$).

Personal Involvement in Harm to Civilians or Prisoners (Central Question 3b)

Personal involvement in harm to prisoners (7.1%) and/or harm to civilians (9.5%) are also strongly related to PSS, with an onset rate of 76.1% among men reporting harming prisoners and 53.9% for those harming civilians. To increase statistical power, the two

Table 5.4 DISTRIBUTION OF VULNERABILITY VARIABLES AND ASSOCIATION
WITH RISK OF WAR-RELATED PSS ONSET AND CURRENT PSS

		PSS Onset			Current PSS		
	%(n)[a]	Risk	RR	95% CI of RR	Risk	RR	95% CI of RR
Whole Sample	100% (248)	21.7%			10.9%		
Age at Entry to Vietnam (Military record)							
25 or older	18.4% (33)	3.7%	ref		2.9%	ref	
Under 25	81.6% (215)	25.8%	6.98	(1.84–26.49)	12.8%	4.48	(0.85–25.58)
Previous Military Experience (Military record)							
Yes	20.9% (38)	6.9%	ref		3.2%	ref	
No	79.1% (210)	25.6%	3.70	(1.37–9.99)	13.0%	4.05	(1.01–16.19)
Score on AFQT (Military record)							
Better than Category III	45.0% (69)	14.1%	ref		7.3%	ref	
Category III or worse	55.0% (165)	28.1%	1.99	(0.94–4.23)	15.4%	2.12	(0.85–5.30)
Education at Entry (Military record)							
More than high school	30.9% (61)	16.3%	ref		4.7%	ref	
High school or less	69.1% (187)	24.1%	1.48	(0.70–3.13)	13.7%	2.91	(0.88–9.62)
Childhood Experiences[b] (NVVRS Interview)							
Physical abuse	18.2% (55)	38.9%	2.17	(1.16–4.07)	28.8%	4.15	(1.94–8.87)
Family member arrested	7.1% (28)	38.4%	1.87	(0.88–4.01)	14.2%	1.34	(0.38–4.73)
Family member with substance abuse	19.9% (48)	32.2%	1.68	(0.88–3.22)	25.3%	3.44	(1.61–7.36)
Pre-War[b] (NVVRS Interview)							
Psychiatric disorder (except PTSD)	17.2% (55)	34.3%	1.79	(0.93–3.44)	18.2%	1.94	(0.82–4.59)
Conduct disorder	14.6% (50)	38.7%	2.06	(1.09–3.88)	22.1%	2.45	(1.10–5.45)

[a]All percentages are weighted to represent population estimates. Unweighted sample *n*'s are in parentheses. Total *n* does not always add up to 248 due to missing values on vulnerability variables.

[b]Reference ("No") categories not shown.

Table 5.5 RELATIONSHIP OF TOTAL VULNERABILITY LOAD
WITH PSS: ONSET AND CURRENT

Percentile[a] of predictor	*n*	Predictor: Total Vulnerability Count	
		Onset (%)	Current (%)
Below 10th	10	4.3	0.0
Below 25th	38	7.4	0.5
Below 50th	84	10.1	3.8
Above 50th	164	31.6	17.1
Above 75th	85	53.8	35.0
Above 90th	45	67.0	49.6
Above 99th	6	89.4	75.4

Note: Percentages are weighted to the population from which the subsample was drawn. N's are unweighted subsample numbers.

[a]Categories are not mutually exclusive (e.g., veterans above 90th percentile on the Total Vulnerability Count are a subset of those above 75th percentile).

measures were combined into a single dichotomous indicator of harm to civilians or prisoners (harm). An estimated 13.3% of soldiers (harmers) reported personal involvement in inflicting harm on prisoners or civilians on these closed questions. Almost two thirds of the harmers (63.2%) had PSS onsets, compared with only 15.3% of the non-harmers. The rate of current PSS was 39.9% among the harmers, compared with only 6.2% among the non-harmers.

Independent Effects of Combat Exposure, Vulnerability Load, and Involvement in Harm to Civilians or Prisoners

Table 5.6 presents the results of regression analyses assessing the independent contributions of combat exposure, vulnerability, and harm to PSS. The CESS and the vulnerability load measure are both standardized, so the odds ratios represent the effects of an increase of one standard deviation in either scale.

Model 1 in Table 5.6 shows that the contributions of the two factors, CESS and vulnerability load, to the onset of PSS were both substantial and about equal. Model 2, with harm added to the equation, shows that the independent contributions of combat exposure and vulnerability were still substantial, and that there was also a large independent contribution of harm, as represented by an odds ratio of 4.78. It should be noted that the independent impacts of CESS and vulnerability load are directly comparable because both are on continuous scales; in contrast, the measure of harm is dichotomous. To produce an equivalent odds ratio to that of being a harmer compared to a non-harmer, a soldier's combat exposure would have to increase by 2.6 standard deviations, $\ln(4.78)/\ln(1.83)$. This could occur in several ways; for example, going from less than

Table 5.6 ADJUSTED ODDS RATIOS (95% CONFIDENCE INTERVALS)
OF PSS ONSETS AND CURRENT PSS

	Onset		Current	
Variable	Model 1[a]	Model 2[b]	Model 1	Model 2
Combat Exposure	2.29	1.83	4.41	3.47
Severity Scale	(1.35, 3.88)	(1.10, 3.03)	(2.10, 9.25)	(1.55, 7.77)
Total vulnerability	2.33	2.31	2.67	2.60
load	(1.51, 3.58)	(1.49, 3.60)	(1.70, 4.19)	(1.65, 4.10)
Harmed civilians/	—	4.78	—	2.70
prisoners		(1.84, 12.45)		(0.78, 9.37)[ns]

Note: These analyses take into account the complex subsample design.
[a]Model 1 simultaneously includes standardized Combat Exposure Severity Scale and standardized total vulnerability load as continuous predictors, as well as racial/ethnic group.
[b]Model 2 adds to Model 1 by including an indicator of whether the soldier reported harming civilians or prisoners.

two life-threatening experiences up to seven or more of such experiences. Alternatively, the veterans' vulnerability load would have to increase by 1.9 standard deviations, equivalent to adding approximately three more vulnerability factors. Suffice it to say that the effects of all three factors, especially harm, on the onset of PSS are very substantial.

For current PSS, both combat exposure and vulnerability have strong independent effects. The odds ratio for harm is appreciable, but it does not represent a statistically significant independent effect.

We investigated interactions among the three risk factors. Only the additive interaction between combat exposure and vulnerability as predictors of current PSS was statistically significant. The interaction contrast (i.e., difference in risk differences) was 9.3% ($SE = 1.6\%, p < .0001$), indicating a positive or super-additive synergistic effect between exposure and vulnerability on current PSS.

We also investigated an additional model, Model 3, to allow for the possibility of a break point along the continuum of exposure, at which point the odds ratio could increase or decrease. Model 3 showed superior fit for PSS onset compared to Models 1 and 2. For current PSS, Model 3 did not show superior fit to Model 1 or 2. The optimal break point along the combat exposure continuum for predicting PSS onset was found with Model 3 to be 0.98, or approximately one standard deviation above the mean, corresponding to approximately the 75th percentile of the CESS in this sample. Model 3 finds for PSS onset that the odds ratio associated with changes in combat exposure in the range below 1 is not significant (OR = 1.25, 95% CI = 0.72, 2.18) but is dramatically large and statistically significant in the range above 1 (OR = 13.00, 95% CI = 1.34, 125.0; the wide CI is due in part to the limited sample size above the 75th percentile and to the large value of the OR in this region). The odds ratio for vulnerability load in Model 3 for PSS onset is also significant (OR = 2.34, 95% CI = 1.47, 3.72), and the odds ratio of harm remains significant (OR = 3.85, 95% CI = 1.44, 10.28).

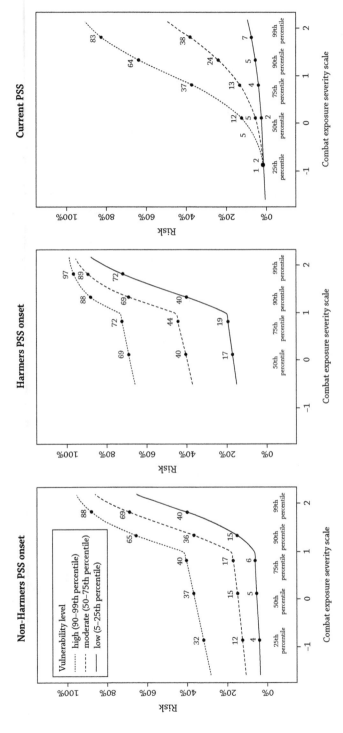

Figure 5.1 Estimated risk of PTSD symptom syndrome (PSS) onset (*left* and *middle* by harmer status) and current PSS (*right*) as a function of both combat exposure severity and vulnerability load. Estimated risks are obtained from best-fitting logistic regression models for PSS onset and current PSS. For PSS onset, the best model was Model 3, including an indicator of harm and a change point in increased log odds risk at +1 standard deviation on the CESS (approximately the 75th percentile). For current PSS, the best-fitting model was Model 1, additionally including a cross product between combat exposure severity and vulnerability. Estimated risks presented are for fixed values of vulnerability and exposure corresponding to low, moderate, and high percentiles of each variable. To avoid extrapolation to combinations of predictors with no observations, no estimates are given for PSS onset among harmers at the low end of combat exposure.

The left and middle panels of Figure 5.1 portray the regression estimated risk of PSS onset (from Model 3) in non-harmers and harmers as a function of combat exposure and vulnerability load. The right panel portrays the estimated risk of current PSS (from Model 1 with interaction) as functions of combat exposure and vulnerability load.

As the left-hand panel of Figure 5.1 shows, both combat exposure and vulnerability contribute to PSS onset. However, the effect of combat exposure is most pronounced above the 75th percentile of severity for both non-harmers and harmers. Because there was no significant interaction between vulnerability and combat exposure in predicting PSS onset, the effect of vulnerability is specified as constant here in terms of odds ratios from one vulnerability value to the next. Comparing this constant effect with the effects of combat exposure below and above the break point, we see that, below the 75th percentile, the impact of vulnerability is higher (significant odds ratios of about 2) than the impact of combat exposure (odds ratio of about 1.3 and not significant), but that above the 75th percentile, exposure matters much more (odds ratio of 13.0) than vulnerability (with odds ratio remaining at about 2). Even at low levels of vulnerability, an estimated 40% of the non-harmers and 72% of the harmers who were highly exposed developed PSS.

It is striking that, as the central panel of Figure 5.1 shows, the predicted rates of PSS onset are shifted markedly upward for harmers compared to non-harmers in the left panel, even for those with low vulnerability load. The veterans with both high combat exposure and high vulnerability have a very high risk (88%) of developing PSS if they were not harmers and a nearly sufficient risk (97%) if they were harmers.

The positive additive interaction found between combat exposure and vulnerability for current PSS is portrayed in the estimated rates plotted in the right-hand side of Figure 5.1. The effect of vulnerability on current PSS increases with combat exposure. For those with combat exposure below the 25th percentile, the estimated rate of current PSS is only around 1.0%, regardless of vulnerability. In contrast, at the 99th percentile, the range is from an estimated current PSS rate of 7% for those with the lowest vulnerability load to 83% for those in the most vulnerable group.

Relationships Among Combat Exposure, Vulnerability, and Harming

Vulnerability was positively correlated only .20 with harming, in contrast with a positive correlation of .41 between harming and combat exposure. The import of this difference can be seen in Table 5.6, which shows that adjusting for harm reduces the effects of combat exposure on PSS onset and current PSS but does not substantially alter the effects of vulnerability.

SUMMARY AND CONCLUSIONS

The central assumption in the DSM-III, DSM-III-R, and DSM-IV that potentially traumatic stressors are more important than personal vulnerability in causing PTSD is controversial. We tested this assumption with data from a rigorously diagnosed sub-sample of men from the NVVRS. Combat exposure, vulnerability, and personal involvement in harming civilians or prisoners were examined, with only combat exposure proving necessary for disorder onset. Though none of the three factors proved sufficient, estimated PSS onset reached 97% for veterans high on all three, with harm to civilians or prisoners showing the largest independent contribution. Severity of combat exposure proved more important than vulnerability in onset; vulnerability was at least as important in long-term persistence. These results have conceptual implications for the primacy of the stressor assumption in the diagnosis of PTSD, and they raise questions that require further research. Moreover, they have policy implications that need consideration.

Even the most severe combat stressors that we measured were not sufficient to bring about the onset of PSS in all or almost all such exposed veterans. The reason may be that the types, severities, and duration (with tours typically lasting about a year) of exposure in the NVVRS sample of Vietnam veterans do not cover the entire variety, intensity, and duration of stressful events that have been found in other research to approach near sufficiency for onset. For example, only two veterans in the subsample reported being prisoners of war, and neither described situations nearly so prolonged or severe as the experiences of U.S. prisoners of war of the Japanese during World War II. As systematic research with a carefully selected and rigorously diagnosed sample found, the PTSD onset rate was 84% in these World War II surviving prisoners of the Japanese; 59% still met criteria 40 to 50 years after capture (Engdahl, Dikel, Eberly, & Blank, 1997).

There is, nevertheless, support for the primary role of combat exposure compared with vulnerability in our results for these factors in the onset of PSS. Most important is that, unlike vulnerability, Criterion A combat stressors were necessary for the occurrence of war-related PSS. We were able to investigate the necessity of Criterion A exposure because of the NVVRS procedure of asking about the symptoms of PTSD in the diagnostic examination regardless of whether the clinicians judged that the veteran satisfied Criterion A. In addition, an estimated 40% of the most severely exposed and least vulnerable men who did not personally harm civilians or prisoners had onsets of PSS (Figure 5.1). Consistent with the primacy assumption, this suggests that PSS can occur in individuals who show little personal vulnerability when stressor exposure is especially severe, as may have been the case for some veterans in our highest-severity exposure category.

In contrast with its role in onset, pre-Vietnam personal vulnerability appears to be at least as important as combat exposure in the adverse course of the disorder represented by current PSS (i.e., present at the time of data collection, 11–12 years after the war). Unlike PSS onset, and contrary to our prediction under the primacy assumption, we found a positive rather than negative interaction between vulnerability and combat exposure for current PSS; that is, the greater the severity of combat exposure, the greater (rather than lesser) the contribution of vulnerability load to highly chronic current PSS (Figure 5.1, right panel). For those with low severity of combat exposure (the 25th percentile), the estimated rate of current PSS is less than 5% regardless of vulnerability load. In contrast, vulnerability makes a huge difference for those with the highest level of combat exposure (99th percentile), ranging from an estimated rate of 7% for the least vulnerable to 83% for those in the most vulnerable group (Figure 5.1).

The full psychological impact of the Vietnam war on U.S. forces cannot be understood without considering the role of the involvement of a substantial minority of the veterans (an estimated 13%) in personally harming civilians or prisoners. We found that such involvement showed a large independent contribution to PSS onset. It is striking that, as the central panel of Figure 5.1 shows, the predicted rates of PSS onset are shifted markedly upward for harmers compared to non-harmers in the left panel, even for those with low vulnerability load. For many reasons, it is important to learn more about the harmers—who they were and why they inflicted harm. We pursue these matters further in our Chapter 6.

Meanwhile, the results reported in this chapter provide a compelling test of the primacy of the stressor assumption as it applies to male U.S. Vietnam veterans whose adjustment problems were so influential in giving rise to the PTSD diagnosis. By doing so, these results have important conceptual implications for the diagnosis of war-related PTSD and the theoretical assumptions that underlie it. The finding that severity of combat exposure is more important than pre-Vietnam vulnerability load in PSS onset is consistent with the formulations in all the DSMs, going back to the 1952 DSM-I and the 1968 DSM-II. The finding that vulnerability factors are more important in long-term course, however, may be more consistent with the role of prior vulnerability set forth in the DSM-I and DSM-II than in subsequent DSMs. As noted at the outset, in these earlier DSMs, the effects of stressor exposure are assumed to be transient unless there is prior vulnerability.

In the controversy over whether to narrow or broaden the types of stressful experience included under Criterion A, our results support narrowing the definition. As we pointed out, it is only in veterans experiencing very severe combat exposure that PSS onset rates are sharply elevated regardless of vulnerability load (Figure 5.1). This suggests that it was the very severe stressors that are important for defining Criterion A for war-related PTSD.

As noted, we will explore questions about who the harmers were and why they engaged in harming civilians or prisoners in our next chapter.

ACKNOWLEDGMENT

This chapter expands on the following article: Dohrenwend, B. P., Yager, T. J., Wall, M. M., & Adams, B. G. (2013), The roles of combat exposure, personal vulnerability, and involvement in harm to civilians or prisoners in Vietnam-war-related posttraumatic stress disorder. *Clinical Psychological Science, 1*(3), 223–238. Publisher: Sage, for the American Psychological Society.

REFERENCES

American Psychiatric Association. (1952). *Diagnostic and statistical manual of mental disorders.* Washington, DC: Author.

American Psychiatric Association. (1968). *Diagnostic and statistical manual of mental disorders* (2nd ed.). Washington, DC: Author.

American Psychiatric Association. (1980). *Diagnostic and statistical manual of mental disorders* (3rd ed.). Washington, DC: Author.

American Psychiatric Association. (1987). *Diagnostic and statistical manual of mental disorders* (3rd ed., rev.). Washington, DC: Author.

American Psychiatric Association. (1994). *Diagnostic and statistical manual of mental disorders* (4th ed.). Washington, DC: Author.

Breslau, N. (2002). Epidemiologic studies of trauma, posttraumatic stress disorder, and other psychiatric disorders. *Canadian Journal of Psychiatry, 47*, 923–929.

Brewin, C. R., Lanius, R. A., Novac, A., Schnyder, U., & Galea, S. (2009). Reformulating PTSD for DSM-V: Life after Criterion A. *Journal of Traumatic Stress, 22*, 366–373. doi:10.1002/jts.20443

Dohrenwend, B. P. (1998). Overview of the evidence for the importance of adverse environmental conditions in causing psychiatric disorders. In B. P. Dohrenwend (Ed.), *Adversity, stress, and psychopathology* (pp. 523–538). New York: Oxford University Press.

Dohrenwend, B. P., Turner, J. B., Turse, N. A., Adams, B. G., Koenen, K. C., & Marshall, R. (2006). The psychological risks of Vietnam for U.S. veterans: A revisit with new data and methods. *Science, 313*, 979–982. doi:10.1126/science.1128944

Dohrenwend, B. P., Turner, J. B., Turse, N. A., Adams, B. G., Koenen, K. C., & Marshall, R. (2007). Continuing controversy over the psychological risks of Vietnam for U.S. veterans. *Journal of Traumatic Stress, 20*, 449–465.

Engdahl, B., Dikel, T. N., Eberly, R., & Blank, A. (1997). Posttraumatic stress disorder in a community group of former prisoners of war: A normative response to severe trauma. *American Journal of Psychiatry, 154*, 1576–1581.

Friedman, M. J. (2005). Veterans' mental health in the wake of war. *New England Journal of Medicine, 352*, 1287–1290. doi:10.1056/NEJMp058028

Friedman, M. J., Resick, P. A., & Keane, T. M. (2007). PTSD: Twenty-five years of progress and challenges. In M. J. Friedman, T. M. Keane, & P. A. Resick (Eds.), *Handbook of PTSD: Science and practice* (pp. 3–18). New York: Guilford Press.

Greenland, S. (2004). Model-based estimation of relative risks and other epidemiologic measures in studies of common outcomes and in case-control studies. *American Journal of Epidemiology, 160*, 301–305. doi:10.1093/aje/kwh221

Kessler, R. C., Sonnega, A., Bromet, E., Hughes, M., & Nelson, C. B. (1995). Posttraumatic stress disorder in the National Comorbidity Survey. *Archives of General Psychiatry, 52*, 1048–1060. doi:10.1001/archpsyc.1995.03950240066012

Kline, R. (2010). *Principles and practice of structural equation modeling* (3rd ed.). New York: Guilford Press.

Kulka, R. A., Schlenger, W. E., Fairbank, J. A., Hough, R. L., Jordan, B. K., Marmar, C. R., et al. (1990). *Trauma and the Vietnam War generation.* New York: Brunner/Mazel.

Laufer, R. S., Gallops, M. S., & Frey-Wouters, E. (1984). War stress and trauma: The Vietnam veteran experience. *Journal of Health and Social Behavior, 25*, 68–72. doi:10.2307/2136705

Lidz, B. T., Stein, N., Delaney, E., Lebowitz, L., Nash, W. P., Silva, C., & Maguen. (2009). *Clinical Psychology Review,29*, 695–706. doi:10.1016/cpr.07,003.

Maier, T. (2007). Weathers' and Keane's "The Criterion A problem revisited: Controversies and challenges in defining and measuring psychological trauma." *Journal of Traumatic Stress, 20*, 915–916.

McNally, R. J. (2003). Progress and controversy in the study of posttraumatic stress disorder. *Annual Review of Psychology,54*, 229–252. doi:10.1146/annurev.psych.54.101601.145112

Rothman, K. J., Greenland, S., & Lash, T. L. (2008). *Modern epidemiology* (3rd ed.). Philadelphia, PA: Lippincott Williams & Wilkins.

Schwartz, S. (2006). Appendix E: Modern epidemiologic approaches to interaction. Applications to the study of genetic interactions. In L. M. Hernandez & D. G. Blazer (Eds.), *Genes, behavior, and the social environment: Moving beyond the nature/nurture debate* (pp. 310–337). Washington, DC: National Academies Press.

Smith, R. (2007). *The utility of force*. New York: Knopf.

Thayer, T. (1985). *War without fronts*. Boulder, CO: Westview Press.

Turse, N. (2013). *Kill anything that moves: The real American War in Vietnam*. New York: Metropolitan Books, Henry Holt.

Weathers, F. W., & Keane, T. M. (2007). The Criterion A problem revisited: Controversies and challenges in defining and measuring psychological trauma. *Journal of Traumatic Stress, 20,* 107–121.

Yehuda, R., & McFarlane, A. C. (1995). Conflict between current knowledge about posttraumatic stress disorder and its original conceptual basis. *American Journal of Psychiatry, 152,* 1705.

CHAPTER 6

ᴄᴧᴐ

Harming Civilians or Prisoners

Characteristics of Persons and Situations

BRUCE P. DOHRENWEND, THOMAS J. YAGER, ROBERTO
LEWIS-FERNÁNDEZ, BEN G. ADAMS, AND NICK TURSE

[U.S. troops in Vietnam] were put into situations of moral stress significantly more complex than those experienced by soldiers in wars where opposing armies fought using conventional battle tactics. . . . American soldiers on the ground were placed in deep moral jeopardy. (Appy, 1993, p. 8)

It's a strange feeling. In retrospect you look back on it and wonder how you yourself could have done it. Twenty years later, when you look back at things that happened, things that transpired, things you did, you say: Why? Why did I do that? That is not me. Something happened to me. (Bilton & Sim, 1992, p. 80)

I felt a sickness in my heart for what we had done. The young innocent man who went to Vietnam died that night. After that night, I no longer had any illusions or objectivity about the war. I had become someone I did not recognize. I had been in Vietnam for five weeks and this was my first firefight. It had not ended in the heroic way I had expected. (Kerrey, 2002, p. 185)

As we showed in Chapter 5, the psychological impact of Vietnam on U.S veterans cannot be understood without giving attention to the role of participation in acts of harming civilians or prisoners by a substantial minority of the veterans. We inquire here into who the harmers were and the situations in which the harm took place, and, perhaps, why participation in such harm proved to be so strongly related to the development of PTSD.

The notion of an increased risk of "moral injury" (Litz et al., 2009) resulting from fighting "wars amongst the people" (Smith, 2007, p. 226) is not new to the literature of the Vietnam war. In 1971, William Gault, an Army psychiatrist who evaluated recently returned Vietnam veterans, speculated that there were six psychological, social, and technical variables specific to the Vietnam experience that readied relatively normal young men to participate in the "slaughter" of defenseless Vietnamese. He hypothesized that the universalization of the enemy (i.e., the idea the enemy was everywhere), the dehumanization of the Vietnamese, a dilution of responsibility, a pressure to act, the natural dominance of the psychopath in the war zone, and the ready availability of massive firepower had the effect of psychologically preparing American men to commit atrocities (Gault, 1971, p. 451). Haley (1974) pointed out that while such illegal acts have occurred in all wars, the conflict in Vietnam was different because of "the concentration of atrocities (due in part to the guerrilla nature of the war, superior firepower, and the phenomenon of the 'body count') and the exposure [by the media to the American public] of these atrocities" (Haley, 1974, p. 194).

Vivid accounts of the experiences of over 80 journalists, most of whom spent time in Vietnam, appeared 23 years after the end of the war in *Reporting Vietnam* (two volumes compiled by a five-member advisory board, Bates et al., for the Library of America and published by Literary Classics of the United States in 1998). Some of these reports describe the involvement by U.S. forces in harm to civilians and prisoners. Notable among them are accounts of the rape and murder of a young Vietnamese peasant girl by four American enlisted men (Lang, 1969); the destruction from the air of dwellings in two rural provinces in South Vietnam (Schell, 2000); and a landmark account of the My Lai massacre of scores of women and children (Hersh, 1969).

Prior to our research, however, there have been no investigations using representative samples of U.S. veterans of the war in Vietnam of the rates of personal involvement in harm to civilians and prisoners. Moreover, there has been very little systematic research on the relationship between veterans' involvement in harm and war-related PTSD. Indeed, the results we report in Chapter 5 are the first, as far as we know, to be based on rigorous diagnoses of PTSD by experienced clinicians. As we report there, about 13% of the Vietnam veterans said in response to closed questions with fixed response alternatives that they were personally involved in harming prisoners or civilians, a figure that rises to about one-third among veterans with the highest risk of combat exposure according to our military-historical measure (MHM). Our purpose now is to inquire further into who these veterans were, the situations in which they harmed civilians or prisoners, and some possible reasons why the veterans' experiences in these situations may have contributed to their increased likelihood of developing war-related PTSD.

HISTORICAL BACKGROUND

Throughout the war, all across South Vietnam, the U.S. military worked to drive villagers out of territory controlled by the Viet Cong and into areas controlled by the Saigon government. These efforts were commonly known as "pacification," but their true aim was to depopulate the contested countryside.

In September 1965, top U.S. commander General William Westmoreland issued MACV [Military Assistance Command, Vietnam] Directive No. 525-3. While ostensibly concerned with "minimizing non-combatant casualties," what this document actually did was allow vast swaths of South Vietnam to be transformed into lethal free-fire zones. It decreed, "Free strike zones should be configured to eliminate populated areas *except those in accepted VC bases* [our italics]" (U.S. Army War College, 1965). A month later, a second MACV document expanded on the first: "Except for accepted VC war zones and base areas, free strike zones are being reconfigured to eliminate populated areas" (U.S. Army War College, 1965). While the emphasis in these directives was on the protection of populated areas, the areas exempted from this protection, because they were believed to be under enemy control or influence, were so vast that, in effect, much of rural South Vietnam became a free-fire zone.

According to Secretary of Defense Robert McNamara's 1964 figures on territory "under Viet Cong control or predominant influence," population centers in 40% of the countryside were fair game, and in 22 of 43 provinces in the Republic of [South] Vietnam (RVN), a full 50% of the land area was theoretically open to unrestrained attack (McNamara & VanDeMark, 1995, p. 501). McNamara later said that since Westmoreland's "attrition strategy relied heavily on firepower," U.S. "[s]hells and napalm rained down on so-called enemy 'base areas'" (McNamara & VanDeMark, 1995, p. 243). This policy would continue, even as the directives on free-fire zones were updated over the course of the war (Dolvin, 1971; Greiner, 2009).

A confidential message that accompanied MACV Directive No. 525-3 granted that "a civilian's presence in a VC or GVN [Government of Vietnam] controlled hamlet depends on factors beyond his control," but offered no more assurance than that warnings of impending attacks would be issued "whenever possible" (U.S. Army War College, 1965). Sometimes such announcements, broadcast from loudspeakers on aircraft, could not be heard or understood (Appy, 1993; Gibson, 2000; Schell, 2000). Other times, leaflets would rain down on illiterate villagers, announcing: "Soon Naval gunfire is going to be conducted on your village to destroy . . . Vietcong supplies. We ask that you take cover as we do not wish to kill innocent people" (Appy, 1993, pp. 196–197; Gibson, 2000, p. 283; Schell, 2000, pp. 204–213). In some cases, however, villagers may have had only an hour's notice before their village was bombarded (Pilger, 1976). Other times, the leaflets drifted off-course. Many times, no warning came at all.

Often air strikes or artillery were unleashed on villages as a means of driving the population from the countryside and breaking their connection with the revolutionary forces. Sometimes most or all of the villagers had been cleared from homes; oftentimes, however, they were not. Many villagers were killed or wounded directly by heavy firepower. Others died when it caused underground bunkers in which they had taken shelter to collapse. In many instances, villagers were killed or wounded when Americans tossed grenades into the bomb shelters where they had taken refuge. Villages were also regularly burned, frequently by ground troops using cigarette lighters ("Zippos") (Turse, 2013, p. 96).

While some attacks on villages may have been carried out on the initiative of low-level officers, most village destruction occurred as a result of the official policy of clearing the population from large areas regarded as enemy territory—areas where anyone might be subject to attack as a presumed enemy. (See Chapter 1 for vivid examples of specific incidents involving harm to civilians and prisoners.) Against this background, we study here who the harming veterans were and, insofar as the data permit, their experiences in the situations in which harm occurred.

CHARACTERISTICS OF HARMERS IDENTIFIED BY CLOSED-QUESTION MEASURES

Fully 35.8% of the veterans involved in harming civilians or prisoners (identified by the closed question measures described in Chapter 3) had one or more disciplinary actions recorded in their military records, compared to only 17.2% of those who were not involved in such personal harm ($p = .048$). However, these harmers were no more likely to say they volunteered for one or more of a list of dangerous activities (19.5% of harmers compared with 22.1% of non-harmers) or to say that they found the excitement of combat at least a "somewhat satisfying" experience, even when the comparison was restricted to veterans in the most severe 25% of combat exposure (27.5% of the harmers compared with 30.3% of non-harmers). Moreover, the harmers were at least as likely to receive combat medals for valor (19.1%) as the non-harmers (13.3%) ($p = .28$); statistical control of severity of combat exposure brings these figures on combat medals closer together but leaves the general finding of little or no difference unchanged.

The morale of the harmers, as measured by their perception of unit cohesion (see Chapter 10 for a description of this measure), did not differ from that of non-harmers; harmers had a mean score of 12.2, as compared to 11.3 for non-harmers, on a scale with possible values ranging from 0 to 20 ($p = .16$).

Vulnerability load was correlated only .20 with harming. Among the individual vulnerability factors, the highest correlation, between harm and the veteran's having experienced physical abuse as a child, was .36. There were small to moderate correlations (.20–.27) of harm with younger age, having no more than a high school education, and the veteran's having had a family member arrested when he was a child. The correlation with lower AFQT score was only .085. The correlations were negligible between harm and childhood conduct disorder (.03) and pre-war psychiatric disorder (−.03).

In contrast, the correlation between severity of combat exposure and harming was twice as high (.41) as that between vulnerability load and harming. Correlations between harm and the individual combat exposure measures were moderate to high (.28–.66), with the scale of life-threatening experiences, killing the enemy, and witnessing the death of a friend in the unit all having correlations greater than .50.

As a corollary of their greater exposure, the two minorities tended to be more likely to report personal involvement in harming civilians or prisoners (whites, .12; Hispanics, .16; and blacks, .23) with the black versus white difference statistically significant ($p = .046$). This difference is greatly reduced when severity of combat exposure is controlled. Specifically, for blacks versus majority whites, the unadjusted odds ratio is 2.32 ($p = .046$); this is reduced to 1.71 when MHM exposure is controlled ($p = .25$), and 1.45 when the composite scale of severity of exposure is controlled ($p = .40$); the difference between Hispanics and majority whites is reduced from an unadjusted odds ratio of 1.41

($p = .48$) to 1.20 when MHM exposure is controlled, and 1.02 when the larger scale of severity of combat exposure is controlled in a parallel analysis.

Clearly, the strongest factor differentiating harmers from non-harmers is their greater severity of combat exposure. The likely reason is that, in this war amongst the people, combat activity brought soldiers into contact with civilians under circumstances that often led to acts of harm. The record-based MHM, with its reliance on type of military unit and military occupational specialty, is the measure of exposure that most clearly differentiates among those veterans whose job was more or less likely to involve seeking combat with enemy forces. Fully half (50.4%) of the veterans in the *high* and *very high* severity categories of the MHM reported that they often or very often "had trouble identifying who the enemy was." Only 15.2% of the veterans in these high-exposure categories said that they never had this problem, compared to 45.2% in the *moderate* and *low* categories. Moreover, 66.4% of those in the two high-exposure MHM categories, compared with 42.7% in the two lower-exposure categories, answered "yes" to the question "Were you ever in a situation in Vietnam where women, children, or old people were either injured or killed by American or South Vietnamese (ARVN) soldiers?" Against this background, it is reasonable to expect the proportions of harmers to be highest in the *very high* and *high* probable exposure categories of the MHM, and this expectation is confirmed. The proportions of harmers at each level of the MHM are as follows: *very high* 33.9% and *high* 27.9%, but *moderate* only 14.7% and *low* only 4.7%.

EXPERIENCES OF HARMERS USING MEASURES BASED ON OPEN-ENDED QUESTIONS

To get more immediate details of the complex circumstances in which harm to civilians and prisoners took place, we extracted narrative accounts that some veterans provided of their actions and of the circumstances surrounding them. This qualitative information is derived mainly from open-ended follow-up questions in the NSVG, but also from events listed by the respondent in a Traumatic Events Booklet and by the clinicians who conducted the diagnostic interviews. Two questions and open-ended follow-up probes were particularly important sources of information. The first asks whether there were "some things you wish you had not chosen to do or had not been assigned to do" in Vietnam. The second asks if the respondent was "ever in a combat situation . . . where you participated in any kind of injury or destruction that seemed necessary then, but that you would consider unnecessary now." A third, even more personal question also yielded a few reports. The respondent was asked whether anything had happened in Vietnam that he felt he couldn't discuss with anyone else. If he answered "yes," he was asked, "Could you tell us about it now?"

In reviewing all these sources of information, we found 63 distinct reports of harm to civilians, prisoners, or essential property. In 55 of these reports, the respondent indicated that he had participated in the harm; but in 21 of these 55 reports, the harm was to property—usually villages or houses—with no indication of bodily harm to people. Three reports were of harm to civilians or prisoners, but it isn't clear which. Of the remaining reports, 25 were of harm to civilians, six of harm to prisoners. These 31 reports of personal harm in which the respondent himself participated are the main focus of our analysis of this material. Because many of the harm responses were elicited by questions premised on the respondent's regret for his own actions or on his later judgment that they were unnecessary, these 31 events are hardly a representative sample of all such harm. But they serve as examples of certain kinds of events that occurred in Vietnam and are, in fact, particularly useful because of the light they cast on the respondents' feelings and judgments about them.

Some reports were of a specific event. For instance, one respondent said he had shot two children. Another said he had physically abused a civilian woman whose unexpected presence had frightened him at a tense moment. Other reports described actions that had occurred on unspecified multiple occasions. For example, in response to the question about injury or destruction that now seemed unnecessary, one respondent simply mentioned going through villages and "destroying" them.

Box 6.1 shows our coding sheet for rating various aspects of each harm report. Detailed information for most of these ratings is fragmentary at best. Nevertheless, we obtained valuable information. In general, even the most detailed reports were quite short. Few consisted of more than a few sentences. For that reason, we often made inferences about what had happened; we tried to be conservative in doing so. As a further caution, we assigned a level of confidence to each rating. "High confidence" means that we felt reasonably confident of the rating. "Low confidence" means that the rating reflects what we thought most likely happened, though we were far from certain.

Both the substantive and the confidence ratings were arrived at, when possible, by agreement between two raters making independent judgments. When the two raters disagreed, four members of our research team, including the two original raters, discussed the discrepant ratings and arrived at a consensus, which became the final rating. Agreement between the raters who made the initial independent judgments was reasonably good. On whether the respondent participated in the attacking or harm, they agreed 94% of the time (kappa = .80). On who was harmed—civilians, prisoners, or neither—they agreed 81% of the time (kappa = .68). On whether there was harm to a village or houses, the raters again agreed 81% of the time (kappa = .67). And on whether anyone was killed, they agreed 88% of the time (kappa = .71). Once disagreements were resolved, of course, agreement was 100% by definition.

The next example illustrates the rating process and the role that inference plays in it, even when most aspects of the situation are quite clear. In response to the question asking whether he had "participated in any kind of injury or destruction that seemed necessary at the time, but that you would consider unnecessary now," one respondent replied, "Wholesale destruction of villages; shooting anything that moved when you were on a search and destroy mission, not only people but animals." Unlike some reports, this one indicates multiple actions of the same general type. Our rating specifies that civilians had been harmed (high confidence). Because the respondent mentioned "wholesale destruction," our rating specified that persons other than the respondent had also participated in the harm. (For this and similar reports of "destroying" or "invading" villages, we concluded that others had participated simply because one man would not

Box 6.1
CODES FOR RATINGS OF NARRATIVE MATERIAL ON INVOLVEMENT IN HARM TO CIVILIANS AND PRISONERS

A. According to the narrative, who specifically was attacked or harmed?
- 1 = Civilian(s).
  → If selected, rate confidence: 2 = high; 1 = low.
- 2 = Prisoner(s).
  → If selected, rate confidence: 2 = high; 1 = low.
- 3 = Either civilian(s) or prisoner(s)—could have been either.
→ If selected, rate confidence: 2 = high; 1 = low.
- 99 = Not specified. → Skip to item D.

B. What type of person was attacked or harmed? **Select all that apply**:
- 1 = Military-age male.
  → If selected, rate confidence: 2 = high; 1 = low.
- 2 = Old male.
  → If selected, rate confidence: 2 = high; 1 = low.
- 3 = Female.
  → If selected, rate confidence: 2 = high; 1 = low.
- 4 = Child.
  → If selected, rate confidence: 2 = high; 1 = low.
- 5 = Other. Specify: _____
→ If selected, rate confidence: 2 = high; 1 = low.
- 99 = Not specified.

C. Was anyone killed?
- 0 = No.
  → If selected, rate confidence: 2 = high; 1 = low.
- 1 = Yes.
  → If selected, rate confidence: 2 = high; 1 = low.
- 99 = Not specified.

D. Was there harm to a village, houses or "hooches," etc.?
- 0 = No.
  → If selected, rate confidence: 2 = high; 1 = low.
- 1 = Yes.
  → If selected, rate confidence: 2 = high; 1 = low.
- 99 = Not specified.

E. Did the respondent (R) participate in the attacking or harming?
- 1 = Yes.
  → If selected, rate confidence: 2 = high; 1 = low.
- 99 = Not specified (possible that respondent witnessed only).

F. Did others participate in the attacking or harming?
- 0 = No.
  → If selected, rate confidence: 2 = high; 1 = low.
- 1 = Yes.
  → If selected, rate confidence: 2 = high; 1 = low.
- 99 = Not specified.

G. How was the harm inflicted? **<u>Select all that apply</u>**:
- 1 = Bombing (high altitude).
  → If selected, rate confidence: 2 = high; 1 = low.
- 2 = Low-altitude attack from the air.
  → If selected, rate confidence: 2 = high; 1 = low.
- 3 = Artillery.
  → If selected, rate confidence: 2 = high; 1 = low.
- 4 = Gun at close range.
  → If selected, rate confidence: 2 = high; 1 = low.
- 5 = Direct physical contact (e.g., hand or bayonet).
  → If selected, rate confidence: 2 = high; 1 = low.
- 6 = Lighting fire.
  → If selected, rate confidence: 2 = high; 1 = low.
- 50 = Other. Specify: _____
  → If selected, rate confidence: 2 = high; 1 = low.
- 99 = Not specified.

H. Did R see, hear, or guess that he attacked or harmed civilians or prisoners?
- 1 = Saw.
  → If selected, rate confidence: 2 = high; 1 = low.
- 2 = Heard.
  → If selected, rate confidence: 2 = high; 1 = low.
- 3 = Guessed.
  → If selected, rate confidence: 2 = high; 1 = low.
- 99 = Not specified.

I. What was the motivation for the harm?
- 1 = Ordered from above.
  → If selected,
- Rate confidence: 2 = high; 1 = low.
- Rate: Was the harm against R's will at the time?
- 0 = No.
  → If selected, rate confidence: 2 = high; 1 = low.
- 1 = Yes.
  → If selected, rate confidence: 2 = high; 1 = low.
- 99 = Not specified.
  - 2 = Intended retaliation.

→ If selected, rate confidence: 2 = high; 1 = low.
- 3 = Accidental.
  → If selected, rate confidence: 2 = high; 1 = low.
- 4 = Intended cruelty.
  → If selected, rate confidence: 2 = high; 1 = low.
- 5 = Loss of control.
  → If selected, rate confidence: 2 = high; 1 = low.
- 50 = Other. Specify: _____
  → If selected, rate confidence: 2 = high; 1 = low.
- 99 = Not specified.

J. Did the harm include any of the following behaviors beyond the pale? **Select all that apply:**
- 0 = None specified.
- 1 = Torture.
  → If selected, rate confidence: 2 = high; 1 = low.
- 2 = Rape.
  → If selected, rate confidence: 2 = high; 1 = low.
- 3 = Mutilation.
  → If selected, rate confidence: 2 = high; 1 = low.
- 50 = Other. Specify: _____
  → If selected, rate confidence: 2 = high; 1 = low.

normally destroy or "invade" an entire village.) Because the report mentioned no deaths, we did not rate the events described as having involved killing, even though killing may have occurred. Because the respondent used the words "destruction of villages," we rated the actions as having damaged villages or houses (high confidence). We concluded that the action had been "ordered from above" (high confidence), because the veteran's use of the word "mission" implied an action conducted under orders, and because a group action on such a scale was not likely to have been undertaken by a rogue group of soldiers, particularly since the destruction of villages and removal of the inhabitants was official policy in places thought to be under enemy control.

CHARACTERIZING VETERANS' ACTS OF HARM TO CIVILIANS AND PRISONERS

We discussed the coding of individual reports of harm. But veterans—not reports— are the focus of our interest and are our units of analysis. Most respondents made only one open-ended report of participation in harm to civilians or prisoners, although one respondent made eight reports, and another made two. Because some reports were of single incidents of harm, while others were of an indeterminate number of incidents, we could not use the reports to count numbers of incidents in which a respondent said he took part. Instead, we based our analyses on variables indicating whether the respondent *ever* took part in incidents of a given type. Twenty respondents reported having taken part in harming civilians; we rated 14 of these with high confidence. Five respondents reported having taken part in harm to prisoners; we rated four of these with high confidence. We next consider some of the more important aspects of respondents' participation in each type of harm.

Harm to Civilians

We concentrate here on information from reports of harm to civilians that we identify with high confidence. Such reports consist almost exclusively of close-up actions on the ground because respondents describing artillery attacks or aerial bombardments usually could not be sure whether they had harmed civilians. The open-ended material provides 18 high-confidence reports made by 14 respondents. Some of these describe shooting or beating up specifically described civilians. Other reports are more general, often involving the "invasion" or "destruction" of a village or of an unspecified number of villages. Seven of the 14 respondents merely mentioned taking part in harming civilians under circumstances that we rate with high confidence as having occurred in conjunction with the destruction of houses or livestock—always in the context of clearing, attacking, or destroying a village. These reports are of special interest to us in light of the U.S. policy of clearing the population from areas considered to be under enemy control. Other veterans' reports of harm to civilians may or may not have occurred in the context of village clearance; they did not provide enough information for us to know.

We have little evidence of lone acts of aggression against civilians. Only two of the 14 veterans reported events in which the participation of others is not indicated. It appears that, most of the time, the harm was inflicted in concert with other members of the veteran's military unit, presumably in accord with superior officers or non-commissioned officers (noncoms).

Harm to Prisoners

Compared with the narrative material on harm to civilians, fewer veterans gave examples of personal involvement in harm to prisoners in response to open-ended queries. Four men gave five reports of taking part in harm to prisoners in acts that we could rate as such with high confidence. The harm includes "mercy" killing of wounded enemy soldiers, torture to obtain information or for its own sake, and mutilating the bodies of dead soldiers. We see no evidence in the narrative material that any of these events took place during attacks on villages. Rather, they appear to have occurred in military operations with identifiable military combatants.

RELATIONSHIP BETWEEN CLOSED-QUESTION AND OPEN-QUESTION MEASURES IN THE IDENTIFICATION OF HARMERS

The narrative rating of responses to open-ended questions identifies an estimated 5.8% as harming civilians only; 0.5% as harming prisoners only; and just one veteran as harming both civilians and prisoners—for a total of 6.3% harming one or the other. These percentages are based on all reports of participation in harm, regardless of whether we had high or low confidence in them.

While substantially more veterans are identified as harmers by the closed-question measure described in Chapter 3, and used in the research reported in previous chapters, Table 6.1 shows that the narrative coding procedure identified nine veterans as harmers of civilians (none as harmers of prisoners) who were not identified by the previous measure. Those newly identified at high confidence increases the weighted rate of harmers identified by the closed-question measures from our previously estimated rate of nearly 13% to almost 14%. Those identified at any level of confidence by the open-end material increases the rate to 16.0%.

Table 6.1 PROPORTIONS OF MALE THEATER VETERANS WHO PARTICIPATED IN HARM TO CIVILIANS OR PRISONERS ACCORDING TO CLOSED-ENDED RESPONSES TO THE NVVRS AND ACCORDING TO THE NARRATIVE RATINGS

According to the Narrative Ratings	According to Closed-Ended Responses			
	No Harm	Harm	Missing	TOTAL
No harm	80.3%	9.8%	3.7%	93.8%
	180	35	9	224
Harm (low confidence)	2.4%	0.3%		2.7%
	5	2		7
Harm (high confidence)	0.8%	2.8%		3.6%
	4	13		17
TOTAL	83.5%	12.8%	3.7%	100.0%
	189	50	9	248

Note: The sample consists of male Theater veterans who had diagnostic information on PTSD and who had not had PTSD onsets prior to their service in Vietnam. Unweighted sample *n*'s are given below the percentages. Percentages are weighted to the population from which the subsample was drawn.

RELATIONSHIP BETWEEN GUILT AND WAR-RELATED PTSD AMONG MEN WHO HARMED CIVILIANS OR PRISONERS

Some studies of patient samples of Vietnam veterans have found that strong feelings of guilt have been associated with involvement in harm to civilians, and that such feelings are associated with PTSD (Beckham, Feldman, & Kirby, 1988; Hendin & Haas, 1991; Henning & Frueh, 1997; Litz et al., 2009; Marx et al., 2010). We developed a measure of Vietnam-related feelings of guilt or remorse (the "guilt scale") from the NVVRS to determine whether these results would hold in our more representative sample from the general population of Vietnam veterans. The guilt scale consists of the veteran's responses to the three questions set forth in Box 6.2.

The scale score is a simple count of these items, with scores ranging from 0–3. It has an internal consistency reliability of .66. As explained, most of the narrative-based harm codes are derived from open-ended follow-up responses to the same three questions. In contrast, the fixed-response harm measures are based on an entirely different set of questionnaire items. Thus, the fixed-response harm measures are independent of the guilt scale, and we can use them to examine the relationship between guilt and harm.

As we showed in Table 6.1, the closed-question measures identify the large majority of the harmers in this study, and we focus on them in the following analyses rather than mix respondents identified by different procedures. Table 6.2 shows that these harmers score much higher than non-harmers on the guilt scale.

Even with controls on severity of combat exposure and vulnerability load, the difference between harmers and non-harmers on this scale remains statistically significant ($p = .015$).

Box 6.2
ITEMS IN GUILT SCALE

- Now think about your primary duties and the kinds of operations you participated in when you were involved in the Vietnam war. Looking back, were there some things you wish you had chosen not to do or had not been assigned to do? *No/Yes*
- Were you ever in a combat situation in (or around) Vietnam where you participated in any kind of injury or destruction that seemed necessary then, but that you would consider unnecessary now? *No/Yes*
- Was there anything that happened in or around Vietnam that you felt you couldn't discuss with anyone else? *No/Yes*

Table 6.2 DIFFERENCES ON MEAN GUILT SCALE SCORES
BETWEEN HARMERS AND NON-HARMERS

Mean guilt score for harmers*	1.62	
Mean guilt score for non-harmers**	.57	
Unadjusted difference	1.05	(*p* = .000)
Difference adjusted for combat exposure (CESS)	.58	(*p* = .012)
Difference adjusted for combat exposure (CESS) and vulnerability load	.52	(*p* = .015)

Note: These analyses take into account the complex subsample design. Possible scores on the guilt scale range from 0–3.

*Harmers are those who reported on the closed-end items that they harmed civilians or prisoners.

**Non-harmers are those who did not report on the closed-end items that they harmed civilians or prisoners.

As Table 6.3 shows, the guilt scale is strongly associated with current war-related PTSD. Moreover, there is some indication even within the harmer group that current war-related PTSD may be elevated among those (*n* = 19) who scored high on the guilt scale (2 or 3) compared to those (*n* = 31) who scored low (0 or 1); the proportions are 46.9% in the high-guilt group compared with 32.9% in the low group (*p* = .48). The fact that PTSD is the dependent variable in these analyses does not, of course, demonstrate that guilt is causally prior. In fact, causation may run in either direction or both. Nonetheless, Table 6.3 serves to show the strength of the relationship between guilt and PTSD, and it is consistent with the possibility that guilt may contribute importantly to the persistence of the disorder.

Table 6.3 ODDS RATIOS FOR CURRENT PTSD CONTINGENT
ON GUILT SCORE

	Current PTSD
Effect of Guilt	O.R. (p)
Unadjusted	3.56 (.000)
Adjusted for combat exposure (CESS)	2.31 (.003)
Adjusted for combat exposure and vulnerability load	2.32 (.007)

Note: Each odds ratio is produced by a separate model. Guilt, combat exposure, and vulnerability load are measured in standard deviation units. These analyses take into account the complex subsample design.

RELATIONSHIP OF ANGER TO GUILT, HARM
TO CIVILIANS OR PRISONERS, AND WAR-RELATED PTSD

Guilt is not the only emotion associated with involvement in harm to civilians or prisoners. Clinicians report that anger and aggressive behaviors are also prominent (Glover, 1985). (See our Chapter 1, Aftermath, the section *Recognition of Veteran Experiences*, which describes the contribution of anger to veterans' mental health going forward.)

We, therefore, developed from NSVG items a scale measuring anger expression and a scale measuring angry aggression. These are summarized in Box 6.3.

The scale of anger expression has an internal consistency reliability of .79. The similarly calculated reliability is .86 for angry aggression. There is a correlation of .50 between the two scales in the diagnosed subsample as a whole, and a substantial correlation of .70 in the subsample of harmers.

Box 6.3

ITEMS COMPRISING THE ANGER EXPRESSION
AND ANGRY AGGRESSION SCALES

ANGER EXPRESSION

During the past year, when you have gotten angry, how often have you:

... sworn or cursed?
... gotten into an argument?
... yelled or shouted?
... shown an angry expression on your face?
... [did you] take out your anger by kicking things, like a chair, giving a door a good slam, punching the wall, or looking for something to throw or smash?

For each of the above, the respondent was asked to choose one of the following:

Very often
Fairly often
Sometimes
Almost never
Never

The response to each item was assigned a score ranging from 0 (never) to 4 (very often). The scale is the sum of these responses, with possible scores ranging from 0–20.

ANGRY AGGRESSION

During the past year, how often did you:

... threaten to hit or throw something at another person?
... actually throw something at someone?

... push, grab, or shove someone?
... slap another person?
... kick, bite, or hit someone with a fist?
... hit or try to hit anyone with something (an object)?
... beat up someone?
... threaten anyone with a knife or gun?
... actually use a knife or gun on another person?

For each of the above, the respondent was asked to choose one of the following:

Never
Once
Twice
3–5 times
6–10 times
11–20 times
More than 20 times

The response to each item was assigned a score ranging from 0 (never) to 6 (more than 20 times). The scale is the sum of these responses, with possible scores ranging from 0–54.

Table 6.4 shows that the guilt scale and the two anger scales all have at least moderate correlations with harm to civilians or prisoners, as well as with current PTSD and PTSD onset. Not too surprisingly, the two anger scales are more highly correlated with each other, particularly among harmers ($r = .70$). Still looking among harmers, we see that guilt is virtually independent of angry actions ($r = -.02$) and shows only a modest correlation with anger expression ($r = .22$).

Unlike our measure of guilt feelings, the two anger scales are not explicitly tied to experiences in Vietnam. Nevertheless, the measures of anger are, like guilt feelings, strongly associated with the personal involvement in harming civilians or prisoners in Vietnam. Since the anger measures show only modest if any correlation with guilt, it seems reasonable to conclude that there may be different types of harmers, those who react with guilt and those who react with anger. A possible third type might be characterized by reactions of both guilt and anger. If we dichotomize the measures of guilt and anger at the median, we find that 24% would be mainly a guilt type (high on guilt, low on anger), 19% mainly an anger type (high on anger, low on guilt), 25% mixed (high on both) and 31% neither (low on both anger and guilt).

Table 6.5 shows that, not surprisingly given what we have learned so far, rates of PTSD are considerably higher in the first three types than in the fourth (low on both).

There is one partial exception, however. Persistence of PTSD, as represented by the rate of current PTSD, is strikingly low among veterans with high guilt but low anger.

Table 6.4 CORRELATIONS AMONG HARM TO CIVILIANS OR
PRISONERS, GUILT, ANGER EXPRESSION, AND ANGRY AGGRESSION;
AND CORRELATIONS OF THESE VARIABLES WITH PTSD ONSET
AND CURRENT PTSD

In the diagnosed subsample (*n* = 248)

	Angry aggression	Anger expression	Guilt feelings
Anger expression	.50		
Guilt	.13	.26	
Harmed civilians/prisoners	.26	.20	.38
PTSD onset	.30	.34	.41
Current PTSD	.28	.36	.44

Among harmers in the diagnosed subsample (*n* = 50)

	Angry aggression	Anger expression	Guilt feelings
Anger expression	.70		
Guilt	−.02	.22	
PTSD onset	.23	.24	
Current PTSD	.32	.33	.26

Note: These analyses take into account the complex subsample design. *N*'s are unweighted subsample numbers.

Table 6.5 RATES OF PTSD ONSET AND
CURRENT PTSD IN HARMERS ACCORDING
TO LEVELS OF ANGER EXPRESSION
AND GUILT

PTSD Onset

		Guilt	
		Low	High
Anger expression	Low	.19 (9)	.91(13)
	High	.85 (10)	.74 (18)

Current PTSD

		Guilt	
		Low	High
Anger expression	Low	.18 (9)	.28(13)
	High	.57 (10)	.65 (18)

Note: Proportions are weighted to represent the population. *N*'s are unweighted sample numbers.

SUMMARY AND CONCLUSIONS

On the basis of responses to direct, closed questions about personal involvement, we identified 12.8% of the veterans as harmers of civilians or prisoners. Analyses of qualitative information indicate that the figure may be as high as 16%. Our analyses focused mainly on the original 12.8%, all of whom were identified by the same procedure. These consist of 5.9% who harmed civilians only, 3.4% who harmed prisoners only, and 3.3% who harmed both. Other than their much more severe combat exposure, we found very few characteristics of the harmers that differentiated them from veterans who were not directly involved in, or responsible for, inflicting harm on civilians or prisoners.

The qualitative material is most useful in providing clues to the context in which harm took place. It suggests that harm to prisoners may usually have occurred following attacks on clearly identifiable enemy forces. Such acts of harm are clearly contrary to the rules of war and can be reasonably called atrocities. Many incidents of harm to civilians appear to have occurred in attempts by U.S. forces to implement the policy of clearing the population from areas considered to be under enemy control. We would like to know how much of the injury to civilians was discovered after attacks on villages that were supposed to have been vacated already and how much involved civilians as direct and visible targets. The term "collateral damage" might reasonably be used to describe the former. The latter were "atrocities," as were the poorly conceived and implemented policies that led to both inadvertent and advertent harm to civilian villagers.

The situations U.S. combat forces faced in Vietnam, though much more serious in their consequences, nevertheless call to mind the artificial situations contrived by Milgram (1963) and Haney, Banks, and Zimbardo (1973) in their classic social psychological experiments. These investigators created contexts in which normal people, in this case university students, did terrible things in the belief that their actions were called for by respected authorities in the pursuit of legitimate goals. If we had more of the information called for in Table 6.1, we could better differentiate the types of harm that occurred on a hypothetical continuum from "collateral damage" to "atrocity" as these terms apply to the acts of the veterans in these situations.

Whatever these details, veterans classified as harmers scored much higher than nonharmers on our scale of implied guilt, even with severity of combat exposure and pre-war vulnerability load statistically controlled. Guilt, in turn, showed a strong relationship with war-related onsets of PTSD and, especially, current PTSD. Given the strong association of guilt with both harm and PTSD, it seems possible that guilt contributes considerably to the onset of war-related PTSD.

Our measures of veterans' anger show strong associations with their reported harming of civilians or prisoners, as well as with PTSD onset and current PTSD. It is notable that the measures of anger show little correlation with our measure of guilt. In the new DSM-5 (APA, 2013), both anger and guilt are included as persistent emotional states, along with the previously emphasized emotion of fear in Criterion D for PTSD (negative alterations in cognition and mood). Anger also figures prominently in Criterion E (arousal and reactivity) involving expression of verbal or physical aggression towards people or objects. It seems possible that both the guilt and anger aspects of

PTSD are heightened for the veterans who personally participated in harming civilians or prisoners.

REFERENCES

American Psychiatric Association. (2013). *Diagnostic and statistical manual of mental disorders* (5th ed.). Washington, DC: Author.

Appy, C. (1993). *Working-class war: American combat soldiers and Vietnam.* Chapel Hill, NC: University of North Carolina Press.

Beckham, J. C., Feldman, M. E., & Kirby, A. C. (1988). Atrocities exposure in Vietnam combat veterans with chronic posttraumatic stress disorder: Relationship to combat exposure, symptom severity, guilt, and interpersonal violence. *Journal of Traumatic Stress, 11*(4), 777–785. doi:10.1023/A:1024453618638

Bilton, M., & Sim, K. (1992). *Four hours in My Lai.* New York: Penguin Books.

Cohen, R. (2016). *Kerry's Vietnam dilemma. New York Times,* p. A21.

COMUSMACV [Westmoreland - Commander US Military Assistance Command Vietnam] to CINCPAC [Commander in Chief, Pacific Command]. (1965). *Minimizing non-combatant battle casualties.* Carlisle, PA: U.S. Army War College.

Dolvin, W. G. (1971). *MACV Directive No. 525-3: Combat operations: Minimizing non-combatant battle casualties.* Carlisle, PA: U.S. Army War College.

Gault, W. B. (1971). Some remarks on slaughter. *American Journal of Social Psychiatry, 5*, 15–18.

Gibson, J. W. (2000). *The perfect war: Technowar in Vietnam.* Boston, MA: Atlantic Monthly Press.

Glover, H. (1985). Guilt and aggression in Vietnam veterans. *The American Journal of Psychiatry, 148*, 586–591.

Greiner, B. (2009). *War without fronts: The USA in Vietnam.* London: The Bodley Head.

Haley, S. A. (1974). When the patient reports atrocities: Specific treatment considerations of the Vietnam veteran. *Archives of General Psychiatry 30*(2), 191–196. doi:10.1001/archpsyc.1974.01760080051008

Haney, C., Banks, C., & Zimbardo, P. (1973). Interpersonal dynamics in a simulated prison. *International Journal of Criminology and Penology, 1*, 69–97.

Hendin, H., & Haas, A. P. (1991). Suicide and guilt as manifestations of PTSD in Vietnam combat veterans. *The American Journal of Psychiatry, 148*, 586–591.

Henning, K. R., & Frueh, B. C. (1997). Combat guilt and its relationship to PTSD symptoms. *Journal of Clinical Psychology, 53*, 801–808.

Hersh, S. (1998). *An atrocity is uncovered: November 1969, The My Lai massacre.* In M. J. Bates, L. Lichty, P. L. Miles, R. H. Spector, & M. Young (Advisory Board), *Reporting Vietnam, Part Two, pp. 13-27.* New York: Literary Classics of the United States, New York, NY.

Kerrey, J. R. (2002). *When I was a young man.* New York: Harcourt.

Lang, D. (1969). An atrocity and its aftermath: November 1966-October 1969, Casualties of war. In Bates, L., Lichty, P. L. Miles, R. H. Spector, & M. Young (Eds.), *Reporting Vietnam, Part One* (pp. 709–767). New York: Literary Classics of the United States, New York, NY.

Litz, B. T., Stein, N., Delaney, E., Lebowitz, L., Nash, W. P., Silva, C., & Maguen, S. (2009). Moral injury and moral repair in war veterans: A preliminary model and intervention strategy. *Clinical Psychology Review, 29*, 695–706.

Marx, B. P., Foley, K. M., Feinstein, B. A., Wolf, E. J., Kaloupek, D. G., & Keane, T. M. (2010). Combat-related guilt mediates the relations between exposure to combat-related abusive violence and psychiatric diagnoses. *Depression and Anxiety, 27,* 287–293. doi:10.1002/da.20659

McNamara, R. S., & VanDeMark, B. (1995). *In retrospect: The tragedy and lessons of Vietnam.* New York: Times Books.

Milgram, S. (1963). Behavioral study of obedience. *Journal of Abnormal and Social Psychology, 67,* 371–378.

Pilger, J. (1976). *The last day.* New York: Vintage.

Schell. J. (2000). *The real war: The classic reporting on the Vietnam war.* New York: De Capo Press.

Smith, R. (2007). *The utility of force: The art of war in the modern world.* New York: Knopf.

Turse, N. (2013). *Kill anything that moves: The real American war in Vietnam.* New York: Henry Holt & Company.

Westmoreland, W. C. (1965). *MACV Directive No. 525-3: Combat operations: Minimizing non-combatant battle casualties.* Carlisle, PA: U.S. Army War College.

CHAPTER 7

◦◊◦

War-Related PTSD in Black, Hispanic, and Majority White Vietnam Veterans

The Roles of Potentially Traumatic Exposure and Vulnerability

BRUCE P. DOHRENWEND, J. BLAKE TURNER, NICK
TURSE, ROBERTO LEWIS-FERNÁNDEZ, AND
THOMAS J. YAGER

President Truman desegregated the military in 1948.... By the 1960s, many believed the military, for all its hierarchies and its obvious authoritarianism, was functionally the most democratic major institution in the United States. That it was the only reliable employer for many young, disadvantaged men, and the only one to conscript its workers, did not change the fact that it was the one place in America where you could find whites, blacks, Latinos, Asians, and Native Americans all living and working together. (Appy, 2003, p. 354)

Vietnam became the first modern American war fought by an entirely desegregated military. Blacks and Hispanics were the two largest racial/ethnic minorities who served in Vietnam. Fortunately, as we reported previously, they were oversampled in the NVVRS in order to provide adequate numbers for statistical analyses. This chapter reports our inquiry into how they fared psychologically as compared with the white majority (i.e., non-Hispanic whites). We start with some recent historical background on these two minority groups.

BLACK VETERANS

Blacks, for the first time, received the same training as whites, held the same weapons, and served in the same units all the way through the conflict. All things were equal— except when they weren't. During the Vietnam war and since, many have noted that African Americans were disproportionately drafted, assigned to combat, and killed, though the subject has yet to be comprehensively addressed by scholars (Baskir & Strauss, 1978; Gibson, 2000; Helmer, 1974; King, 1967; Moskos, 1970; Polner, 1971; Terry, 1984; Thompson, 1990; Westheider, 1997).

While much remains unknown about military "channeling" efforts (i.e., inducting individuals into the armed forces and assigning them to combat units) in regard to blacks, the available evidence offers telling insights. Levy (1995) points out that a 1966 study demonstrated that African Americans made up only 1.6% of the members of all local U.S. draft boards.

Research by Moskos (1970) revealed that from 1960–1966, 55% of blacks (as opposed to 15% of whites) did not pass the pre-induction mental screenings, thus exempting large numbers of African Americans from service. But this advantage for African Americans in avoiding the draft was negated by the fact that 95% of whites could obtain deferments, while only 5% of blacks deemed fit for military service could do the same, according to 1967 figures. Despite the fact that large numbers of them failed to meet induction standards, blacks were approximately 15% of the draftees from 1960– 1967, a period during which blacks accounted for 12% of the U.S. population (Baskir & Strauss, 1978; Clodfelter, 1995; Moskos, 1970).

In 1966, Secretary of Defense Robert McNamara instituted "Project 100,000," the military's Great Society program that drafted 100,000 men a year who otherwise would have been rejected from service. Blacks constituted 36% of the program's conscripts, and a disproportionate number of these "new standards men" were assigned to the combat arms (e.g., infantry, armor and artillery) (Buckley, 2007). While composing 12.1% of the total recruited personnel in 1967, 28.6% of African Americans were in combat arms (e.g., infantry, armor, and artillery), while the percentage of whites in combat arms was 22.8% (Moskos, 1970).

While African Americans constituted 9.5% of the total armed forces personnel in 1965 (Moskos, 1970), the number serving in high-risk units stood at 31% (Clodfelter, 1995). That same year, blacks suffered 24% of the fatalities (Baskir & Strauss, 1978; Clodfelter, 1995). Statistics like these prompted a number of prominent African American commentators such as Martin Luther King, Jr., Malcolm X, Muhammad Ali, Adam Clayton Powell, Dick Gregory, Eldridge Cleaver, and others to begin to condemn the disparity in the casualty rates of black and white soldiers (Appy, 1993; Cleaver, 1968). (See our Chapter 1, section War, *The Rise of the Civil Rights Movement and Black Power*, describing growing black consciousness and militancy with increasing opposition to the war.)

In a response to these criticisms and growing public awareness of these disparities, the Department of Defense (DoD) began an intensive campaign to lower African

American combat exposure and casualty rates (Baskir & Strauss, 1978). It was carried out, according to Brigadier General John Johns, a Vietnam veteran who served in the office of the Army Chief of Staff in the early 1970s, for public relations purposes. While it is yet unclear exactly how this was accomplished, the DoD was successful in reducing African American combat deaths to 13% in 1968 and below 10% in 1970–1972 (Appy, 1993; Baskir & Strauss, 1978). It should be noted that the reduction in African American casualties was specifically carried out by the Army. The Marine Corps had a stable casualty level of approximately 13% throughout the Vietnam war (Appy, 1993). By the end of the war, blacks accounted for a more representative 12.3–12.7% of all combat deaths during the conflict (Levy, 1995; Lewy, 1978).

HISPANIC VETERANS

Hispanic troops played an outsized role in the Vietnam War. One need look no further than the Vietnam Veterans Memorial in Washington, D.C., where "Rodriguez" is the second most common name etched in the polished granite monument memorializing the war's American military dead (Mariscal, 1999). Yet, even such basic information as the total number of Hispanics who served in the war is unknown, due to methods of military record-keeping during that era (Appy, 1993; Mariscal, 1999). The classificatory category "Hispanic" would not even be used by the military until 1979 (Mariscal, 1999; Trujillo, 1990). The DoD, however, estimates that around 83,000 Hispanics served in Vietnam, while others place the total as high as 170,000 (Daugherty & Mattson, 2001; Trujillo, 1990).

Mirroring the experience of blacks, Hispanics found themselves not just under-represented at draft boards but sometimes completely *un*represented. "In several Rio Grande counties in Texas with populations that were over 50 percent Mexican," writes Terry Anderson (2007), "not one Mexican American sat on the draft board." While Hispanic men constituted 40% of the population of San Antonio, Texas, in 1966, they suffered 60% of that city's casualties (Anderson, 2007). From 1961–1967, around 19% of casualties from Arizona, California, Colorado, New Mexico, and Texas had distinctive Spanish surnames, despite the fact that just 11.8% of the Southwestern population, and 13.8% of military-age males, had such names (Guzman, 1970). (See our Chapter 1, section War, *Nixon's War*, for descriptions of Hispanic anti-war protests and subsequent violent police responses.)

PRIOR RESEARCH REPORTS OF HIGHER PTSD PREVALENCE RATES IN BLACKS AND HISPANICS

Prevalence rates of current PTSD, PTSD-like symptoms, and other psychological problems were found to be significantly higher in black than in white majority veterans many years after the Vietnam war (Centers for Disease Control, 1988; Green, Grace, Lindy, & Leonard, 1990; Koenen, Stellman, Stellman, & Sommer, 2003; Kulka et al.,

1990; Laufer, Gallops, & Frey-Wouters, 1984; Penk et al., 1989). There has been less research comparing Hispanics and majority whites, but the nationwide study by Kulka et al. (1990) found even higher rates of current PTSD in Hispanic than in black Vietnam veterans.

Various possible explanations have been offered for the elevated prevalence rates of PTSD in black and Hispanic Vietnam veterans: greater exposure to war-zone stressors (e.g., Beals et al., 2002; Green et al., 1990; Kulka et al., 1990; MacDonald, Chamberlin, & Long, 1997); differences in pre-war vulnerability factors (e.g., Kulka et al., 1990); ethno-cultural factors, especially subcultural differences in modes of expressing distress that could lead to the over-diagnosis of PTSD (e.g., Ortega & Rosenheck, 2000); post-war stressful events that could contribute to persistence or recurrence of PTSD (e.g., Schlenger & Fairbank, 1996); and experiences with ra-cial/ethnic prejudice and discrimination (Allen, 1986; Cortright, 1990; Graham, 2003; Parson, 1984; Ruef, Litz, & Schlenger, 2000; Terry, 1984; Van Deburg, 1992). However, no compelling or comprehensive explanation of these group differences has emerged from previous research. (cf. Beals et al., 2002; Green et al., 1990; Koenen et al., 2003; Kulka et al., 1990).

For example, while many agreed that differential exposure to war-zone stressors plays a major part in the racial/ethnic differences, others questioned the accuracy of the self-report measures of exposure on which this conclusion is based (e.g., Frueh et al., 2005; McNally, 2003; Wessely & Jones, 2004). Skepticism about these retrospective reports has been stimulated by systematic research on recall bias in reports of such experiences (e.g., Roemer et al., 1998; Southwick, Morgan, & Nicolau, 1997). While there is no evidence that such biases are greater in reports from some racial/ethnic groups than others, the investigations cited suggest that it would be useful to examine whether measures of exposure that do not rely on veterans' recall would yield the same results.

Another problem is the focus of most previous research on the current prevalence of PTSD; that is, on the presence of the disorder, or symptoms of the disorder, many years after the war when the studies were conducted. Prevalence is a function of initial onset or incidence and subsequent course. Risk factors for one may be quite different from risk factors for the other (e.g., Schnurr, Lunney, & Sengupta, 2004; Susser, Schwartz, Morabia, & Bromet, 2006).

These issues are present in previous results from the NVVRS, the study with the largest samples of black and Hispanic Vietnam veterans (Kulka et al., 1990). We use data from the NVVRS and from military records to address these issues.

OUR RESEARCH REGARDING HIGHER PTSD RATES

The problem with the limited assessment of PTSD can be resolved by using detailed di-agnostic histories of PTSD obtained for a subsample of NVVRS veterans (Kulka et al., 1988, 1990; our Chapter 2). The difficulty of measuring exposure can be addressed by using data obtained from military records and data from record-based historical ac-counts (Dohrenwend et al., 2004; Dohrenwend et al., 2006; our Chapter 3).

We previously used these measures to investigate the hypothesis advanced by Ortega and Rosenheck (2000) that the elevation in Hispanic rates of PTSD reported in the NVVRS by Kulka et al. (1990) is an artifact of a subcultural expressive style that led to over-reporting of symptomatology. We found that although self-report symptom scales seem affected by a pattern of Hispanic expressiveness, the clinical diagnoses in the subsample, which also showed an Hispanic elevation, seemed generally free of such problems (Lewis-Fernández et al., 2008).

Our purpose here is to use these diagnoses, the record-based measures of exposure, and other measures developed with data from the NVVRS to investigate the relevance of the remaining substantive hypotheses, summarized, about why black and Hispanic veterans had elevated prevalence rates of PTSD compared with majority white veterans many years after the end of the Vietnam war.

Composition of Subsample

To do so, we again use the NVVRS subsample of male Theater veterans who received psychiatric examinations by experienced clinicians. As noted earlier, diagnoses according to the then-current DSM-III-R criteria were made by 28 doctoral-level clinicians using the Structured Clinical Interview for DSM-III-R Diagnoses (SCID) (Spitzer, Williams, & Gibbon, 1987). Suitably weighted, the demographic distribution of subsample veterans, including the proportional distribution of racial/ethnic groups, is very similar to that in the full 1,200-member sample of NVVRS Theater veterans, except that veterans from rural areas are under-represented (see our Chapter 2, Table 2.1).

Five veterans from minority backgrounds other than black and Hispanic in this subsample had to be removed as too few to analyze. Relevant data on PTSD status or information about sampling weights was missing for three more, thus also omitted. Only four subsample veterans in the three racial/ethnic groups compared here had first onsets of PTSD prior to their service in Vietnam. These rates are too low and the n's on which they are based are too small to provide a basis for evaluating whether pre-war PTSD increased vulnerability to war-related PTSD; these four veterans are, therefore, also omitted from the analyses. The sample for the following analyses now consists of 248 male veterans of the Vietnam war: 94 majority white, 70 black, and 84 Hispanic.

All respondents in the NVVRS identified their racial/ethnic background as American Indian, Alaskan Native, Asian, Pacific Islander, Black, White, Other (specify). They were then asked if they were of Hispanic (Spanish) origin and, if so, which of several groupings (e.g., Puerto Rican, Mexican) described their origin or ancestry. This information was used to cross-check the information in the military records on which the racial/ethnic stratification for sampling purposes was based (Hunt et al., 1994, pp. 21–23).

The large majority of the 84 Hispanic respondents, 63, are Mexican American; 15 are Puerto Rican; and the remaining six are from various other Latin American countries. Because PTSD rates are elevated in all but the last (and smallest) of these three Hispanic subgroups, and because the sample sizes of all but the Mexican-American subgroup are very small, all Hispanics are combined in the present analyses.

Measurement of Combat Exposure

In light of criticisms that previous findings of racial/ethnic differences may have resulted from recall bias in self-report measures of combat exposure, the record-based Military/ Historical Measure (MHM) serves as the main indicator of severity of combat exposure in the analyses that follow. This measure, described in detail in our Chapter 2, is clearly antecedent and cannot be affected by recall bias.

In brief summary, the composite MHM consists of four categories ranging from probable very high to probable low severity of exposure. Veterans in the high and very high categories (11.7%) typically had high-exposure military occupational specialties (MOS's), served in large military units with high casualty rates measured by numbers killed in action (KIA), and served at times of high U.S. KIA rates; men in the very high category (3.2%) were further distinguished by having been in small units (e.g., companies) that suffered 10 or more KIAs during the veteran's tour in Vietnam. By contrast, veterans in the low exposure category (19.8%) typically had low exposure MOS's, served in large units with low KIA rates, served at times of low KIA rates, and were in small units with no KIAs during the veteran's tour of duty in Vietnam. The remaining veterans in the moderate exposure category (68.4%) differed from those in the low category mainly in that most served in Vietnam when KIA rates were moderate or high rather than low.

This MHM is based largely on casualty rates. In addition, we use our most comprehensive measure of severity of combat exposure, consisting of self-reported combat experiences as well as the record-based measures in some of the analyses; this measure is fully described in our Chapter 3.

Race/Ethnicity, War-Zone Stress Exposure, and SCID Diagnoses

The three panels in Table 7.1 display, respectively, racial/ethnic differences in rates of war-related PTSD (first onset incident PTSD and current PTSD), the relationship of PTSD to our MHM of probable war-zone stress exposure, and the distribution of MHM exposure across the three racial/ethnic groups. The first panel (Panel A) shows that blacks and Hispanics are more likely than majority whites to develop onsets of war-related PTSD.

The two minorities also have elevated rates of current PTSD. However, unlike blacks' current rate, Hispanics' current rate accounts for well over half of onsets. In other words, PTSD is more persistent among Hispanics than in either blacks or majority whites.

The second panel of Table 7.1 (Panel B) shows that current PTSD is directly related to MHM severity of exposure. Onset, too, increases with exposure, but the trend falls short of the .05 level of significance. In contrast, past PTSD, consisting of onsets of PTSD that have remitted, appears to be unrelated to severity of exposure. The third panel of Table 7.1 (Panel C) shows that both minorities were more exposed to war-zone stressors than majority whites.

Table 7.1 ASSOCIATIONS BETWEEN RACE/ETHNICITY, MILITARY HISTORICAL MEASURE (MHM) OF SEVERITY OF WAR-ZONE STRESS EXPOSURE, AND RATES OF WAR-RELATED PTSD

A. Rates of War-Related PTSD by Racial/Ethnic Background

PTSD Status	White ($n = 94$) %	Black ($n = 70$) %	Hispanic ($n = 84$) %	Wald χ^2
PTSD Onset	18.7	33.0[b]	32.9[a]	5.52*
Current PTSD	9.0	16.8	22.0[b]	6.82**
Past PTSD	9.7	16.2	10.9	1.22

B. Rates of War-Related PTSD by MHM of War-Zone Stress Exposure

PTSD Status	Low ($n = 38$) %	Moderate ($n = 152$) %	High ($n = 37$) %	Very High ($n = 21$) %	Wald χ^2
PTSD Onset	10.3	23.3	38.6	38.7	6.78*
Current PTSD	0.3	12.3	27.0	33.5	30.32****
Past PTSD	9.9	11.0	11.6	5.2	1.38

C. MHM of Severity of War-Zone Stress Exposure by Racial/Ethnic Background

MHM of Exposure Severity	White ($n = 94$) %	Black ($n = 70$) %	Hispanic ($n = 84$) %	Wald χ^2
Low	29.8	9.7[c]	15.0[b]	9.17**
Moderate	63.6	59.0	65.6	0.50
High	5.3	20.5[b]	12.0	6.22**
Very High	1.3	10.8[c]	7.4[b]	10.61***

Note: Percentages are weighted to the population from which the subsample was drawn. Unweighted subsample *n*'s are in parentheses.

[a]Indicates a trend difference from white majority in pair-wise test; p < .10. [b]Indicates significant difference from white majority in pair-wise test; p < .05. [c]Indicates significant difference from white majority in pair-wise test; p < .01.

* p < .10.

** p < .05.

*** p < .01.

**** p < .001.

We compared the three racial/ethnic groups on our most comprehensive measure of the combat exposure, the Combat Exposure Severity Scale (CESS). This measure includes the MHM as one of its six component measures and, as mentioned, is described in detail in Chapter 3. As we reported there, veterans above the 75th percentile in severity of exposure were particularly likely to develop war-related PTSD. The present results show that 46% of blacks were above the 75th percentile on this measure compared with 34% of Hispanics and 22% of majority whites. These overall group differences are statistically significant ($p = .01$), as is the difference between whites and blacks ($p = .003$); Hispanics appear to be intermediate between majority whites and blacks, although Hispanics do not show a statistically significant difference from either ($p = .13$ from majority whites; $p = .24$ from blacks). These results are consistent with those obtained with the MHM exposure alone.

The next set of analyses examines the extent to which racial/ethnic differences in war-zone combat exposure account for minority elevations in war-related PTSD. Because past war-related PTSD, unlike current PTSD, is not associated with exposure level and racial/ethnic background, these regression analyses focus on veterans with current war-related PTSD contrasted with veterans with no onsets of PTSD.

Table 7.2 compares unadjusted odds ratios for the racial/ethnic differences in current PTSD with odds ratios adjusted for controls on MHM severity of exposure. Consistent with previous NVVRS research with a measure of exposure based on self-report and the NVVRS algorithmic approximation of current PTSD (Kulka et al., 1988, 1990), the Table 7.2 results show that controlling MHM exposure comes close to accounting for the difference between blacks and majority whites, but less so for the difference between Hispanics and majority whites. The logistic regression coefficient for blacks is reduced by 73.5% when exposure is added to the model. This compares with a reduction of 25.9% for Hispanics.

Table 7.2 ODDS RATIOS (ORs) AND CONFIDENCE INTERVALS (CIs) FOR RACIAL/ETHNIC CONTRASTS IN WAR-RELATED PTSD UNADJUSTED AND ADJUSTED FOR MILITARY HISTORICAL MEASURE OF PROBABLE SEVERITY OF EXPOSURE TO WAR-ZONE STRESSORS

Racial/Ethnic Contrasts (*n*)	Unadjusted OR (95% CI)	OR Adjusted for Exposure (95% CI)
Majority White (94)	Ref	Ref
Black (70)	2.23	1.24
	(0.95–5.23)	(0.45–3.38)
Hispanic (84)	2.95	2.23
	(1.27–6.82)	(0.90–5.52)

Note: These analyses take into account the complex sampling design. *N*'s are unweighted subsample numbers.

Other Risk Factors

The result in Tables 7.1 and 7.2 suggest that differences between blacks and majority whites in rates of PTSD onset and current PTSD are largely explained by blacks' greater severity of combat exposure. But the results raise other questions: What are the factors in addition to combat exposure that explain the elevated PTSD rates of Hispanics compared with PTSD rates of majority whites? And why do rates of current PTSD tend to be higher for Hispanics than blacks despite the fact that Hispanics experienced less severe combat than blacks?

We considered a number of possible additional risk factors. Most, however, did not qualify. For example, some of the risk factors for PTSD, such as pre-war psychiatric disorders, are unrelated to race/ethnicity. Other omitted factors are elevated among the minorities, but the elevations in blacks are at least equal to, and often greater than, the elevations in Hispanics and thus cannot help explain why Hispanics have higher rates of current PTSD than blacks. These other factors include involvement in harm to civilians or prisoners, disciplinary actions during the war, post-war adversities like marital separation/divorce and unemployment, and lack of treatment by members of the mental health professions. Blacks also report having experienced more prejudice and racial discrimination in Vietnam and more adverse reactions from others upon homecoming than do Hispanics. Clearly, these factors cannot explain the higher rates of current war-related PTSD in Hispanics compared with blacks.

We are, however, able to identify seven pre-Vietnam risk factors that (a) differentiate Hispanics from majority whites, and (b) show a positive association with current PTSD that might, together with exposure, help explain elevated rates of current PTSD in Hispanics compared with majority whites. These factors include having one or more family members who were arrested and charged with offenses more serious than traffic violations; lower educational level prior to Vietnam; lower scores on the Armed Forces Qualifications Test (AFQT); being younger; and, related to age, going to Vietnam as an enlisted man in a rank below sergeant; having no prior military tours; and reporting no prior exposure to enemy fire.

Of the seven, the three that are least susceptible to recall bias and most strongly related to current PTSD are pre-Vietnam educational level, AFQT score, and pre-Vietnam age (especially the difference between those under 25 and those 25 and over). Pre-Vietnam educational level and AFQT scores are lower in both blacks and Hispanics than in majority whites, and Hispanics' age as well as their lower educational level and lower AFQT scores differentiate them from blacks.

Table 7.3 gives inter-ethnic contrasts in the form of relative odds of current PTSD—first unadjusted, then adjusted for MHM exposure, and finally adjusted for MHM exposure, education and AFQT, and (in the case of Hispanics) age at entry to Vietnam.

This table shows that including pre-war vulnerability factors in the model reduces the odds ratio to .80 for Hispanics as compared to majority whites and .82 for Hispanics as compared to blacks, completely accounting for the Hispanic elevation in both cases.

Table 7.3 ADJUSTED AND UNADJUSTED ODDS RATIOS (ORs) AND
CONFIDENCE INTERVALS (CIs) FOR RACIAL/ETHNIC CONTRASTS
IN CURRENT WAR-RELATED PTSD

Contrast	OR	95% CI
Black vs. White		
Unadjusted	2.23	0.95–5.23
Adjusted for exposure	1.24	0.45–3.38
Adjusted for exposure & pre-war risk factors	1.16	0.37–3.64
Hispanic vs. White		
Unadjusted	2.95	1.27–6.82
Adjusted for exposure	2.23	0.90–5.52
Adjusted for exposure & pre-war risk factors	0.80	0.25–2.59
Hispanic vs. Black		
Unadjusted	1.35	0.57–3.20
Adjusted for exposure	1.72	0.69–4.31
Adjusted for exposure & pre-war risk factors	0.82	0.30–2.25

Note: These analyses take into account the complex subsample design. Pre-war risk factors for the Black vs. White contrast include Armed Forces Qualification Test categories and pre-war educational attainment levels. Pre-war risk factors for the Hispanic vs. White and Hispanic vs. Black contrasts include these same two variables plus age at entry to Vietnam.

Sources of Racial/Ethnic Differences in Severity of Combat Exposure

In view of the major role of severity of combat exposure in these racial/ethnic differences, the question arises: Why was the combat exposure of blacks and, to a lesser degree, Hispanics, more severe than that of majority whites? The main answer lies in differences in how each group entered the military and in the branches in which they served. The men who served in Vietnam were there either because they enlisted or because they were drafted. If they enlisted, they could have their choice of branch of service. If they were drafted, they went into the Army. Only about a fifth (20.4%) were drafted; a similar percent (19.7%) said they enlisted to avoid the draft. A substantial majority of the

Table 7.4 PERCENTAGES OF VETERANS WHO EXPERIENCED HIGH LEVELS OF COMBAT EXPOSURE ACCORDING TO THE MHM AND THE CESS, BY BRANCH OF SERVICE

Branch of Service	Percentages at High Risk (MHM Levels 3 and 4)	Percentages with High CESS Scores (75th Percentile or Above)
Army	11.7%	34.0%
Marines	48.3%	48.5%
Navy	2.2%	6.1%
Air Force	0.0%	7.2%
All branches	10.8%	25.5%

Note: Percentages are weighted to the population from which the subsample was drawn.

veterans (59.9%) enlisted voluntarily. Overall, 57.5% served in the Army; 20.6% in the Navy, 14.3% in the Air Force, and 7.5% in the Marines.

Severity of combat exposure varied with branch of military service.

As Table 7.4 shows, veterans who served in the Marines and, to a lesser extent, the Army, were much more likely than those who served in the Air Force or Navy to be in the two high exposure categories of the MHM and the high exposure category of the CESS.

Substantial majorities of the majority whites (62.1%) and Hispanics (59.1%) enlisted voluntarily. Only a minority (40.7%) of blacks did so. Unlike the other two groups, the majority of blacks were drafted. Among the men who enlisted voluntarily or to avoid the draft, majority whites were much more likely to choose the Navy or Air Force compared with blacks. Hispanics who voluntarily enlisted were similar to majority whites in choosing these two low combat severity branches, but also, unlike majority whites, Hispanics had a substantial proportion who enlisted in the Marines. The net result of these choices and chances is summarized in Table 7.5.

Table 7.5 PERCENTAGES OF MAJORITY WHITES, BLACKS, AND HISPANICS WHO SERVED IN EACH BRANCH

Racial/Ethnic Group	Army	Marines	Navy	Air Force	Total
Majority Whites (94)	56.6%	5.3%	23.4%	14.6%	100%
Blacks (70)	69.5%	15.7%	7.5%	7.3%	100%
Hispanics (84)	44.6%	17.5%	13.3%	24.6%	100%
All Three Groups (248)	57.5%	7.5%	20.6%	14.3%	100%

Note: Percentages are weighted to the population from which the subsample was drawn. Unweighted subsample *n*'s are in parentheses.

As Table 7.5 shows, blacks have the largest proportion in the two higher-combat branches of service—the Marines and the Army; Hispanics are similar to blacks in the Marines but differ from them in having much lower proportions in the Army. The majority white men differ from blacks in having much lower proportions in the two higher-combat branches and from Hispanics in having a lower proportion in the Marines. These racial/ethnic differences in branch of service appear to go far in accounting for the group differences in severity of exposure to combat.

Table 7.6 shows, however, that even within each branch of service, blacks, and to a lesser extent Hispanics, were exposed to more severe combat than whites. It seems possible that individual behaviors following entry into one of the service branches are related to severity of combat exposure and also contribute to the racial/ethnic

Table 7.6 PERCENTAGES OF VETERANS WHO EXPERIENCED HIGH LEVELS
OF COMBAT EXPOSURE ACCORDING TO THE MHM AND THE CESS, BY ETHNIC/
RACIAL GROUP, BRANCH OF SERVICE, AND WHETHER ENLISTED OR DRAFTED
INTO THE ARMY

Racial/Ethnic Group, Branch of Service, and Whether Drafted or Enlisted	Percentage at High Risk (MHM Levels 3 and 4)		Percentage with High CESS Scores (75th Percentile or Above)	
	Percentage	(n)	Percentage	(n)
Majority White				
Army (drafted)	11.5%	(20)	34.4%	(20)
Army (enlisted)	5.9%	(39)	28.0%	(38)
Marines	32.5%	(7)	32.5%	(7)
Air Force or Navy	1.4%	(30)	7.1%	(29)
Total	6.6%	(94)	21.5%	(94)
Black				
Army (drafted)	25.3%	(28)	56.2%	(26)
Army (enlisted)	37.0%	(21)	46.0%	(21)
Marines	68.0%	(14)	68.8%	(14)
Air Force or Navy	0.0%	(9)	0.0%	(8)
Total	32.4%	(69)	47.3%	(69)
Hispanic				
Army (drafted)	19.7%	(24)	59.0%	(23)
Army (enlisted)	9.5%	(19)	22.0%	(19)
Marines	71.3%	(19)	71.1%	(19)
Air Force or Navy	1.8%	(22)	3.6%	(22)
Total	19.8%	(83)	32.3%	(83)

Note: Percentages are weighted to reflect the population from which the subsample was drawn. *N*'s are unweighted sample numbers.

differences in severity of exposure. One of the types of behavior we consider is volunteering for dangerous assignments. We measure this variable by responses to the question, "Did you ever volunteer for any special jobs, such as medic, special forces, long range reconnaissance patrols (LRRP), or something else? (If "yes"), What kind of special jobs?" On the basis of the latter information, it was possible to limit positive responses to jobs that were indeed dangerous. We also investigated whether heroic action measured by a military record of having received one or more medals for valor in combat played a part. It seems possible, as well, that pre-war college education and above average AFQT score qualified some veterans for skilled clerical and technical support roles.

As Table 7.7 shows, none of these additional variables have independent effects nearly so large as branch of service on MHM exposure or on severity of exposure measured by the composite scale. Nor do they have nearly so much impact on the racial/ethnic differences in exposure.

Is it possible that racial/ethnic discrimination played a part in the group differences in severity of exposure? We do not have an objective measure of discrimination. We do, however, have a measure of perceived racial and ethnic prejudice and discrimination. Minority veterans answered five questions about their perceptions of whether they were discriminated against because of their ethnic or racial background with reference to being (a) sent to Vietnam, (b) demoted or denied a promotion, (c) given an unpleasant duty assignment, (d) given a dangerous duty assignment, and (e) in some other way treated unfairly. These items formed an additive scale with internal consistency reliabilities of .80 for blacks and .79 for Hispanics. blacks with a mean of 1.55 scored much higher on this scale than Hispanics, with a mean of .41; $p < 000$ for the difference.

This measure was not administered to majority whites, so we must limit the analysis to blacks and Hispanics. Table 7.8 shows that blacks' odds of high combat exposure as measured by the CESS and of high exposure risk as indicated by the MHM are higher than the odds for Hispanics. (Odds ratios are 1.633 and 1.895, respectively, with each exposure measure.) When differences in branch of service and method of entry (whether drafted or enlisted if in the Army) are controlled, these odds ratios are reduced (to 1.244 and 1.698, respectively). Adding the scale of reported discrimination to the model further reduces these odds ratios only slightly (to 1.064 and 1.537, respectively). So the role of reported or perceived discrimination in explaining blacks' higher exposure is small if not negligible. One further test is in order. The discrimination scale encompasses a broad range of forms of possible discrimination, but one item is clearly related to exposure to life-threatening danger. This item asks, "Do you think you were ever given dangerous duty assignments while you were in (or around) Vietnam because you're (black/Hispanic)?" Once military entry is held constant, this item does little or nothing to reduce blacks' greater odds of severe combat exposure as compared to Hispanics.

Table 7.7 LOGISTIC REGRESSION MODELS PREDICTING COMBAT EXPOSURE ACCORDING TO TWO MEASURES

A. Dependent Variable Is High MHM (Level 3 or 4)

Contrasts and Independent Variables	OR	(p)	OR	(p)	OR	(p)
Racial/Ethnic Group						
Black vs. White	6.55	(.000)	4.74	(.008)	4.27	(.046)
Hispanic vs. White	3.41	(.013)	2.66	(.049)	2.58	(.077)
Black vs. Hispanic	1.92	(.13)	1.78	(.22)	1.65	(.077)
Military Service Category						
Army (drafted)			10.22	(.025)	10.39	(.029)
Army (enlisted)			7.52	(.055)	8.56	(.052)
Marines			53.37	(.000)	44.71	(.000)
Air Force or Navy (ref. gp.)			---	---	---	---
Overall Significance				(.001)		(.003)
Other Factors (all dichotomous)						
Medals for Valor					2.79	(.068)
Volunteered for Dangerous Duty					0.73	(.68)
H.S. Graduate or Less					1.39	(.61)
Lower AFQT Score					1.01	(.99)

B. Dependent Variable Is High CESS Score (75th percentile or higher)

Contrasts and Independent Variables	OR	(p)	OR	(p)	OR	(p)
Racial/Ethnic Group						
Black vs. White	3.06	(.003)	2.23	(.047)	1.74	(.21)
Hispanic vs. White	1.88	(.12)	1.66	(.16)	1.08	(.85)
Black vs. Hispanic	1.63	(.24)	1.34	(.45)	1.62	(.22)
Military Service Category						
Army (drafted)			8.90	(.001)	10.58	(.000)
Army (enlisted)			5.98	(.005)	6.93	(.003)
Marines			11.10	(.001)	9.64	(.003)
Air Force or Navy (ref. gp.)			---	---	---	---
Overall Significance				(.003)		(.003)
Other Factors (all dichotomous)						
Medals for Valor					1.28	(.54)
Volunteered for Dangerous Duty					1.003	(.996)
H.S. Graduate or Less					1.80	(.30)
Lower AFQT Score					1.47	(.44)

Note: These analyses take into account the complex subsample design.

Table 7.8 ODDS OF COMBAT EXPOSURE BY TWO MEASURES FOR BLACKS AS COMPARED TO HISPANICS: UNADJUSTED, ADJUSTED FOR MILITARY ENTRY, FOR MILITARY ENTRY AND PERCEIVED DISCRIMINATION, AND FOR MILITARY ENTRY AND PERCEIVED DISCRIMINATION IN DANGEROUS ASSIGNMENTS

Effect of Being Black (vs. Hispanic)	High CESS (>75%) O.R. (p)	High MHM O.R. (p)
Unadjusted	1.633 (.18)	1.895 (.12)
Adjusted for MilEntryTypology	1.244 (.60)	1.698 (.27)
Adjusted for MilEntryTypology and Prej/Discrim	1.064 (.89)	1.537 (.39)
Adjusted for MilEntryTypology and Dangerous Assignments*	1.134 (.78)	1.809 (.28)

Note: These analyses take into account the complex subsample design.

Diagnosed subsample: Blacks and Hispanics only.

*This is one item in the five-item Prejudice/Discrimination scale.

SUMMARY AND CONCLUSIONS

Consistent with the results of previous research that found higher rates of PTSD-like symptoms and other psychological problems in black Vietnam veterans than in majority white veterans, Kulka et al. (1990) reported higher prevalence rates of current PTSD in blacks in the NVVRS. These investigators also found Hispanic rates of current PTSD that were even higher than black rates. However, unlike the elevated rate in blacks, the elevated rate in Hispanics could not be accounted for by the greater severity of exposure to war-zone stressors reported by the two minorities compared with majority whites. And the finding of a higher rate of current PTSD in Hispanics than in blacks posed an additional puzzle because the Hispanics reported less severe exposure to war-zone stressors than did the blacks in the NVVRS.

Apart from these unsolved substantive questions, there were methodological problems with these previous results. The exposure measure was based on retrospective reports by veterans that were open to recall biases and on a measure of current PTSD that left it unclear whether the racial/ethnic differences were due to risk factors for the onset of PTSD, for adverse course, or both; and the measure of current PTSD may have had other limitations (see our Chapter 4).

We attempted to resolve these methodological and substantive problems by using record-based measures of exposure to war-zone stressors and diagnostic histories in a subsample of NVVRS veterans. Since the record-based measure of exposure was less than fully comprehensive of war-zone combat experiences, we cross-checked the results with a more comprehensive measure that adds self-report indicators to the MHM. It is of interest that the racial/ethnic differences, while replicated, are less on the composite measure of exposure than on the MHMs alone. This may be due to some racial/ethnic response bias in the self-report indicators added to the composite measure; or, alternatively, to under-representation in the MHM of combat experiences that were more widespread than those that correlated highly with the MHM; for example, casualties from sapper and mortar attacks on rear-echelon military headquarters and bases. Nevertheless, the results are similar with the two measures of severity of exposure.

Breaking new ground, we found that both blacks and Hispanics had higher rates of war-related first onsets of PTSD and current PTSD than majority whites. However, while blacks and Hispanics had similar rates of PTSD onset to each other, PTSD course was more chronic for Hispanics, resulting in higher rates of current PTSD in Hispanics than in blacks.

Unlike current PTSD, past PTSD showed no association with racial/ethnic background and exposure. For this reason, we focused on current PTSD in our investigation of why previous research found that exposure accounted for most of the elevation in black but not for the even greater elevation in Hispanic rates of current PTSD. We replicated with our new record-based measure of exposure the finding with self-reported exposure by Kulka et al. (1990) that Hispanics, and even more so blacks, experienced more severe war-zone stressors than majority whites. Also consistent with the previous results of Kulka et al. (1990), we found that, while control of severity of exposure nearly eliminated the difference in rates of current PTSD between black veterans and majority white veterans, it did not come close to eliminating the difference between Hispanics and majority whites. Nor did control of exposure account for the higher rate of current PTSD in Hispanics than in blacks.

To address these continuing puzzles, we investigated a variety of other possible explanations. On the basis of findings by Lewis-Fernández et al. (2008), we discounted the possibility that an ethno-cultural factor of greater expressivity in Hispanics contributed to an over-diagnosis of PTSD. Moreover, the prime vulnerability candidate of pre-war psychiatric disorder did not show differences in rate among the three racial/ethnic groups. Nor did Hispanics report more personal involvement than blacks in harming civilians or prisoners, a variable that is strongly associated with war-related PTSD. We also investigated and discounted the possibilities that Hispanics (a) experienced more prejudice and discrimination in Vietnam than blacks; (b) were met with more adverse reactions upon homecoming than blacks or majority whites; and/or (c) had more adverse post-war events such as marital separations/divorces and periods of unemployment.

We found, rather, that a set of pre-war vulnerability factors was critically important. Hispanics were younger than black veterans when they went to Vietnam, and they had less pre-war education and lower AFQT scores than majority whites, and, to a lesser degree, than blacks. Focusing on these variables, we found that controlling their lower education, lower AFQT scores, and greater exposure accounted for the higher rates of current PTSD in Hispanics compared with majority whites. Moreover, controlling age, education, and AFQT scores accounted for the higher rates of current PTSD in Hispanics than in blacks, despite the greater exposure of blacks to war-zone stressors. These greater vulnerabilities in Hispanics may override in importance other factors, such as blacks' more severe exposure to war-zone stress and blacks' reports of experiencing more prejudice and negative homecoming reactions.

These results have important historical and contemporary implications. As we noted at the outset, Vietnam was the first war in which blacks were fully integrated into U.S. military units. The change resulted, however, in blacks going from near exclusion from combat roles in World War I and World War II, with only the beginnings of change in the Korean conflict (Bogart, 1969), to being more exposed to war-zone stressors than men from majority white backgrounds in Vietnam. Blacks did more than their share of the fighting, and paid a greater psychological price that was wholly commensurate with that excess of combat.

Hispanics were also more exposed to war-zone stressors than majority whites and paid more of a psychological price, but Hispanics were less exposed than blacks. The additional factors of younger age, less pre-war education, and lower AFQT scores appear to have put them at greater psychological risk than either black or white majority veterans. The reason may be that younger age than blacks was the critical vulnerability factor for Hispanics.

Because of the major role of severity of combat exposure in the racial/ethnic differences, we investigated the question of why the combat exposure of blacks and, to a lesser degree, Hispanics, was more severe than the combat exposure of majority whites. We found little evidence that pre-Vietnam educational level, AFQT score, or possible psychological predispositions indicated by volunteering for dangerous assignments, or even being awarded medals for valor in combat played substantial parts in the group differences in severity of combat exposure.

Rather, the main reason for the group differences in severity of exposure appears to be racial/ethnic contrasts in the military branches in which the veterans served. The majority of veterans enlisted in the military, although a substantial minority were drafted. Those who enlisted could express a choice of branch of service. Majority whites who enlisted tended to choose the Navy or Air Force, where relatively few men served in severe combat compared to those in the Marines and the Army. In contrast, blacks were the group most likely to be drafted into the Army and, like Hispanics, to be more likely than majority whites to enlist in the Marines. These are the main factors in the group differences in severity of combat exposure. They are not, however, the only factors. Within branches of services, there were also racial/ethnic differences in severity of combat exposure. Taken singly, individual differences in behaviors, such as volunteering for dangerous assignments, did not account for these differences. It is, therefore, possible that accumulations of such factors or some unmeasured variables, such as actual prejudice and discrimination, were also involved.

ACKNOWLEDGMENT

This chapter expands on the following article: Dohrenwend, B. P., Turner, J. B., Turse, N. A., Lewis-Fernández, R. and Yager, T. J. (2008), War-related posttraumatic stress

disorder in black, Hispanic, and majority white veterans: The roles of exposure and vulnerability. *Journal of Traumatic Stress, 21*(2), 133–141.
  Publisher: International Society for Traumatic Stress Studies: Wiley InterScience.

REFERENCES

Allen, I. M. (1986). Posttraumatic stress disorder among black Vietnam veterans. *Hospital and Community Psychiatry, 37*, 55–61.
Anderson, T. H. (2007). Vietnam is here: The anti-war movement. In D. L. Anderson & J. Ernst (Eds.), *The war that never ends: New perspectives on the Vietnam war*. Lexington, KY: University Press of Kentucky.
Appy, C. G. (1993). *Working class war: American combat soldiers and Vietnam*. Chapel Hill, NC: University of North Carolina Press.
Baskir, L. M., & Strauss, W. A. (1978). *Chance and circumstance: The draft, the war and the Vietnam generation*. New York: Alfred A. Knopf.
Beals, J., Manson S. M., Shore J. H., Friedman M., Ashcraft M., Fairbank, J., & Schlenger W. (2002). The prevalence of posttraumatic stress disorder among American Indian Vietnam veterans: Disparities and context. *Journal of Traumatic Stress, 15*, 89–97.
Bogart, L. (1969). *Social research and desegregation of the U.S. Army*. Chicago, IL: Markam.
Buckley, K. (2007). "'The Graham Greene argument": A Vietnam parallel that escaped George W. Bush. *World Policy Journal, 24*(3), 89–98.
Centers for Disease Control. (1988). Health status for Vietnam veterans: 1. Psychosocial characteristics. *Journal of the American Medical Association, 259*, 2701–2707.
Cleaver, L. E. (1968). *Soul on ice*. New York: McGraw-Hill.
Clodfelter, M. (1995). *Vietnam in military statistics: A history of the Indochina wars, 1772-1991*. Jefferson, NC: McFarland and Co.
Cortright, D. (1990). Black GI resistance during the Vietnam war. *Vietnam Generation, 2*(1), 51–64.
Daugherty, L. J., & Mattson, G. L., 2001. *Nam: A photographic history*. Metro Books.
Dohrenwend, B. P., Neria, Y., Turner, B. J., Turse, N., Marshall, R., Lewis-Fernández, R. et al. (2004). Positive tertiary appraisals and posttraumatic stress disorder in U.S. male veterans of the war in Vietnam: The roles of positive affirmation, positive reformulation, and defensive denial. *Journal of Consulting and Clinical Psychology, 72*, 417–433.
Dohrenwend, B. P., Turner, J. B., Turse, N. A., Adams, B. G., Koenen, K. C., & Marshall, R. (2006). The psychological risks of Vietnam for U.S. Veterans: A revisit with new data and methods. *Science, 313*, 979–982.
Frueh, B. C., Elhai, J. D., Grubaugh, A. L., Monnier, J., Kashdan, T. B., Sauvageot, J. A., et al. (2005). Documented combat exposure of U.S. veterans seeking treatment for combat-related post-traumatic stress disorder. *British Journal of Psychiatry, 186*, 467–472.
Gibson, J. W. (2000). *The perfect war: Technowar in Vietnam*. Boston, MA: Atlantic Monthly Press.
Graham, H., III. (2003). *The brothers' war: Black power, manhood, and the military experience*. Gainesville, FL: University Press of Florida.
Green, B. L., Grace, M. C., Lindy, J. D., & Leonard, A. C. (1990). Race differences in response to combat stress. *Journal of Traumatic Stress, 3*, 379–393.
Guzman, R. (1970). *Mexican American casualties in Vietnam*. Santa Cruz, CA: University of California at Santa Cruz.
Helmer, J. (1974). *Bringing the war home: The American soldier in Vietnam and after*. New York: Free Press.

Hunt, P. N., Schlenger, W. E., Jordan, B. K., Fairbank, J. A., LaVange, L. M., & Potter, F. J. (1994). *NVVRS public use analysis file documentation: Analysis variables from the National Vietnam Veterans Readjustment Study.* Research Triangle Park, NC: Research Triangle Institute.

King, M. L., Jr. (1967, April 4). Beyond Vietnam (speech). Riverside Church, New York, NY.

Koenen, K. C., Stellman, J. M., Stellman, S. D., & Sommer, J. F. (2003). Risk factors for course of posttraumatic stress disorder among Vietnam veterans: A 14-year follow-up of American Legionnaires. *Journal of Consulting and Clinical Psychology, 71,* 980–986.

Kulka, R. A., Schlenger, W. E., Fairbank, J. A., Hough, R. L., Jordan, B. K., Marmar, C. R., et al. (1988). *National Vietnam Veterans Readjustment Study (NVVRS): Description, current status, and initial PTSD prevalence estimates.* Washington, DC: Veterans Administration.

Kulka, R. A., Schlenger, W. E., Fairbank, J. A., Hough, R. L., Jordan, B. K., Marmar, C. R., et al. (1990). *Trauma and the Vietnam war generation.* New York: Brunner/Mazel.

Laufer, R. S., Gallops, M. S., & Frey-Wouters, E. (1984). War stress and trauma: The Vietnam veteran experience. *Journal of Health and Social Behavior, 25,* 68–72.

Levy, D. W. (1995). *The debate over Vietnam* (2nd ed.). Baltimore, MD: Johns Hopkins University Press.

Lewis-Fernández, R., Turner, J. B., Marshall, R., Neria, Y., & Dohrenwend, B. P. (2008). Elevated rates of current PTSD among Hispanic veterans in the NVVRS: True prevalence or methodological artifact? *Journal of Traumatic Stress, 21,* 123–132.

Lewy, G. (1978). *America in Vietnam.* New York: Oxford University Press.

MacDonald, C., Chamberlin, K., & Long, N. (1997). Race, combat, and PTSD in a community sample of New Zealand Vietnam war veterans. *Journal of Traumatic Stress, 10,* 117–124.

Mariscal, G., ed. (1999). *Aztlan and Vietnam: Chicano and Chicana experiences of the war.* Berkeley, CA: University of California Press.

McNally, R. J. (2003). Progress and controversy in the study of posttraumatic stress disorder. *Annual Review of Psychology, 54,* 229–252.

Moskos, C. C. (1970). *The American enlisted man: The rank and file in today's military.* New York: Russell Sage Foundation, distributed by Basic Books. Abridged and reprinted in Bernard Rosenberg, ed., Analysis of Contemporary Society (NY: Thomas Y. Crowell, 1974, pp. 74–150).

Ortega, A. N., &Rosenheck. R. (2000). Posttraumatic stress disorder among Hispanic Vietnam veterans. *American Journal of Psychiatry, 157,* 615–619.

Parson, E. R. (1984). The gook-identification syndrome and posttraumatic stress disorder in black Vietnam veterans. *The Black Psychiatrists of America Quarterly, 13,* 14–18.

Penk, W. E., Robinowitz, R., Black, J., Dolan, M., Bell, W., Dorsett, D., et al. (1989). Ethnicity: Post-traumatic stress disorder (PTSD) differences among black, white, and Hispanic veterans who differ in degrees of exposure to combat in Vietnam. *Journal of Clinical Psychology, 45,* 729–735.

Polner, M. (1971). *No victory parades: The return of the Vietnam veteran.* New York: Holt, Rinehart & Winston.

Roemer, L., Litz, B., Orsillo, S., Ehlich, P. J., & Friedman, M. J. (1998). Increases in retrospective accounts of war-zone exposure over time: The role of PTSD symptom severity. *Journal of Traumatic Stress, 11,* 597–605.

Ruef, A. M., Litz, B. T., & Schlenger, W. E. (2000). Hispanic ethnicity and risk for combat-related PTSD. *Cultural Diversity and Ethnic Minority Psychology, 6,* 235–251.

Schlenger, W., & Fairbank, J. (1996). Ethnocultural considerations in understanding PTSD and related disorders among military veterans. In A. J. Marsella, M. J. Friedman, E. T. Gerrity, & R. M. Scurfield (Eds.), *Ethnocultural aspects of PTSD: Issues, research, and clinical application* (pp. 529–538). Washington, DC: American Psychological Association.

Schnurr, P. P., Lunney, C. A., & Sengupta, A. (2004). Risk factors for the development versus maintenance of posttraumatic stress disorder. *Journal of Traumatic Stress, 17,* 85–95.

Southwick, S. M., Morgan, C. A., & Nicolau, A. L. (1997). Consistency of memory for combat-related traumatic events in veterans of Operation Desert Storm. *American Journal of Psychiatry, 154,* 173–177.

Spitzer, R., Williams, J., & Gibbon, M. (1987). *Structured clinical interview for DSM-III-R, version NP-V.* New York: New York State Psychiatric Institute, Biometrics Research Department.

Susser, E., Schwartz, S., Morabia, A., & Bromet, E. J. (2006). *Psychiatric epidemiology: Searching for the causes of mental disorder.* New York: Oxford University Press.

Terry, W. (1984). Bloods: An oral history of the Vietnam war by black veterans. New York: Random House.

Thompson, L. (1990). *The U.S. Army in Vietnam.* New York: Sterling Publishing Co.

Trujillo, C. (1990). *Soldados: Chicanos in Viet Nam.* San Jose, CA: Chusma House Publications.

Van Deburg, W. (1992). *New day in Babylon: The black power movement and American culture, 1965–1975.* Chicago, IL: University of Chicago Press.

Wessely, S., & Jones, E. (2004). Psychiatry and the "lessons of Vietnam": What were they, and are they still relevant? *War & Society, 22,* 89–103.

Westheider, J. E. (1997). *Fighting on two fronts: African Americans and the Vietnam war.* New York: New York University Press.

CHAPTER 8

࿏

PTSD in Women Who Served as Nurses in Vietnam

THOMAS J. YAGER AND BRUCE P. DOHRENWEND

It was a wonderful, horrible experience. I felt that everything that I had ever learned in my career, I put to use in Vietnam. I felt that I was in control. I wasn't a subservient individual. Vietnam gave me a feeling of accomplishment. I actually had the power to do what I wanted to do. In the states, you don't have that. (Nurse quoted in Freedman & Rhoads, 1987, p. 68)

On the basis of the nationally representative NVVRS sample, Kulka et al. (1990, p. 18) estimate that 7,166 women served in the Vietnam theater. We estimate, based on military records and self-reports, that 85% of those women were nurses. A substantial proportion of them developed war-related PTSD. That disorder's very definition arose in response to symptoms suffered by men with combat experience in the Vietnam war, but nurses did not have combat roles in Vietnam. However, the bases and hospitals where they served were subject to shelling and, perhaps more importantly, the very nature of their work was often highly stressful. On the other hand, their work could also be highly rewarding, and many found a sense of comradeship and professional effectiveness in Vietnam that exceeded anything they had experienced in civilian life.

Our purpose here is to identify stressful experiences and personal vulnerabilities associated with PTSD, as well as factors that may have protected against it, among the nurses in our sample, all of whom were women.

As explained in Chapter 4, we have found limitations and problems with the NVVRS Projected Probability algorithm, so we rely on the psychiatric diagnoses made by clinician interviewers in the NVVRS's diagnosed subsample. We concentrate on nurses rather than women in general for the very practical reason that, in that subsample, women who served in other capacities are too few to analyze separately ($n = 12$). But the exclusion of non-nurses from our analysis also offers a fortuitous benefit for the possible generalizability of our results to later wars. Military nurses' duties have certainly changed less since Vietnam than have the duties of other women soldiers, who are now eligible to serve in combat roles and have done so in Afghanistan and Iraq.

COMPARISON WITH MALE VETERANS

Based on the NVVRS diagnostic interview, an estimated 16.8% of nurses serving in Vietnam had onsets of war-related PTSD, with 5.2% having cases that persisted until the time of the interview ("current" PTSD). Because most women veterans served as nurses, estimated rates of PTSD are similar for women veterans as a whole. As Table 8.1 shows, these rates fall roughly midway between those for male veterans with low and those with moderate probable combat exposure on our military historical measure (MHM).

But nurses differed from male veterans on at least three demographic variables. By virtue of their professional training, they were more highly educated on average than the men, and they were older when they arrived in Vietnam. Also unlike the men, they were nearly all white—all were white in the diagnosed subsample. Any of these demographic variables might plausibly have accounted for at least part of the gap between nurses' rates

Table 8.1 RATES OF PTSD ONSET AND CURRENT PTSD IN MALE AND FEMALE VIETNAM VETERANS, DISTINGUISHING NURSES FROM NON-NURSES (WOMEN) AND EXPOSURE LEVELS (MEN)

	PTSD Onset	Current PTSD	N
A. Male and Female Veterans			
Male	21.6%	10.9%	248
Female	16.0%	5.0%	73
Male vs. Female	$(p = .30)$	$(p = .06)$	
B. Female Veterans			
Nurses	16.8%	5.2%	61
Non-nurses	12.1%	4.0%	12
Nurses vs. Non-nurses	$(p = .64)$	$(p = .80)$	
C. Male Veterans by Exposure Level (MHM)			
Low	10.3%	0.3%	38
Moderate	23.3%	12.3%	152
High	38.6%	27.0%	37
Very high	38.7%	33.6%	21
Overall comparison	$(p = .08)$	$(p = .00)$	

Note: Percentages are weighted to the population from which the subsample was drawn. N's are unweighted sample numbers.

of PTSD and those of highly-exposed male veterans. In fact, however, they make relatively little difference and do not substantially change the picture.

The first column of Table 8.2 repeats what we presented in Table 8.1; again, nurses (the reference group, with odds ratio [OR] = 1 by definition) fall between low exposure and moderate exposure male veterans. The second column adds demographic variables to the model as controls. The odds ratios are somewhat smaller, but again, nurses fall between low exposure and moderate exposure male veterans.

In the first two columns of Table 8.2, the results on current PTSD are roughly consistent with those found by members of our research group in a comparison of male and female veterans in the full NVVRS sample (Turner, Turse, & Dohrenwend, 2007). That study used the NVVRS Projected Probability algorithm whose utility we now question, as noted.

The last column in Table 8.2 gives odds ratios adjusted, not only for demographic variables, but also for four vulnerability factors—childhood family member arrested,

Table 8.2 ODDS RATIOS FOR PTSD IN MALE VETERANS AT DIFFERENT LEVELS OF PROBABLE WAR-ZONE EXPOSURE RELATIVE TO NURSE VETERANS (ALL OF WHOM WERE WOMEN)

	Control Variables		
	No Control	Demographic Variables	Demographic Variables and Vulnerability Factors
A. PTSD Onset			
Nurses (reference group)			
Low exposure men	.565	.436	.524
Moderate exposure men	1.504	1.532	1.354
High exposure men	3.112	2.669	240.800*
Very high exposure men	3.122	2.100	1.858
Overall comparison	$(p = .14)$	$(p = .21)$	$(p = .000)$
B. Current PTSD			
Nurses (reference group)			
Low exposure men	.056*	.037*	.003
Moderate exposure men	2.543	1.974	.259
High exposure men	6.726*	4.646	20.545
Very high exposure men	9.170*	4.992	1.530
Overall comparison	$(p = .000)$	$(p = .000)$	$(p = .096)$

Note: These analyses take into account the complex sampling design. Controls in column 2 are race/ethnicity, age at entry to Vietnam, and pre-military education. The latter two variables take the multi-categorical form used by Turner et al. (2007). Controls in column 3 are race/ethnicity, age at entry to Vietnam, pre-military education (dichotomized this time: nurses and persons with some college vs. all others), childhood family member arrested, childhood family member abused alcohol or drugs, pre-Vietnam conduct disorder, and any other pre-Vietnam psychiatric disorder.

*This group differs significantly from nurse veterans, $p < .05$.

childhood family member abused alcohol or drugs, childhood conduct disorder, and any other pre-Vietnam psychiatric disorder. We chose these particular vulnerability factors because we had found them to discriminate male veterans diagnosed as having had PTSD onsets or current PTSD from those not so diagnosed, and because they were available for both men and women. This last column shows odds ratios comparing nurses to men with various levels of probable combat exposure. For PTSD onset, nurses fall once more between low exposure and moderate exposure male veterans. For current PTSD, however, they fall between moderate exposure and high exposure male veterans. With or without controls, nurses' rates of PTSD onset and current PTSD are considerably higher than those of low exposure male veterans.

POSSIBLE RISK AND PROTECTIVE FACTORS

What accounts for the high incidence of war-related PTSD among nurses? While they did not serve in combat, they were exposed to some of the personal risks associated with a war zone that had no fixed fronts. Moreover, in the course of their work, nurses were confronted with not only the physical presence of many freshly and severely wounded soldiers, but also the sometimes overwhelming responsibility of caring for them. While the challenge of their work was stressful, it was often highly rewarding as well. Shared responsibility under stress could forge bonds of comradeship among nurses. Some women (nurses and non-nurses alike) were subjected to sexual harassment and even rape by fellow American soldiers. Finally, personal vulnerabilities the nurses brought with them when they arrived in Vietnam may have made some of them more susceptible to PTSD than others.

A number of researchers have studied women veterans of the Vietnam war using data from the NVVRS (King et al., 1996; Fontana et al., 1997; Turner, Turse, & Dohrenwend, 2007). In this chapter, we expand on previous studies by introducing a measure of war stress reflecting the nature of nurses' demanding work that is based on the military record rather than personal recollection, examining the effects of nursing specialty, focusing on the possible role of a supportive work environment, and investigating their on-going exposure to sexual harassment and assault. In addition, using clinical diagnoses of the subsample, we look at individual nurses' periods of service during the war, their assignment to duties in the operating room, and their pre-Vietnam vulnerability to assess both the onset of war-related PTSD and its persistence years later at the time of the nurses' interviews. Our ability to distinguish PTSD onset from current PTSD allows us to analyze separately the factors associated with each.

Nature of Nursing in Vietnam

Any study of PTSD in war veterans begins, quite naturally, by assessing the stressful conditions inherent in the war itself. Nurses were generally assigned to base camp areas where their primary combat exposure took the form of stand-off attacks, usually from mortars and rockets, and, to a lesser extent, sapper raids on the camps. During the 1968 Tet Offensive, large military bases, such as those at Tan Son Nhut and Bien Hoa, were also subject to enemy attack by battalion-sized forces. (For more on the various forms of base attacks, see Fox, 1979.) Seventy-six percent of nurses in the full NVVRS sample (77% in the diagnosed subsample) reported having come under enemy fire at least once in Vietnam, yet only one American military nurse is believed to have died as the result of enemy attack during the entire war. Lieutenant Sharon Lane died from shrapnel wounds when the 312th Evacuation Hospital at Chu Lai was hit by rockets on June 8, 1969 (Memorial to Lt. Sharon Ann Lane at the "Virtual Wall" website; Norman, 1990).

While the proportion of male veterans who experienced hostile fire in base camps may not have been any higher, women in the war zone would not normally have faced enemy ambushes, mines and booby traps, or firefights with enemy forces, as combat soldiers did. But nurses' work did bring them into frequent and intimate contact with wounded and dying soldiers. The nature and psychological consequences of this contact are a central concern of this chapter.

Nursing was a stressful but rewarding job. Both aspects of wartime nursing are encapsulated in a personal experience described by Jacqueline Navarra Rhoads (Freedman & Rhoads, 1987, pp. 19–21). She had been in Vietnam about seven months when a soldier was brought in who had been shot in the face.

> It was the middle of the night and I was on duty with a medical corpsman, no doctors around at all. . . . I told the corpsman that the only time I'd ever done a trach [tracheotomy] was on a goat back in basic training at Fort Sam Houston. The corpsman said, "If you don't do it, he'll die." So he put my gloves on for me, and handed me the scalpel. I was shaking so badly I thought I'd cut his throat.

She made the incision, inserted the tube, and the man began breathing easily. He was sent on to Da Nang within minutes, where Rhoads happened to see him three months later. He tapped her on the shoulder in the mess hall. Despite his injuries, he had gotten a good look at her during the tracheotomy, and he recognized her then and said, "I'll never forget you."

> I wanted to go back to the hospital and tell the others, "Hey, you remember what's-his-name? He's from Arkansas and he's doing fine." We always wanted to put names to faces, but we rarely got a chance to do it. You kept believing that everyone who left the hospital actually lived. When you found out someone actually had survived, it helped staff morale. (Freedman & Rhoads, 1987, pp. 19–21)

Conditions were often difficult, but American soldiers in Vietnam received more effective medical care than in earlier wars. In an official medical-military history, Neel (1991, p. 172) concludes that:

> The wounded soldier in Vietnam received better care more quickly than in any previous conflict. This was possible because . . . relatively small numbers of helicopters

with an exclusive medical mission could evacuate large numbers of patients to centrally located medical facilities. As the years went by, equipment was updated, more powerful helicopters were used . . . , radio communications were refined . . . , and air ambulance crews were given sufficient basic medical training to enable them to evaluate a patient's condition, to recommend the most suitable destination, and to provide resuscitative care en route.

More effective transport was enormously helpful to wounded soldiers, but it made doctors' and nurses' work more difficult, as "rapid helicopter evacuation brought into the hospital mortally wounded patients who, with earlier, slower means of evacu- ation, would have died en route" (Neel, p. 51). As a result, more catastrophically wounded patients were able to reach hospitals, and nurses were exposed to more gruesome injuries and witnessed the deaths of patients who, in the past, would have died before they reached the hospital. Furthermore, efficient transport could do nothing to prevent the fact that nurses sometimes had to deal with exceptionally large numbers of patients at one time. A nurse assigned to a mobile Army surgical hospital recalled:

During Operation Attleboro in November 1966, we treated more than 300 patients during a 96-hour period. We each had three hours of sleep. The casualties began coming in . . . on Thursday. We finally finished on Sunday afternoon. The helicopter pad was designed to hold one helicopter at a time. When I looked out on Friday, there were four helicopters landing with patients at the same time. (Hartl, 1991, p. 1198)

Even in the absence of such mass-casualty incidents, everyday work could be ex- ceptionally taxing. "We worked a six-day week with 12-hour shifts. Any nurse that has worked 12-hour shifts knows it isn't 12 hours, it's 14 to 16 hours. In the 365 days that I was in Vietnam, I may have gotten off early 10 times," a male nurse recalled (Seymour, 2002, p. 13).

In addition, nurses had duties in Vietnam, such as closing wounds, which were re- served for doctors in civilian hospitals (Freedman & Rhoads, 1987). These duties could be a shock and a surprise when nurses first confronted conditions in the war zone. An Army nurse recalled:

I had to amputate the leg of one patient. That was the first time I ever had to do that. His leg was hanging by a tissue band. I was new there, and the doctor yelled at me to "get the damn thing off." . . . I took out my pocket knife, and I cut it off. . . . I'm holding this leg, and the doctor, with a few choice words, says "Get rid of the leg, and come up here and help me." I didn't know what to do with the leg, so I threw it in the trash can. I have felt guilty ever since. (Scannell-Desch, August 2000, pp. 533–534)

The bullet wounds that nurses dealt with were typically made by high-velocity, lightweight rounds from AK-47 assault rifles and M-16 automatic rifles. These weapons left larger temporary and permanent cavities and more severe tissue damage . . . and their easy deflection by foliage resulted in tumbling and spinning and the generation of even larger entrance wounds. . . . These rapid fire weapons increased the chances of multiple wounding, which complicated resuscitation and treatment. (Neel, 1991, p. 53)

In addition to treating especially challenging gunshot wounds and injuries due to shrapnel from rockets and mortars, nurses also dealt with complex and grotesque injuries caused by mines and booby traps (Neel, 1991, p. 54). They encountered men who had lost limbs, genitals, or their sight.

I had never seen shrapnel wounds, just like I had never seen a traumatic amputation. . . . I didn't know what to do, so I just quit functioning. . . . But I knew I had eleven months to go. . . . I couldn't just sit there folded up in a chair not functioning. (LeVasseur, 2003, p 32)

Injuries caused by mines and booby traps frequently not only resulted in catastrophic bodily damage, but also caused dirt, shrapnel, and debris to contaminate the wound, making treatment even more difficult. The proportion of these injuries increased as the war advanced (Neel, 1991, p 53).

The wounded men were unusually young, as noted in Chapter 2. In World War II, the average American soldier was 26 years old. During the Vietnam war, the average draftee or enlistee was only 19. Marines as young as 17 fought and died in Vietnam (Appy, 1993; Clodfelter, 1995). "What got to me the most was the youth of the patients and the terrible injuries they sustained. It was very hard to deal with; they were just kids," recalled an Air Force intensive care unit (ICU) nurse who served in Vietnam (Scannell-Desch, 2000, p. 533). Another nurse remembered, "I looked down and saw this guy who was about 17 years old. He had both eyes out, and he was clutching a Purple Heart. I remember standing there and thinking, 'My God, that Purple Heart means nothing'" (LeVasseur, 2003, p. 33). An Army nurse recalled that, "Amputations were a common procedure. Sometimes, a patient would have two or three amputations at the same time. Emotionally, those were very difficult for me to deal with because the patients were so young" (Hartl, 1991, p. 1201).

All of these aspects of the stressful nature of nurses' work appear in a letter home written by an Army nurse who served during 1969 and 1970. After relating the story of a patient who endured two surgeries to save his leg, only to have it amputated on Christmas Eve due to the onset of gangrene, she wrote:

I've been working nights for a couple of weeks and have been spending a great deal of time in post-op. They've been incredibly busy. . . . This is now the seventh month of death, destruction, and misery. I'm tired of going to sleep listening to outgoing and incoming rockets, mortars and artillery. I'm sick of facing, every day, a new bunch of children ripped to pieces. They're just kids—eighteen, nineteen years old! It stinks! Whole lives ahead of them—cut off. I'm sick to death of it. I've got to get out of here. . . . (Edelman, 1985, p. 190)

Nurses working under such enormous pressure sometimes had to triage their patients, leaving aside men who were expected to die in order to treat those with better prospects (Freedman & Rhoads, 1987; Rogers & Nickolaus, 1987). Though circumstances and military protocol required it, the decision not to treat a severely injured patient was contrary to the nurses' civilian training, and the experience was understandably difficult for them (Freedman & Rhoads, 1987). Norman (1990, p. 38) writes:

> The women learned to measure death and soothe the way. These expectant soldiers were strangers. Military "dog tags" were their only identification. For the nurses, it was crucial that these anonymous soldiers not die alone or unattended. "When the end was near," said a former army nurse who cried as she remembered these scenes, "I would just stand near them. I felt that his mother would feel better knowing someone was standing with her son when he died."

Despite the stressful challenge of trauma medicine in Vietnam, many nurses also found it enormously fulfilling. Many missed their war-zone work when they returned to civilian life. Some even found their civilian roles so confining that, after a return to civilian nursing, they quit the profession altogether. Others stayed in the military to avoid a loss of professional authority (Freedman & Rhoads, 1987; Steinman, 2000).

Teamwork and Supportive Work Environment

We and others have identified not only traumatic experiences in Vietnam that are associated with subsequent PTSD, but also factors that may have moderated or exacerbated the effect of the traumatic experience itself. A comprehensive meta-analysis of risk factors for PTSD found that lack of social support exhibited a mean effect size larger than that for any other risk factor (Brewin, Andrews, & Valentine, 2000). Fontana et al. (1997) found that low social and material support when women veterans returned home were both risk factors for PTSD, but they did not examine the effects of teamwork, morale, or the social environment during the women's tours of duty in Vietnam.

A group confronted by a stressful situation may respond either by dissolving into a collection of disputing factions and uncooperative individuals or by pulling together to deal effectively with the common challenge. When danger evokes a collective positive response, stress-induced symptoms may be reduced. The groundbreaking sociologist Émile Durkheim (1951, pp. 166–167) argued that in circumstances such as war that call for widespread social solidarity, the rate of suicide declines in the general population. The "stronger integration of society," he suggested, was "due not to the crisis but to the struggles it occasions. As they force men to close ranks and confront the common danger, the individual thinks less of himself and more of the common cause." Durkheim's focus was on large populations, but the same principle might plausibly apply to smaller groups engaged in meeting a common challenge.

While the stress inherent in seeing and treating wounded and dying men may have produced psychiatric symptoms, the sense of significance nurses experienced in their work may sometimes have mitigated or prevented those symptoms. The highly coordinated teamwork and mutual support required by their job may have reinforced this sense of significance and may also have been protective in its own right.

This essentially social, cognitive, and emotional process may even have a hormonal parallel. In a broadly theoretical article, Taylor et al. (2000) argue that researchers studying reactions to stress may have focused too narrowly on the fight-or-flight response observed in their predominantly male subjects, missing a tend-and-befriend response that may be more typical of women. Evolution, they suggest, may have prepared women and females of other mammalian species to respond to danger by protecting their young ("tending") and affiliating with other adults ("befriending"). Citing animal studies, they suggest that, like fight-or-flight, this response may be mediated by a hormonal mechanism. "Oxytocin and endogenous opioid mechanisms may be at the core of the tending response," they say, citing the work of Panksepp, Nelson, and Bekkedal (1999). Oxytocin "may serve both to calm the female who is physiologically aroused by a stressor and also to promote affiliative behaviors, including maternal behavior toward offspring" (Taylor et al., 2000, pp. 415–416). They add that, like fight-or-flight, this response may occur in both sexes.

It is not necessary to accept their suggestion that this hormonal reaction is biologically more typical of females in order to recognize its possible relevance to the stress responses of nurses serving in Vietnam, whose work entailed not only tending to patients and, when possible, befriending them, but also intense cooperation with the medical team, which amounted to collegial befriending. If the tend-and-befriend response is a calming one, it may reduce symptomatic reactions—not only at the time of stress but, conceivably, years later. Whatever the mechanism—cognitive, emotional, or hormonal—we must seriously consider the possibility that military nurses' work in wartime has the potential both to produce symptoms and to protect against them, and that the strength of each effect may vary with circumstances.

Nurses' own accounts suggest that they responded collectively and cooperatively to the demands of their work. In a study of 50 Vietnam veteran nurses, Norman reports that more than half said their friendships in Vietnam were among the most intimate of their lives. One nurse said,

I don't think I have ever been as close to people as I was in Vietnam. I became friends with people I probably wouldn't have met at home. I couldn't have made it through the year without them. (Norman, 1990, p. 48)

Based on open-ended responses to four very general questions posed to a nonprobability sample of 24 women who had served in Vietnam as military nurses, Scannell-Desch reports that, "Many nurses described their colleagues as 'family.' There was a strong sense of teamwork characterized by people working together in the face of danger and uncertainty." One nurse stated, "There was a type of camaraderie that you just can't explain." Another added:

I have never been in a situation so professionally satisfying, even though you have to separate out that we never got used to seeing men blown apart. The people were always willing to help their colleagues. I've never seen this happen to that degree since Vietnam. It was professionalism at its best. (Scannell-Desch, 1996, p. 121)

We propose here the hypothesis that such teamwork helped to protect the nurses against symptoms induced by stress.

Good leadership may also be crucial to a satisfactory group experience. A survey conducted during the Gulf War provides a rare glimpse of nurses' responses to war-zone stress as reported at the time, rather than retrospectively. Dahl and O'Neal helped to establish a combat support hospital in Saudi Arabia ten miles from the Iraqi border and close enough to the front line that it was subject to missile attack. While serving in the hospital, which treated battle casualties during the war and for several days afterward, they distributed a brief open-ended questionnaire to their colleagues ($n = 43$, 70% female) concerning the rewards and stresses of their work. Of particular interest to our inquiry is the finding that, among the "stressors most reported to have a negative effect on working conditions," the "single most agreed-upon stressor was 'lack of leadership responses' " (Dahl & O'Neal, 1993, p. 18).

Sexual Harassment and Attack

Women serving in Vietnam, whether nurses or not, were subject to the stress of sexual harassment, even rape. In her 1971 end-of-tour report, Patricia Murphy, the chief nurse in Vietnam, wrote that:

Very few female nurses worry or fear enemy attacks, rocket, sapper or a real attack. The females are more fearful of assault by our own troops and with good reason from experience.... In the history of Vietnam, allowing enlisted men in the nurses' quarters has led to nothing but trouble including assaults and rape. (Vuic, 2009, pp. 143–144)

On some bases, curfews for nurses were instituted for their own protection, and guards were posted outside their quarters to defend them from fellow American personnel (Vuic, 2009, p. 144).

Anecdotal evidence and analyses of nonprobability samples support Murphy's view that sexual assault was a serious problem in Vietnam. One nurse reported that:

The executive officer for the squadron paid me a visit late at night. When I would not let him in, he went away, only to return later banging on my door, [saying], "it will only take a few minutes and it will mean everything to me" [which was] the nicest thing he said.

Filthy invectives and demands followed. I sat sobbing on the floor enforcing the door with my back until . . . morning. (Rushton, 2011, p. 616)

Interviewing a nonprobability sample of 137 Vietnam nurse veterans, Paul (1985) found that most reported some form of sexual harassment. As officers and valued members of a medical team, nurses may often have been protected from such pressures. One Army nurse who served in Vietnam said:

In the military sexual harassment was very common. But I'd say—because we were nurses—we were kind of on a little bit of a pedestal . . . so I think we got the least of it as far as being women in the military compared to women who were maybe enlisted or in another field. (Steinman, 2000, p. 51)

But another nurse reported that the protection could end as soon as they left their work:

When we were on duty, acting as nurses, I really felt we were treated as queens or as angels. I mean, the guys really respected us, I felt, and treated us well. Step out of that role and you were a piece of meat, and that was always difficult for me. . . . I told off more than one senior officer because he was out of line and [was] always wondering what the repercussions were going to be. . . . Would I be charged with insubordination? Could I be court-martialed because of it? (Steinman, 2000, pp. 132–133)

During the Vietnam war and the years immediately following it, sexual harassment and assault in the military received little attention from the military or the general public, leaving us with far-from-perfect data to estimate their prevalence. Other than the NVVRS, which presents its own methodological problems, we are aware of no representative survey that has been used to estimate rates of sexual harassment or rape among Vietnam veterans. However, a number of surveys have been conducted among women treated or seeking treatment at health facilities of the Department of Veterans Affairs. These studies suggest that rape in particular has been a serious problem in the military for decades and that the Vietnam war period did not differ significantly from other periods (Sadler et al., 2003; Skinner et al., 2000).

Period of Service

Any comprehensive review of the Vietnam war must take into account the fact that both the war itself and the political context in which it was fought changed every few years. As we report in Chapters 1 and 10, the experiences of the men and women who served in Vietnam changed, too. The number of nurses was not reduced as markedly as the number of troops in the final years of the war. Nurses who served toward the end of the war were often engaged mainly in the work of treating soldiers for drug addiction, seeing few or none who had been wounded in action. We therefore review the experiences of the nurses taking into account when they served in Vietnam.

Service in the Operating Room

The military record enables us to distinguish among nurses according to their military occupational specialty (MOS). In particular, we can identify nurses whose MOS's indicate that they worked in the operating room, a duty that may have been especially stressful since it often entailed minute-by-minute responsibility for the lives of severely wounded soldiers.

Pre-Vietnam Vulnerability

In Chapter 4, we concluded that male veterans' pre-war vulnerabilities were an important factor in the risk of both PTSD onset and current PTSD. We include them among the risk factors to be investigated in the nurses.

HYPOTHESES FOR INVESTIGATION

Our purpose is to inquire into the etiology of PTSD onsets and current PTSD in women veterans of the Vietnam war who served as nurses. We follow Fontana et al. (1997) in distinguishing between war trauma and sexual trauma. War trauma here takes two very different forms—the stress of treating wounded soldiers and the stress of personal risk in the war zone. In addition to the effects of trauma, as noted, we investigate the possible protective effect of teamwork and social support or unit cohesion in the medical team.

Unfortunately, reported sexual trauma is too infrequent in the diagnosed subsample to permit an analysis of its effects on the nurses. However, compelling anecdotal reports of sexual harassment and attack in Vietnam lead us to ask a simpler question: Just how frequent was it? Because answering that question does not require psychiatric diagnoses, we address it later in this chapter using the full sample of women veterans.

Meanwhile, we propose the following five hypotheses concerning factors that may have influenced rates of onset of war-related PTSD in women who served as nurses and its persistence as current PTSD at the time of the diagnostic interview:

(1) Onset and persistence will increase with the numbers of wounded soldiers in the nurses' patient load.
(2) Onset and persistence will be elevated among nurses whose MOS indicates that they worked in the operating room.
(3) Onset and persistence will increase with the degree of nurses' exposure to personal risk from enemy attack.
(4) Onset and persistence will decrease with the social cohesion of the nurse's unit.

(5) Onset and persistence will be elevated among nurses who had pre-Vietnam vulnerabilities.

DATA SOURCES AND PARTICIPANTS

The NVVRS interviews and questionnaires were administered to a national probability sample in which women were over-represented (Kulka et al., 1990). Their responses are supplemented by data from military records.

In most cases, we were able to determine from the MOS given in the military record whether a woman served as a nurse. However, when the record was insufficient, we relied on the veteran's own report of her primary duties for this purpose. The military record identified 280 women as nurses, to whom we added another 62 based on self-reports. Of these 342 nurses, 64 were given a diagnostic interview. Three of these had had onsets of PTSD before their service in Vietnam. Because they were too few to permit an assessment of the effect of preexisting PTSD on war-related PTSD, these three women were excluded from our analysis, leaving a sample of 61 nurses.

PTSD DIAGNOSES

Clinician interviewers made a broad range of diagnoses based on the Structured Clinical Interview for Diagnosis (SCID) (Spitzer, Williams, & Gibbon, 1987). As explained in Chapter 2, the SCID interview distinguishes between lifetime and current PTSD. The time of PTSD onset was used to determine whether it was war-related. As in other chapters, the outcome measures used here will be whether the nurse had an onset of war-related PTSD and whether the nurse's PTSD was current at the time of her diagnostic interview.

MEASURES OF VIETNAM EXPERIENCE
Casualty Load

It is a central goal of this study to assess nurses' challenging work as a possible risk factor for PTSD. Ideally, we would know the number of wounded soldiers for whom each nurse was responsible on a typical day, but that information is unavailable. The closest we can come is an indirect indicator of the workload typical of *all* nurses during a particular nurse's tour of duty—an indicator that, we believe, has good face validity.

The U.S. Department of Defense provides, in an online database, the official numbers of combat-related deaths and the numbers of wounded who were hospitalized and returned to duty during each month from January 1966 through December 1971 (Comptroller, Secretary of Defense, 2008). These two statistics are highly inter-correlated (r = .95, with the 72 months as units of analysis), which leads us to suspect that a third, unavailable statistic—the numbers of wounded who were hospitalized each month and *not* returned to duty—may be highly correlated with the other two. Given the high correlation between the two available statistics, either would serve equally well as the starting point for constructing a measure of nurses' workload.

We have chosen U.S. combat-related deaths as possibly the best reflection of the numbers of seriously wounded soldiers admitted to American military hospitals in Vietnam. Any stress associated with treating the wounded should increase with the number of wounded a nurse is responsible for. This would have been a function not only of the number of wounded, but also of the number of nurses available to care for them. For this reason, we have used the number of combat-related deaths divided by the number of American military nurses in Vietnam as an indicator of nurses' wounded-patient load during each month. This figure is averaged across all the months of a nurse's tour in Vietnam to yield an indicator of her personal wounded-patient load. For the sake of brevity, we call this the variable casualty load.

We estimate the number of nurses serving in Vietnam during each month using the NVVRS sample itself, since we were unable to find monthly or even yearly data elsewhere. The number of nurses in Vietnam did not closely track the numbers of casualties, as one might expect it to do, so casualty load scores vary considerably from one period of the war to another. Toward the end of the war, for instance, the number of those wounded in combat declined sharply, but the number of nurses did not follow suit. As a result, the number of war casualties per nurse was much lower during that period.

Personal Risk

Of course, exposure to and responsibility for the wounded and dying were not the only war-related traumas to which nurses were exposed. Many were also subject to the violence and personal risk of enemy attack. Lacking an objective measure of the levels of violence at the places where nurses were stationed, we rely on their responses to the questionnaire, which, fortunately, includes a number of questions on exposure to enemy attack that are both relevant to nurses' experience and worded with unusual precision.

The NVVRS uses measures of war-zone stressor exposure, which are constructed differently for men and women. Both include a broad variety of stressors. The female version is derived from scores on clusters of items representing, among other things, exposure to wounded and dead, exposure to enemy fire, loss of meaning and control, and deprivation. A complex weighting of these cluster scores is dichotomized so that the highest-scoring 25% of women are classified as having received high exposure, the remainder low exposure.

But our interest here is the narrower one of personal risk, which is covered by the NVVRS "exposure to enemy fire" cluster. Some of the 27 items in that cluster require the nurse to make subjective evaluations such as how unpleasant a given experience was for her. However, several items asking nurses how often an experience occurred provide concrete definitions of *very often, often, sometimes*, and so on. For instance, for receiving

---

Box 8.1

THE PERSONAL RISK SCALE

Five items, scored as indicated here. Proportions reporting that they ever had each experience are shown after the item (weighted to reflect the population).

J37–J37A. Were you ever under enemy fire? [If yes] How often? (76.4%)

J40. How often were you *near* combat situations, but were not actually involved in combat? (Near = within a mile or so.) (89.4%)

J43. During your tour(s) in or around Vietnam, how often (if ever) . . .

    A.   . . . did you receive small arms fire from the enemy? (53.2%)

    B.   . . . did you receive incoming fire from enemy artillery, rockets, and/or mortars? (76.6%)

    D.   . . .did your unit receive sniper fire and/or sapper attacks? (48.0%)

Note: These five questions are numbered here as in the NVVRS. The responses to these five questions are specified and coded as follows: very often—more than 50 times (4), often—13–50 times (3), sometimes—3–12 times (2), rarely—1–2 times (1), never (0).
Items J43A, B, and D further specify that very often may also mean nearly daily for a shorter period of time and that often may also mean more often for a shorter period.
The scale score is the sum of the item scores.

---

small arms fire from the enemy *very often* is defined as "weekly or more (more than 50 times) during my tour(s), or nearly daily for a shorter period of time."

We constructed a scale of personal risk by summing six items that are anchored in this way and that record events that nurses sometimes experienced. In the full sample, this scale is highly correlated with the 27-item cluster (r = .92 among nurses) and is reasonably well correlated with the much broader NVVRS measure of war-zone stressor exposure (r = .59). Our personal risk scale and scoring appear in Box 8.1.

Sexual Trauma

We follow the definition of harassment used by De Roma, Root, and Smith (2003, p. 400) in their study of sexual trauma in women veterans—namely, "any unwanted or uninvited pressure for dates or sex, touching, sexual gestures or body language, sexual teasing, jokes, remarks, whistles, hoots, or yells of a sexual nature." We identified instances of sexual harassment based on open-ended material in the NVVRS. We also identified instances of sexual attack. Female theater veterans responding to the NVVRS were asked, "While serving in or around Vietnam, were there any ways you were treated unfairly or badly because you are a woman?" Those who answered "yes" were asked, "In what ways were you treated unfairly or badly?" The NVVRS also includes a list of traumatic events including physical assault, torture, rape, abuse, mugging or similar assault. Respondents were asked to indicate which, if any, they had experienced at any time during their lives.

Among the 64 nurses who were given a diagnostic interview, open-ended responses to these questions identified four (a weighted 4.6% of nurses) who reported being harassed in Vietnam and only one (1.5%) who reported being attacked. However, the sample used in our analysis is a bit smaller. Three of the 64 nurses were diagnosed as having had pre-war onsets of PTSD. As we have throughout this monograph, we excluded respondents with pre-war onsets from our analysis as too few to analyze. As a result, our working sample consists of 61 nurses. Only one of these reported being sexually attacked and only one reported being harassed without having been attacked. Feeling that these two cases were too few to provide the basis for any conclusion about the association between sexual trauma and PTSD, we reluctantly dropped attack and harassment from our statistical analysis. We note, however, that neither of these nurses had an onset of war-related PTSD.

Service in the Operating Room

Most of the nurses had MOS's with very general titles like medical surgical nurse or clinical nurse. Nurses in Vietnam typically worked under high pressure and did whatever was needed at the moment, so their MOS's are of limited value in identifying the work they actually did. However, one group is clearly identified—those whose MOS's indicate that they worked in the operating room; namely, operating room nurses and nurse anesthetists.

Clinician's Record of Stressful Events

The SCID provides a place for the clinician to record stressful events throughout the respondent's lifetime, including events in Vietnam, that are elicited by a question loosely modeled on Criterion A in DSM III-R. The record of these events, and of responses to questions about specific types of stressful events in Vietnam, provides a useful indication of the evidence used by the clinician to determine whether the respondent's experiences in Vietnam satisfied Criterion A. Three items inquiring about particular events are of particular interest:

> Were you ever under enemy fire?
> Did you see people being killed or wounded or people who had been killed or
>   wounded? (If yes: How frequently?)
> Were you ever in danger of being injured or killed? (If yes: How frequently?)

Sometimes the interviewer recorded specific words offered by the respondents in response to these questions. For instance, when asked the second question, one nurse replied "Every day as a nurse." In response to the third question, she said, "Four times."

Box 8.2

THE UNIT COHESION SCALE

The scale score is the sum of five items, scored as indicated:

J21. In your opinion, how competent were the people in charge of your unit— would you say *highly competent and able* (4), *fairly competent* (3), *about average* (2), *somewhat incompetent* (1), *totally incompetent* (0)?

J21A. How much did you trust the people you served with in (or around) Vietnam—*completely* (4), *a great deal* (3), *somewhat* (2), *not very much* (1), or *not at all* (0)?

J22. How many of the people you served with in your unit were the kind who looked out for the welfare of others—would you say *none* (0), *a few* (1), *about half* (2), *most* (3), or *all* (4)?

J22A. How often did you feel that members of your unit understood you and your problems while in (or around) Vietnam—*very often* (4), *often* (3), *sometimes* (2), *rarely* (1) or *never* (0)?

J23. And how close or tight were you with the people in your unit—would you say *extremely close* (4), *very close* (3), *fairly close* (2), *not very close* (1), or *not close at all* (0)?

Unit Cohesion

Our scale of unit cohesion is based on veterans' own recollections and evaluations as reported in response to five questions in the NVVRS. Four items bear directly on the matter of collegial support. Three of these ask about the women's personal experience, while the fourth asks about members of the unit in general. While they do not explicitly exclude superiors, we believe these four items are more likely to evoke perceptions of the nurses' relationships with colleagues in Vietnam. The fifth item asks the respondents to assess the competence of the people in charge of their units. It is worth noting that the nurses had a high level of confidence in the competence of their leaders. In the full sample, 58.6% thought they were *highly competent and able*, while another 23.5% thought they were *fairly competent*. The five questions appear in Box 8.2, which also shows the scores assigned to each response. The scale has possible scores ranging from 0–20 and is internally consistent (Cronbach's alpha = .93 in our sample of nurses, data weighted or not).

Pre-Vietnam Vulnerability Factors

As described in Chapter 3, 15 possible indicators of pre-Vietnam vulnerability were extracted from the NVVRS based on male veterans' self-reports, military records, or retrospective diagnoses made in the clinical interview. Nine of these differentiated male veterans with onsets of war-related PTSD or current war-related PTSD from their colleagues with relative risks of 1.5 or more, or with statistical significance at the .10 level or better, and were subsequently used to create a total vulnerability load score. Two of these indicators were unavailable or unusable in the sample of nurses.

We applied the same criteria to the remaining seven indicators as we had applied in the sample of male veterans. Table 8.3 lists these seven factors, giving their frequencies, the relative risks of PTSD onset and current PTSD associated with each, and the statistical significance of these risks. Four of the seven meet our criteria for selection as a vulnerability factor to be included in regression models: one or more family members with alcohol or drug abuse problems, childhood conduct disorder, any other pre-Vietnam disorder, and no pre-Vietnam military experience. All four had relative risks over 1.5 for PTSD onset. By far the highest relative risk for onset (5.45) was associated with pre-Vietnam disorder. Because all nurses who had current PTSD also had pre-Vietnam disorders, the relative risk for current PTSD was effectively infinite and represented in Table 8.3 by the ∞ sign. All but one of the remaining vulnerabilities had relative risks of zero for current PTSD, which reflects the fact that none of the nurses having any of these risk factors also had current PTSD.

Period of Service

As we did for the male veterans (see Chapter 4), we divided the war into four periods. As with the men, we classified nurses according to the period when their service in Vietnam

Table 8.3 FREQUENCIES OF SEVEN POSSIBLE VULNERABILITY FACTORS FOR PTSD AND ASSOCIATED RELATIVE RISKS ("RR") OF WAR-RELATED PTSD ONSET AND WAR-RELATED CURRENT PTSD

Vulnerability Factor	Frequency	PTSD Onset RR (p)	Current PTSD RR (p)
Childhood family member arrested	6.1% (3)	0.00 (.41)	0.00 (.65)
Childhood family member abused alcohol or drugs	13.2% (8)	**2.35** (.18)	0.00 (.48)
Physically abused in childhood	10.3% (6)	.80 (.83)	0.00 (.54)
Childhood conduct disorder	2.8% (2)	**2.09** (.49)	0.00 (.75)
Other pre-Vietnam disorder	14.9% (10)	**5.45** (**.001**)	∞ (**.000**)
Younger than 25	60.4% (10)	.94 (.92)	.84 (.87)
No pre-Vietnam military experience	6.9% (4)	**1.86** (.51)	0.00 (.62)

Note: Proportions are weighted to represent the population, with unweighted sample *n*'s in parentheses. P-values are for test of independence (Pearson chi-square). Figures in **bold** are relative risks or p-values that meet our criterion for inclusion in our models as a vulnerability factor. The infinity sign indicates that relative risk is effectively infinite because the denominator is zero—in this case because every respondent with current PTSD had had a disorder before serving in Vietnam.

began. This classification served to distinguish those who left Vietnam before the Tet Offensive from those who were in Vietnam during the Offensive or at a later time when this major turning point had redefined the nature of the war for many Americans.

None of the nurses in our sample of 61 served in the first period. The large number who served late in the war leaves a substantial portion of the sample in each of the two last periods. We hoped the distinction between periods 3 and 4 would help us to discover any trends that might have resulted from progressive deterioration of the American effort during the period of Vietnamization and gradual withdrawal from the war. (See Chapter 1: section War, *Nixon's War* and *The Final Years*, which discuss increasing drug use and discipline issues affecting nurses' responsibilities in Vietnam.)

DATA ANALYSIS PLAN AND STATISTICAL PROCEDURES

The purpose of our statistical analysis was to identify sources of variation in rates of PTSD onset and of current PTSD. First, we examined bivariate relationships between the Vietnam experience variables and PTSD, eliminating any variable whose association with PTSD onset or current PTSD was not at least marginally significant; that is, any having a *p*-value greater than .10. Then, we used multivariate logistic regression models consisting of the variables thus selected to test the hypotheses listed that were testable with these variables. We used separate models to estimate effects on PTSD onset and on current PTSD. In each case, our first model consisted exclusively of variables representing nurses' experience in Vietnam. A second model included pre-war vulnerability factors in addition to the Vietnam experience variables. In all of these models, a *p*-value of .05 or less was our standard of statistical significance, but we considered any substantial effect whose *p*-value was .10 or less to be of interest. We also examined rates of PTSD onset and current PTSD among nurses who served in each of three later periods of the war.

RESULTS

A statistical overview of the war will help to set the context before we present the results of our formal analysis. Figures 8.1 through 8.3 are based on monthly statistics that were averaged over six-month periods. Figures 8.1 and 8.3 are derived in part from the Department of Defense statistics mentioned, which cover 1966 through 1971. Figure 8.2 is based on the full NVVRS sample of 342 nurses. For ease of comparison, it was restricted to the same six-year period as Figures 8.1 and 8.3.

Combat deaths varied with the vagaries of war, but Figure 8.1 shows that they peaked at the time of the Tet Offensive in early 1968 and declined after that, reaching their lowest level toward the end of the war. Figure 8.2 shows that the number of nurses serving in Vietnam increased steadily until the months following the Tet Offensive, remained high for about two years, and, even after that, declined much less sharply than combat deaths. Figure 8.3 shows that, as a result, combat deaths per

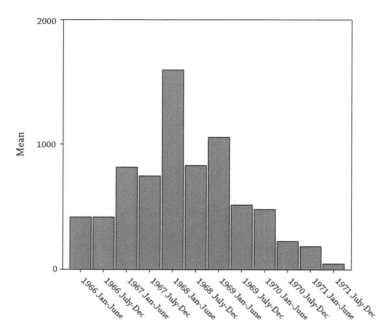

Figure 8.1 Mean Monthly Combat Deaths 1966–1971

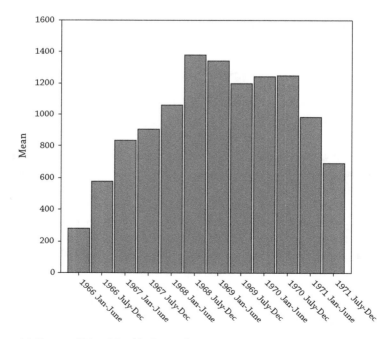

Figure 8.2 Estimated Mean Monthly Count of Nurses in Vietnam 1966–1971

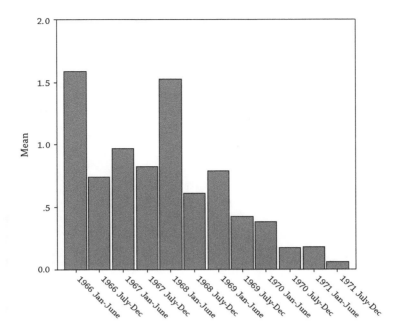

Figure 8.3 Monthly Combat Deaths Per Nurse 1966–1971

nurse declined from a peak at the time of Tet and reached unprecedented low levels by the end of 1971.

If the risk of PTSD increased with the numbers of wounded soldiers a nurse cared for, we would expect rates of PTSD to be highest among nurses who served in the periods of highest combat and lowest nurse staffing. Table 8.4 shows again, this time in the smaller diagnosed subsample, the sharp decline in nurses' casualty load toward the end of the war that we have just seen in figures based on all nurses and all combat deaths. The table shows only a modest decline in onsets of PTSD in nurses toward the end of the war, but it shows a much sharper decline in current cases—which suggests that patient load may have played an important part in the persistence of PTSD years after the war.

These figures also suggest that stressors other than patient load are associated with PTSD onset in nurses. Table 8.4 shows that personal risk does not decline with period of the war, which is surprising given the lower level of combat. Sexual harassment and attack increased at the end of the war—a finding that is consistent with the breakdown of military discipline occurring at that time. These latter figures are based on the full sample, since the diagnosed subsample had too few cases of harassment and attack to analyze meaningfully.

Table 8.4 RATES OF PTSD ONSET AND CURRENT PTSD, MEAN CASUALTY
LOAD, MEAN PERSONAL RISK, AND PROPORTION OF NURSES REPORTING
SEXUAL HARASSMENT OR ATTACK BY PERIOD OF THE WAR

			Diagnosed Subsample			Full Sample	
Service in Vietnam Began	Rates of PTSD		Casualty Load	Personal Risk	N	Sexual Harr/Att	N
	Onset	Current					
Before July 28, 1965	--	--	--	--	--	.000	2
July 28, 1965 to Jan 29, 1968	.181	.074	1.082	5.10	13	.030	99
Jan 30, 1968 to Nov 30, 1969	.171	.056	.563	7.05	27	.040	137
On or after Dec 1, 1969	.158	.000	.167	6.22	21	.132	104
TOTAL	.168	.052	.527	6.40	61	.067	342

Note: Percentages are weighted to the population from which the samples were drawn. N's are unweighted sample numbers.

Rates of Sexual Harassment and Attack

As explained, women who had experienced sexual harassment or attack were
identified based on open-ended responses to a question about mistreatment as a
woman and to an item in the NVVRS Traumatic Events Booklet asking respondents
to report instances of physical assault, torture, rape, abuse, mugging, or similar assault. In the full sample of 404 women Vietnam veterans (nurses and non-nurses), five
women reported having been sexually attacked in Vietnam—that is, subjected to rape,
attempted rape, or "sexual assault" in one woman's words. Responses to the mistreatment question identified 19 additional women who reported sexual harassment short
of physical attack, including seven women who themselves used the phrase "sexual
harassment" to characterize their mistreatment. When weighted to reflect the population, these numbers represent 1.4% who reported attacks and 5.1% who reported
harassment but no attack. Rates are similar among the 342 nurses in the full sample.
Three nurses (1.0%) reported sexual attacks, and 18 (5.7%) reported harassment but
not attack.

Were women serving in the Vietnam war at an unusually high risk of sexual harassment and attack? We do not know of any population surveyed at that time using a probability sample that might serve as an instructive comparison group. However, the military
now conducts surveys to estimate the prevalence of sexual harassment and rape in its
ranks. In a 2012 survey (Defense Manpower Data Center, 2013), 23% of women in the
military reported having been sexually harassed in the previous 12 months, while 6.1%
reported experiencing "unwanted sexual contact" in that period. Nearly a third of the
latter group (1.89%) reported having been raped. These rates are higher than the ones
we found in the NVVRS. The time span covered in the two studies is nearly the same: in

the NVVRS, tour lengths varied, but most women served 12 months in Vietnam, which was almost exactly the average tour as well. The proportion of rapes reported in the 2012 survey is somewhat higher than the proportion of attacks we found, and the latter were not all rapes. A much higher proportion of women reported being harassed in the 2012 survey than in our analysis of the NVVRS.

However, the rates found in both studies may be underestimates. The 2012 survey had an abysmal completion rate—only 29%. The reason for this low rate may have been a reluctance to report sexual harassment or attack on the part of the active-duty women interviewed. Nonetheless, that survey was at least designed for the purpose of eliciting reports of harassment and attack. Not so the NVVRS, which lacked the careful framing and sequencing of questions that would no doubt have been useful in eliciting sensitive personal information.

If the rates of harassment and attack elicited by both surveys are likely to be underestimates, it is hard to say which population—women who served in the Vietnam war, or women serving in the military in 2012—actually suffered higher rates of harassment and attack. However, we can at least say that neither the VA-based studies cited (Sadler et al., 2003; Skinner et al., 2000) nor the 2012 survey provide any evidence that rates of harassment and attack were higher in Vietnam than in other military or veteran populations.

Associations of Vietnam Experience and Pre-Vietnam Vulnerability Factors with PTSD

As stated previously, lack of sufficient cases prevents sexual harassment and attack from being included in this analysis. Period of the war is not included either, for the simple, if regrettable, reason that our sample was too small to enable us to analyze risk factors separately in each period.

Table 8.5 gives odds ratios for the bivariate relationship between each Vietnam experience variable and PTSD-onset, then current. Service in the operating room is dichotomous. The other variables shown are continuous; their odds ratios are expressed in standard deviation units.

Unit cohesion showed essentially no association with PTSD onset or current PTSD. For that reason, we dropped it from further analysis and concentrated on the remaining three variables—personal risk, casualty load, and service in the operating room.

Looking first at these variables' associations with PTSD onset, we see that personal risk and service in the operating room both show substantial statistical effects, although their p-values fall a bit short of the .05 standard. Casualty load shows essentially no effect. But this pattern is reversed when current PTSD is the outcome. Now casualty load shows a substantial and statistically significant effect, while personal risk and service in the operating room can be said to have essentially no effects, particularly given their outsized p-values.

Table 8.6 shows the independent effects of these three variables in multivariate models. The pattern shown in the left-hand column is similar to the one shown in Table 8.5.

Table 8.5 BIVARIATE ASSOCIATIONS OF PTSD ONSET
AND CURRENT PTSD WITH MEASURES OF VIETNAM
EXPERIENCE (ODDS RATIOS [O.R.])

	PTSD	Onset	Current	PTSD
	O.R.	(p)	O.R.	(p)
Personal risk*	2.00	(.07)	1.38	(.57)
Casualty load*	1.14	(.71)	2.04	(.04)
Service in the OR	4.39	(.08)	1.49	(.75)
Unit cohesion*	0.84	(.69)	1.28	(.77)

Note: These analyses take into account the complex subsample design.

*Continuous variable expressed in standard deviation units. Service in the Operating Room (OR) is dichotomous, scored 0–1.

Again, both personal risk and service in the operating room show substantial effects on PTSD onset that nonetheless fall short of the .05 standard; and again, casualty load shows a substantial and significant effect on current PTSD but not on PTSD onset.

A certain caution is in order here. Unsurprisingly, casualty load is highest among nurses who served at the peak of the war (defined in Table 8.6 as the period from July 28, 1965 to Jan 29, 1968) and declines after that. So we may wonder whether the casualty load variable reflects some more general aspect of each historical period, such as the climate of opinion about the war. Fortunately for the sake of clarity, this appears not to be the case. The statistical effect of casualty load on current PTSD is not reduced when we control period of the war, as represented by the categories shown in Table 8.6.

The potentially traumatic events recorded in the SCID by the clinical interviewers are consistent with the associations shown in Tables 8.5 and 8.6. That part of the SCID is available for 11 of the 13 nurses who were diagnosed with onsets of war-related PTSD. Most of the Vietnam events elicited by the question relevant to Criterion A are of two types. They describe either occasions when the nurse was exposed to personal danger, or experiences she had with wounded patients. For two nurses, both kinds of events were recorded. One said she "never slept above ground" and that she "saw a lot of kids not as whole as [they] should be." The other reported four distinct occasions on which she was exposed to personal danger and one event related to nursing care; namely, the death of a soldier in intensive care. A third nurse reported a pair of events that were unique in this small group—seeing the destruction of a "sampan village" and seeing the stillbirth of a baby. The clinician apparently felt that all of these events, or at least one of them for each of these three nurses, satisfied Criterion A. For two additional nurses, only events related to nursing care were recorded—five events in one case, a single event in the other, and all but one of these events involving the loss of body parts.

If no particular traumatic event could be singled out, but the interviewer nonetheless wished to indicate that the respondent had had experiences in Vietnam that satisfied Criterion A, he or she was instructed simply to enter "Vietnam" as the traumatic event.

Table 8.6 MULTIVARIATE LOGISTIC REGRESSION MODELS PREDICTING PTSD ONSET AND CURRENT PTSD FROM THREE SOURCES OF POSSIBLE STRESS IN VIETNAM, AND FROM THOSE THREE SOURCES IN COMBINATION WITH VULNERABILITY FACTORS

PTSD Onset Is Dependent Variable:

	O.R.	(p)	O.R.	(p)
Stress in Vietnam				
Personal risk*	1.82	(.09)	2.53	(.07)
Casualty load*	1.29	(.54)	1.20	(.69)
Service in the OR	3.62	(.09)	4.97	(.15)
Vulnerability Factors				
Childhood family member abused drugs or alcohol	—	—	8.62	(.06)
Childhood conduct disorder	—	—	1.10	(.93)
Other pre-Vietnam disorder	—	—	23.16	(.015)
No pre-Vietnam mil. experience	—	—	.55	(.64)

Current PTSD Is Dependent Variable:

	O.R.	(p)	O.R.	(p)
Stress in Vietnam				
Personal risk*	1.40	(.53)	1.29	(.70)
Casualty load*	2.31	(.016)	2.20	(.34)
Service in the OR	1.62	(.71)	1.09	(.96)
Vulnerability Factors				
Childhood family member abused drugs or alcohol	—	—	.94	(.996)
Childhood conduct disorder	—	—	0	
Other pre-Vietnam disorder	—	—	∞	
No pre-Vietnam mil. experience	—	—	0	

Note: These analyses take into account the complex subsample design.

*Continuous variable expressed in standard deviation units. All other independent variables are dichotomous, scored 0–1.

The infinity sign indicates an odds ratio that is effectively infinite because the denominator is zero – in this case because every respondent with current PTSD had had a disorder before serving in Vietnam.

Three interviewers entered "Vietnam" or simply "war." In all three of these cases, the nurse responded in the affirmative both to the items inquiring about personal risk and to the item inquiring about exposure to the sight of injured, dying, or dead people. We can only assume that, in each of these cases, the interviewer relied on one or both of these responses. In fact, the interviewer who wrote "war" drew an arrow pointing to the next page, where the affirmative responses about danger and witnessing appeared. All 11 nurses endorsed the witnessing item, and all but one endorsed the personal danger item. The exception was a nurse who worked onboard a ship and was therefore removed from the fighting.

The clinicians did not record a single incident of sexual harassment or attack as a possible precipitating cause of war-related PTSD, nor did any of the 13 nurses diagnosed with war-related PTSD onsets report an incident of sexual harassment or attack in the non-diagnostic interview. This does not mean that such incidents did not in fact occur and contribute to the onset of PTSD in some nurses; but if they did, the nurses did not report them. On the basis of the evidence we have, it is quite clear that both our statistical analysis and the events recorded in the clinical interview indicate that the most important, if not the only, traumatic experiences leading to the onset of PTSD were exposure to personal danger and witnessing of injured, dying, or dead people in the course of the nurses' work. For many of the nurses, both types of experience may have contributed to the syndrome.

Hypotheses Findings

In light of these results, we can review the first four hypotheses that we set out to test:

(1) *Onset and persistence will increase with the numbers of wounded soldiers in the nurses' patient load.* This hypothesis is supported only in the case of current PTSD.

(2) *Onset and persistence will be elevated among nurses whose MOS indicates that they worked in the operating room.* This hypothesis is supported, but only at the .10 significance level, and only in the case of PTSD onset.

(3) *Onset and persistence will increase with the degree of nurses' exposure to personal risk from enemy attack.* This hypothesis is supported, but only at the .10 significance level, and only in the case of PTSD onset.

(4) *Onset and persistence will decrease with the social cohesion of the nurse's unit.* This hypothesis is not supported.

The right-hand column of Table 8.6 adds vulnerability factors to the model. The three effects that are substantial and statistically significant or marginally so in the left-hand column are not greatly reduced when vulnerability factors are controlled, although their statistical significance is seriously degraded in two of the three cases—a degradation that appears to be due mainly to an increase in the number of degrees of freedom caused by the introduction of new variables to the model. What is most impressive about these results is the fact that effect sizes remain about the same even when pre-war vulnerability factors are controlled.

Equally interesting are the statistical effects of the vulnerability factors themselves. Alcoholism or drug abuse in the respondent's childhood home has a large effect on PTSD onset, even if the statistical significance of that effect falls just short of the .05 standard; but the effect of the same variable disappears completely when we look at current PTSD. Most striking, however, is the fact that onset of a psychiatric disorder (other than conduct disorder) prior to Vietnam has a very large statistical effect on PTSD onset—an odds ratio of 23 ($p = .015$). That effect persists until the time of the interview, when it is unquantifiable but effectively infinite—because of the simple fact that every one of the four respondents with current PTSD had had a psychiatric disorder before serving in Vietnam. On the basis of this result, we can say this of our final hypothesis:

(5) *Onset and persistence will be elevated among nurses who had pre-Vietnam vulnerabilities.*
   This hypothesis is confirmed for both PTSD onset and current PTSD, particularly with respect to pre-war psychiatric disorders.

The strong association of pre-Vietnam disorders with both PTSD onset and current PTSD raises the obvious question "What disorders?" Of nine nurses who had PTSD onsets that did not persist until the interview, only two (25.9%) were diagnosed as having had psychiatric disorders before Vietnam. The four nurses whose PTSD did persist until the interview present a starker picture. All four had had psychiatric disorders before Vietnam. Two of the four had had social phobias, one had had a simple phobia, and the fourth had abused both drugs and alcohol. Of course, a history of psychiatric disorder is not sufficient to give rise to PTSD, let alone persistent war-related PTSD. By definition, all four of these nurses endured stresses in the war zone that qualified for Criterion A in the clinical interviewer's opinion. The narrative extractions reveal that three reported that they had worked in the operating room or in intensive care at bases that were frequently targets of enemy attack. While one worked in the safety of a hospital ship, all four reported working either in intensive care or with severely injured patients—men who had lost limbs or other body parts, were severely burned, or had suffered head trauma.

LONG-TERM IMPACT OF THE WAR ON NURSES' LIVES

Between July 3, 2012, and May 13, 2013, a number of the NVVRS investigators undertook a follow-up study of the NVVRS sample of veterans, especially those who had served in the Vietnam theater of operations. The follow-up was called the National Vietnam Veterans Longitudinal Study (Longitudinal Study), and, like the NVVRS, it was mandated by Congress and conducted with funds from the Veterans Administration (now the Department of Veterans Affairs [VA]). The design and methods of the Longitudinal Study have been described in detail by Schlenger et al. (2015).

The Longitudinal Study enables us to follow the nurses decades after their service in Vietnam. As in our analysis of the NVVRS data, we concentrate here on nurses who were given diagnostic interviews. The Longitudinal Study attempted to interview as many veterans from the original survey as possible, but some could not be found, or declined to participate, and some had died. Table 8.7 shows the distribution of key variables among nurse veterans in each of three Longitudinal Study groups: responders, non-responders, and those who had died. We see first that responders had much higher rates of PTSD onset and of current PTSD in the original survey than the non-responders did. They also had higher rates of three risk factors whose associations with PTSD we examined—namely, alcohol or drug abuse in the nurse's childhood family, conduct disorder in her own childhood, and exposure to personal risk in Vietnam. However, three risk factors were more prevalent among the non-responders—namely, any psychiatric disorder other than conduct disorder or PTSD, casualty load in Vietnam, and service in the operating room in Vietnam. The dead also differ substantially from responders on most variables shown, but the small number who died ($n = 9$) precludes statistical analysis of these differences.

Table 8.7 DISTRIBUTION OF PTSD ONSET, CURRENT PTSD, AND RISK FACTORS FOR PTSD IN THE NVVRS, AMONG LONGITUDINAL STUDY NURSE RESPONDERS, NON-RESPONDERS, AND NVVRS RESPONDENTS WHO DIED BEFORE THE LONGITUDINAL STUDY

NVVRS Variable	Alive			Dead mean/ prop	Grand Total mean/ prop
	Responders mean/ prop	Non- responders mean/ prop	Total Alive mean/ prop		
PTSD onset	.214	.112	.184	.055	.168
Current PTSD	.070	.033	.059	.000	.052
Childhood family alc/drug	.157	.079	.134	.119	.132
Conduct disorder (as child)	.045	.000	.032	.000	.028
Any other pre-Viet disorder	.119	.237	.154	.119	.149
No previous mil. experience	.082	.071	.079	.000	.069
Personal risk (mean)*	.026	−.226	−.044	.313	.000
Casualty load (mean)*	-.009	.034	.004	−.031	.000
Served in OR	.045	.294	.118	.119	.118
N	37	15	52	9	61

Means and proportions (prop) are weighted to represent the population. N's are unweighted sample n's but are occasionally slightly smaller than shown, owing to missing data.

*Continuous variables expressed in standard deviation units with mean = 0.

All other variables are dichotomous.

Because the number of nurses who were assessed for PTSD and other disorders in both the NVVRS and the Longitudinal Study is quite small (n = 37), the scope of our analysis is limited. Also because of the small sample size, we have not attempted to compute weights to adjust for discrepancies between responders and non-responders, as we did in analyzing follow-up data in male veterans (see Chapter 12), but we have decided instead to use only the population weights that were used in the original NVVRS survey.

Has the rate of current PTSD among women who served as nurses increased, decreased, or remained about the same since the NVVRS? An attempt to answer that question is complicated by the fact that the NVVRS and the Longitudinal Study used different interview instruments, based on different editions of the DSM. As noted earlier and as reported in Chapter 2, the NVVRS used an instrument called the SCID (Spitzer, Williams, & Gibbon, 1987), whose diagnostic criteria were based on the then-current DSM-III-R. Diagnoses in the Longitudinal Study were made according to DSM-5, using a new diagnostic instrument called the Clinician-Administered PTSD Scale for DSM-5 (CAPS-5) (Weathers et al., 2013).

Table 8.8 shows that, based on these two instruments, the rate of PTSD may have increased slightly in our sample of 37 nurses—from 7.0 to 7.8%. However, this increase may be due to the different criteria and symptoms used in the instruments and in the editions of the DSM upon which each is based. Because all but one of the SCID symptoms also appear in the CAPS-5, we were able to construct a simulated SCID diagnosis based on CAPS-5 items in the Longitudinal Study. That simulated diagnosis yields a rate of 6.2% at the time of the Longitudinal Study. While this is somewhat lower

Table 8.8 RATES OF CURRENT PTSD AT THE TIMES OF THE NVVRS AND THE LONGITUDINAL STUDY INTERVIEWS BY VARIOUS MEASURES IN NURSES WHO WERE ASSESSED IN BOTH INTERVIEWS

1. PTSD at the NVVRS interview	mean/prop (95% CI)
a. SCID diagnosis – based on *DSM-III-R* (rate)*	.070 (.000, .156)
b. Number of PTSD symptoms common to *DSM-III-R* and *DSM-5* (mean) range 0-15	2.26 (1.18, 3.34)
2. PTSD at the Longitudinal Study interview	
a. CAPS diagnosis – based on *DSM-5* (rate)	.078 (.000, .162)
b. Simulated SCID diagnosis using CAPS items (rate)	.062 (.000, .141)
c. Number of PTSD symptoms common to *DSM-III-R* and *DSM-5* (mean) range 0-15	1.19 (.425, 1.95)

Percentages are weighted to reflect the population. Unweighted sample size is 37.

*One SCID item ("foreshortened future") does not appear in the CAPS. However, removing that item makes no difference to the SCID diagnosis in this sample of 37 nurses.

Statistical significance of differences in proportions between the two interviews was tested using a sampling weighted version of McNemar's test – namely, testing whether the weighted proportion of discordant pairs across time that indicate an increase versus a decrease is different from 50%, using the Rao-Scott (RS) Chi-square obtained from the SAS procedure PROC SURVEYFREQ. Two differences in estimated rates of PTSD were tested: for 1a vs. 2a, p = 0.896; for 1a vs. 2b, p = 0.884. Statistical significance of the difference in mean numbers of symptoms (1b vs. 2c) was tested using a paired t-test using the SAS procedure PROC SURVEYMEANS, p = .070.

than the original rate of 7.0%, the difference is remarkably small. However, a second approach to comparing the NVVRS and the Longitudinal Study interviews shows a more marked decrease. A simple count of PTSD symptoms included in both interviews shows that a mean of 2.26 symptoms at the NVVRS interview decreased to only 1.19 in the Longitudinal Study—only slightly more than half the original number. None of the differences tested in Table 8.8 is statistically significant at the .05 level, but the decrease in the number of symptoms comes fairly close ($p = .07$).

As we have noted, the rate of current PTSD decreases only slightly between the NVVRS and the Longitudinal Study when the most comparable measures are used, but this should not lead us to believe that most of the nurses who had current PTSD at the first interview still had it at the follow-up. In fact, Table 8.9 shows that two of the three nurses who had current PTSD at the time of the NVVRS did not have it at the time of the Longitudinal Study. Similarly, two of the three nurses who had current PTSD at the time of the Longitudinal Study had not been diagnosed with it at the time of the NVVRS. These two women may have had recurrences in later life of disorders that had remitted at the time of the earlier assessment. The large proportional turnover in Table 8.9 suggests that, at least in this small sample of nurse veterans, PTSD may have persisted as an underlying disorder that flared up and subsided from time to time.

This view gains support if we expand the inquiry to include nurses who had onsets of war-related PTSD regardless of whether the disorder was current at either the NVVRS or the Longitudinal Study interview. Of the 37 nurse veterans in our sample, seven (16.9%) had onsets of PTSD before the NVVRS interview that had remitted by the time of the Longitudinal Study interview—that is, they did not have current PTSD at the Longitudinal Study interview according to either the CAPS or the simulated SCID. All but one of the seven (13.7%) had at least one CAPS symptom at the time of the Longitudinal Study. Thus, there appears to have been a long-term residue of the disorder in nearly all of those who no longer met criteria for the diagnosis.

Table 8.9 TURNOVER IN CURRENT PTSD BETWEEN THE TIMES OF THE NVVRS AND THE LONGITUDINAL STUDY, BASED ON THE MOST COMPARABLE MEASURES

	Current PTSD in the Longitudinal Study (Simulated SCID Using CAPS Items)		
	NO	YES	Total
Current PTSD in the NVVRS (SCID)			
NO	88.1% (32)	4.9% (2)	93.0% (34)
YES	5.7% (2)	1.4% (1)	7.0% (3)
TOTAL	93.8% (34)	6.2% (3)	100.0% (37)

Note: Percentages are weighted to reflect the population. N's are unweighted sample *n*'s.

Table 8.10 NURSE VETERANS' EMPLOYMENT STATUS
IN THE NVVRS INTERVIEW AND THE LONGITUDINAL
STUDY INTERVIEW

Employment Status	NVVRS	Longitudinal Study
Employed	73.6% (26)	19.2% (7)
Unemployed	3.3% (1)	—
Retired	10.2% (5)	74.4% (27)
In school or training	2.9% (1)	—
Keeping house	8.9% (3)	—
Disabled (unable to work)	1.1% (1)	3.3% (1)
Other	—	3.1% (2)
TOTAL	100.0% (37)	100.0% (37)

Note: Percentages are weighted to reflect the population. *N*'s are unweighted
sample *n*'s.

The Longitudinal Study inquired as to how many of the nurse veterans were currently employed. Table 8.10 compares their employment status in the NVVRS and
Longitudinal Study. In the NVVRS, 73.6% were employed. A minority of 10.2% reported that they had already retired. Another 8.9% said they were keeping house, and
2.9% were in school or training. Perhaps not surprisingly, given their ages, most of the
nurses (74.4%) had retired by the time of the Longitudinal Study. However, 19.2% were
still employed.

When the nurse veterans were in Vietnam, only one of them was married, according
to the military record. (When the data are weighted to reflect the population, she
represents 1.3% of those from which the full diagnosed subsample of nurses was drawn
and 2.6% of those who were clinically assessed in both the NVVRS and the Longitudinal
Study.) By the time of the NVVRS, most of the nurse veterans had been married. Table
8.11 shows that a weighted 65.2% were married and another 9.7% were divorced or

Table 8.11 NURSE VETERANS' MARITAL STATUS IN THE
NVVRS AND THE LONGITUDINAL STUDY INTERVIEWS

Marital Status	NVVRS	Longitudinal Study
Married	65.2% (22)	56.2% (19)
Separated	3.4% (1)	—
Divorced	6.3% (2)	17.9% (6)
Widowed	—	4.5% (2)
Never married	25.2% (12)	21.3% (10)
TOTAL	100.0% (37)	100.0% (37)

Note: Percentages are weighted to reflect the population. *N*'s are unweighted sample *n*'s.

separated. In the Longitudinal Study, slightly fewer (56.2%) were married, but 17.9% were divorced and 4.5% were widowed. Those who were never married declined slightly from 25.2% to 21.3%.

In both the NVVRS and the Longitudinal Study, veterans were asked questions about the impact of their military experience on their present lives. We consider responses to three questions here. In our sample of 37 nurses, only 34 answered these questions in the Longitudinal Study, so this part of the analysis is based on that slightly reduced sample.

Veterans were asked, "Tell me how closely [this] statement matches your feelings: Being in the Vietnam War was the biggest event in my life up until now." Possible responses were *very closely, somewhat closely, not too closely*, and *not at all*. In the NVVRS, 42.9% responded "very closely" or "somewhat closely." The corresponding proportion in the Longitudinal Study was slightly smaller (40.1%). However, Table 8.12 shows that the most extreme positive response ("very closely") was much more frequent in the NVVRS than in the Longitudinal Study. This reduction in the war's perceived importance should not necessarily be surprising, since the war was much further in the past by the time of the Longitudinal Study, and the veterans could have experienced other important events since then.

Veterans also were asked, "What effect has military service had on your life?" This question had fixed alternative responses: *entirely positive effects, mostly positive effects, an equal balance of positive and negative effects, mostly negative effects*, and *entirely negative effects*. Table 8.13 shows nurses' responses to this question in both the NVVRS and the Longitudinal Study. In the NVVRS, 80.3% said the effect was entirely or mostly positive. In the Longitudinal Study, this proportion was slightly lower (76.2%). However, as Table 8.13 shows, the proportion who said the effect was *entirely* positive decreased markedly.

Table 8.12 NURSE VETERANS' RESPONSES TO BEING ASKED IF THE VIETNAM WAR WAS THE "BIGGEST EVENT" OF THEIR LIVES IN THE NVVRS AND LONGITUDINAL STUDY INTERVIEWS

Effect of Vietnam Service	NVVRS	Longitudinal Study
Tell me how closely [this] statement matches your feelings: "Being in the Vietnam War was the biggest event in my life up until now."		
Very closely	15.0% (6)	6.1% (2)
Somewhat closely	27.9% (10)	34.0% (13)
Not too closely	34.5% (10)	37.5% (12)
Not at all	22.6% (8)	22.3% (7)
TOTAL	100.0% (34)	100.0% (34)

Note: Percentages are weighted to reflect the population. *N*'s are unweighted sample *n*'s.

Table 8.13 NURSE VETERANS' APPRAISALS OF THE EFFECT OF MILITARY SERVICE ON THEIR LIVES IN THE NVVRS AND LONGITUDINAL STUDY INTERVIEWS

Effect of Military Service	NVVRS	Longitudinal Study
What effect has military service had on your life?		
Entirely positive	27.6% (9)	11.1% (5)
Mostly positive	52.7% (17)	65.1% (20)
An equal balance of positive and negative	18.0% (7)	15.5% (5)
Mostly negative	1.7% (1)	8.2% (4)
Entirely negative	—	—
TOTAL	100.0% (34)	100.0% (34)

Note: Percentages are weighted to reflect the population. *N*'s are unweighted sample *n*'s.

The proportion who said the effect was mostly negative increased substantially. Current PTSD was much more prevalent among the nurses who reported negative effects or a balance of negative and positive effects of their military service on their lives. Table 8.14 shows that these rates were 39.0% and 28.6% in the NVVRS and the Longitudinal Study, respectively. Rates were much lower among those who reported positive effects (0.0% and 2.2%, respectively).

Table 8.14 RATES OF CURRENT PTSD AMONG NURSE VETERANS IN THE NVVRS AND LONGITUDINAL STUDY INTERVIEWS ACCORDING TO THEIR APPRAISALS OF THE EFFECT OF MILITARY SERVICE ON THEIR LIVES IN EACH STUDY

Effect of Military Service	NVVRS (SCID)	NVVLS (CAPS-5)
Entirely positive	0.0% (9)	0.0% (5)
Mostly positive	0.0% (17)	2.6% (20)
An equal balance of positive and negative	42.7% (7)	23.3% (5)
Mostly negative	0.0% (1)	38.7% (4)
Entirely negative	—	—.
TOTAL	7.7% (34)	8.5% (34)
Combined Responses		
Positive	0.0% (26)	2.24% (25)
Equal balance or negative	39.0% (8)	28.6% (9)
TOTAL	7.7% (34)	8.5% (34)

Note: Percentages are weighted to reflect the population. *N*'s are unweighted sample *n*'s.

Table 8.15 RESPONSES TO THE QUESTION "IN
GENERAL, HOW SATISFYING DO YOU FIND THE WAY
YOU'RE SPENDING YOUR LIFE THESE DAYS?" IN THE
LONGITUDINAL STUDY AND NVVRS

	NVVRS	Longitudinal Study
Completely satisfying	14.3% (6)	24.8% (8)
Pretty satisfying	75.1% (25)	55.0% (19)
Not very satisfying	10.6% (3)	20.2% (7)
TOTAL	100.0% (34)	100.0% (34)

Note: Percentages are weighted to reflect the population. *N*'s are unweighted sample *n*'s.

A broad look at the nurse veterans' lives is provided by a question that asks, "In general, how satisfying do you find the way you're spending your life these days?" As shown in Table 8.15, the great majority in both surveys found their lives "completely satisfying" or "pretty satisfying." However, a small minority (10.6%) responded "not very satisfying" in the NVVRS, a proportion that nearly doubled to 20.2% in the Longitudinal Study.

SUMMARY AND CONCLUSIONS

Most of this chapter analyzes responses and diagnoses recorded in the NVVRS, and we began by reviewing those. We then considered findings from the Longitudinal Study, which offered us an opportunity to evaluate the long-term effects of the Vietnam war on nurse veterans.

Over 7,000 women served in the American military during that war, an estimated 85% as nurses. While women did not serve in combat roles, the bases and hospitals where they served were subject to enemy attack. Perhaps more importantly, the work of treating severely wounded soldiers, sometimes in greater numbers than could be given adequate attention, was stressful in itself. Furthermore, women serving in Vietnam, nurses included, could be subject to sexual harassment, even rape, by fellow American soldiers. But serving as a nurse could also be highly rewarding. Many nurses enjoyed a sense of comradeship and professional responsibility that were greater than anything they had experienced in civilian life.

Male veterans had a somewhat higher rate of war-related PTSD onset (21.6%) than nurses (16.8%). However, we found a higher rate of war-related PTSD onset among nurses serving in Vietnam than among male veterans with low probable combat exposure. The rate of PTSD that persisted until the NVVRS interview was much higher among the nurses than among male veterans with low probable combat exposure (5.0% vs. 0.3%). These differences held even when the effects of demographic variables and vulnerability factors were held constant. In fact, with these variables controlled, the odds of PTSD that persisted until the NVVRS interview were nearly four times higher among the nurses even than among male veterans with *moderate* probable combat exposure.

Numerous personal accounts and informal surveys have identified likely sources of war-related stress in this population. This literature also suggests a possible protective factor—a strong collegial bond among nurses who shared the challenging responsibility of caring for wounded soldiers in the war zone. We assessed the relative importance of these factors. The three main stressors we tested did produce sizeable statistical effects. However, the effect of unit cohesion did not show the protective effect we expected to find.

Service in the operating room and personal risk resulting from enemy attack show strong associations with PTSD onset, although statistical significance is marginal in both cases. Nurses' casualty load is not significantly associated with PTSD onset, but it shows a substantial and highly significant association with the persistence of PTSD until the time of the NVVRS interview. This last finding is particularly impressive, given that the casualty load variable did not characterize individual nurses' experiences but could be estimated only on the basis of general conditions in Vietnam during each nurse's tour of duty. It is puzzling that casualty load is significantly associated with current PTSD but not with PTSD onset. While association is no more than an indicator of possible causation, this finding suggests that a heavy casualty load may have caused the persistence of PTSD, but that its initial role in onsets was small or nonexistent. If this is the case, we should look to other traumatic experiences as possible causes of onset. Our statistical results suggest that both personal risk and service in the operating room are likely candidates for having provoked onset.

Quite different stresses affected women nurses and male soldiers in the war zone. Each was subject to the threat of deadly enemy action, although only male soldiers took part in combat; but nurses experienced stresses that were inherent in the job of caring for wounded soldiers. Both of our measures of nurses' job-related stress are indirect. The mere fact that a nurse served at a time when the average casualty load for all American nurses in Vietnam was high does not automatically establish that she personally was subject to an elevated level of stress, nor does the fact that she served in the operating room. We have interpreted the associations we report here as associations between PTSD and the stresses of caring for wounded soldiers or of experiencing the danger of enemy attack.

That interpretation is supported by the traumatic events and stressful experiences the clinical interviewers elicited from the nurses whom they diagnosed as having suffered onsets of war-related PTSD. Virtually all such experiences occurring in Vietnam that those nurses reported to the interviewer involved either personal risk under enemy attack or seeing wounded, dying, or dead soldiers, with such witnessing often explicitly linked to the job of caring for wounded soldiers. With only one possible exception (the nurse who witnessed both a stillbirth and the destruction of a "sampan village"), the interviewers had no other basis for determining that Criterion A had been satisfied. Thus, both our statistical analysis and the clinical interviewers' determination of Criterion A point to the same conclusion: war-related PTSD was associated with personal risk and the stresses of nursing. In the statistical analysis, this conclusion is indicated mainly by substantial associations that fall short of the .05 level of significance. However, casualty load shows a substantial and statistically significant association with current PTSD. Thus, at a minimum, our analysis supports the hypothesis that PTSD was associated with the stressful nature of nurses' work in the war zone.

Despite the fact that the diagnosed subsample data proved insufficient for testing the effects of sexual harassment and attack, the full NVVRS sample was large enough to yield *rates* of sexual harassment and attack. These are considerably lower than those found among women in a 2012 survey of women in the military. However, both surveys suffer from serious methodological problems. The 2012 survey had a very low completion rate, and it is quite possible that more of the NVVRS nurses would have reported attack or harassment to the interviewer if the line of questioning had been specifically designed to elicit those experiences.

It is well worth noting, however, that the combined rate of reported sexual harassment and attack in Vietnam increased from 3% and 4% in the two middle periods of the war to 13% in the last period, when the intensity of combat had diminished, but military discipline had deteriorated. This may help to explain why rates of PTSD onset among nurses declined only slightly in the last period of the war, when combat showed a sharp decline for U.S. forces.

The effects of war-zone experience were not reduced when pre-war vulnerability factors were controlled, so these effects were statistically independent of vulnerability. All the same, possibly our most striking finding is the apparent importance of pre-war vulnerabilities in determining which nurses, operating in what must have been a stressful environment for most or all of them, actually experienced PTSD onsets—and, even more importantly, which nurses still suffered from the disorder at the time of the interview, years after the war. A childhood in which a family member abused drugs or alcohol was a strong risk factor for PTSD onset but fell just short of statistical significance at the .05 level. Most remarkably, though, having had a psychiatric disorder before serving in Vietnam was an extremely potent and highly significant risk factor for both PTSD onset and current PTSD. Nurses with pre-war psychiatric histories were 23 times more likely than their colleagues to suffer an onset of PTSD, and all four nurses who still had PTSD at the time of the NVVRS interview had such histories. Three of the four had suffered from phobias before arriving in Vietnam. It would be informative to investigate the possible role in PTSD of preexisting psychiatric disorder in general and of phobias in particular in a larger sample than was available to us here.

The Longitudinal Study, conducted in 2012 and 2013, provides useful information about veteran nurses' lives many years after the NVVRS. Thirty-seven nurse veterans constituted the sample used in our analysis of the Longitudinal Study. As might be expected, life circumstances changed as the nurses aged. Nearly three-quarters were retired by the time of the Longitudinal Study. While virtually all had been single during their service in Vietnam, three-quarters had married by the time of the NVVRS, although a few had become separated or divorced. At the time of the Longitudinal Study, the proportion ever married had increased slightly, to about four-fifths, although by this time a fair number were divorced or widowed.

Did the prevalence of current PTSD among the nurses increase, decrease, or remain about the same? While a different diagnostic instrument was used in each survey, measures based on the same diagnostic criteria and symptoms show current PTSD decreasing only slightly, from a rate of 7.0% in the NVVRS interview to 6.2% in the Longitudinal Study interview. However, a simple count of PTSD symptoms included in both instruments shows a much sharper decline. There was considerable turnover between the two interviews in this small sample; only one nurse was diagnosed with current PTSD at both interviews. This turnover suggests that PTSD may have remitted and recurred in some responders—a possibility that is further supported by examining the seven nurse veterans who had onsets of war-related PTSD that had remitted by the time of the Longitudinal Study. All but one of the seven had at least one CAPS-5 symptom at the Longitudinal Study. Thus, there appears to have been a long-term residue of the disorder in nearly all of those who no longer met criteria for the diagnosis.

Slightly over 40% in both studies felt the Vietnam war was the biggest event in their lives. Large majorities in both studies thought the effect of military service on their lives had been entirely positive or mostly positive. In both studies, current PTSD was rare in these two groups. (The rates were 0.0% and 2.2%, respectively.) However, rates were much higher among those who characterized the effect of military service as negative or an equal balance of positive and negative (39.0% and 28.6%, respectively). We do not know to what extent the nurses' appraisals of their military experience may have contributed to the persistence of PTSD, and to what extent the persistence of PTSD may have influenced their appraisals. However, we do know that, among the minority whose appraisals were not positive, a substantial proportion also suffered from current PTSD. All the same, we also know that large majorities (89.4% in the NVVRS, 79.8% in the Longitudinal Study) found their lives either completely satisfying or pretty satisfying. Despite the stresses of their service, and despite the emotional toll of PTSD on some, most of the nurse veterans reported that their experience in Vietnam had a positive effect and that their lives today are satisfying.

REFERENCES

Appy, C. (1993). *Working-class war: American combat soldiers and Vietnam.* Chapel Hill, NC: University of North Carolina Press.

Brewin, C. R., Andrews, B., & Valentine, J. D. (2000). Meta-analysis of risk factors for posttraumatic stress disorder in trauma-exposed adults. *Journal of Consulting and Clinical Psychology, 68*, 748–766.

Clodfelter, M. (1995). *Vietnam in military statistics: A history of the Indochina wars, 1772–1991.* Jefferson, NC: McFarland and Co.

Comptroller, Secretary of Defense. (2008). Vietnam war deaths and casualties by month. http://www.americanwarlibrary.com/vietnam/vwc24.htm

Dahl, J., & O'Neal, J. (1993). Stress and coping behavior in nurses in Desert Storm. *Journal of Psychosocial Nursing and Mental Health Services, 31*, 17–21.

Defense Manpower Data Center. (2013). *2012 workplace and gender relations survey of active duty members.* Arlington, VA: Van Winkle, E.P., Branch Chief.

DeRoma, V. M., Root, L. P., & Smith, B. S., Jr. (2003). Socioenvironmental context of sexual trauma and well-being of women veterans. *Military Medicine, 168,* 399–403.

Durkheim, E. (1951). *Suicide: Astudy in sociology.* New York: Free Press. (Originally published in 1879.)

Edelman, B. (Ed.). (1985). *Dear America: Letters home from Vietnam.* New York: W.W. Norton & Co.

Fontana, A., Spoonster Schwartz, L., & Rosenheck, R. (1997). Posttraumatic stress disorder among female Vietnam veterans: A causal model of etiology. *American Journal of Public Health, 87,* 169–175.

Freedman, D., & Rhoads, J. (Eds.). (1987). *Nurses in Vietnam: The forgotten veterans.* Austin, TX: Texas Monthly Press.

Fox, R. P. (1979). *Air base defense in the Republic of Vietnam, 1961–1973.* Washington, DC: Office of Air Force History.

Hartl, M. A. (1991). Wartime nursing: One nurse's experience in Vietnam, *AORN Journal, 53,* 1193–1208.

King, D. W., King, L. A., Foy, D. W., & Gudanowski, D. M. (1996). Prewar factors in combat-related posttraumatic stress disorder: Structural equation modeling with a national sample of female and male Vietnam veterans. *Journal of Consulting and Clinical Psychology, 64,* 520–531.

Kulka, R. A., Schlenger, W. E., Fairbank, J. A., Hough, R. L., Jordan, B. K., Marmar, C. R., & Weiss, D. (1990). *Trauma and the Vietnam War generation.* New York: Brunner/ Mazel.

LeVasseur, J. J. (2003) The proving grounds: Combat nursing in Vietnam. *Nursing Outlook, 51,* 31–36.

Memorial to Lt. Sharon Ann Lane at http://www.virtualwall.org/women.htm, accessed Nov. 24, 2014.

Neel, S. (1991). *Medical support of the U.S. Army in Vietnam 1965–1970.* Washington, DC: Department of the Army.

Norman, E. (1990). *Women at war: The story of fifty military nurses who served in Vietnam.* Philadelphia, PA: University of Pennsylvania Press.

Panksepp, J., Nelson, E., & Bekkedal, M. (1999). Brain systems for the mediation of social separation distress and social-reward: Evolutionary antecedents and neuropeptide intermediaries. In C. S. Carter, I. I. Lederhendler, & B. Kirkpatrick (Eds.), *The integrative neurobiology of affiliation* (pp. 221–244). Cambridge, MA: MIT Press.

Paul, E. A. (1985). Wounded healers: A summary of the Vietnam Nurse Veteran Project, *Military Medicine, 150,* 571–576.

Rogers, B., & Nickolaus, J. (1987). Vietnam nurses. *Journal of Psychosocial Nursing & Mental Health Services, 25,* 10–15.

Rushton, P. (2011). Protecting and respecting military nurses. *International Journal of Nursing Practice, 17,* 615–620.

Sadler, A. G., Booth, B. M., Cook, B. L., & Doebbeling, B. N. (2003). Factors associated with women's risk of rape in the military environment. *American Journal of Industrial Medicine, 43,* 262–273.

Scannell-Desch, E. A. (1996). The lived experience of women military nurses in Vietnam during the Vietnam War. *Image: The Journal of Nursing Scholarship, 28,* 119–124.

Scannell-Desch, E. A. (August 2000). Hardships and personal strategies of Vietnam War nurses. *Western Journal of Nursing Research, 22,* 526–550.

Schlenger, W. E., Corry, N. H., Kulka, R. A., Williams, C. S., Henn-Haase, C., & Marmar, C. R. (2015). Design and methods of the National Vietnam Veterans Longitudinal Study. *International Journal of Methods in Psychiatric Research 24,* 186–203.

Seymour, R. S. (2002). Vietnam: One nurse's story. *Kansas Nurse, 77,* 13–15.

Skinner, K., Kressin, N., Frayne, S., Tripp, T., Hankin, C., Miller, D., & Sullivan, L. (2000). The prevalence of military sexual assault among female Veterans' Administration outpatients. *Journal of Interpersonal Violence, 15,* 291–310.

Spitzer, R., Williams, J., & Gibbon, M. (1987). Structured Clinical Interview for DSM-III-R, Version NP-V. New York: New York State Psychiatric Institute, Biometrics Research Department.

Steinman, R. (2000). *Women in Vietnam: The oral history.* New York: TV Books.

Taylor, S. E., Klein, L. C., Lewis, B. P., Gruenwald, T. L., Gurung, R. A. R., & Updegraff, J. A. (2000). Behavioral responses to stress in females: Tend-and-befriend, not fight-or-flight. *Psychological Review, 107,* 411–429.

Turner, J. B., Turse, N. A., & Dohrenwend, B. P. (2007). Circumstances of service and gender differences in war-related PTSD: Findings from the National Vietnam Veteran Readjustment Study. *Journal of Traumatic Stress, 20,* 643–649.

Vuic, K. D. (2009). *Officer, nurse, woman: The Army Nurse Corps in the Vietnam War.* Baltimore, MD: Johns Hopkins University Press.

Weathers, F. W., Blake, D. D., Schnurr, P. P., Kaloupek, D. G., Marx, B. P., & Keane, T. M. (2013). *The Clinician-Administered PTSD Scale for DSM-5 (CAPS-5).* Interview available from the National Center for PTSD at http://www.ptsd.va.gov.

CHAPTER 9

⌁

Families of Veterans

The Question of Secondary Traumatization

THOMAS J. YAGER, NICOLE GERSZBERG,
AND BRUCE P. DOHRENWEND

My biggest interest right now is everything that has to do with the Vietnam War. I'm reading a lot
of war books. I watched Full Metal Jacket and Platoon. It makes me see what my dad went through,
and I think, wow, no wonder he was so weird. . . . My dad actually killed people. He was trained to
kill people. You're trained to kill people, you get shot a lot, and then you come home to a regular
family. How weird is that? (Coleman, 2006, pp. 43–44)

The phrase "secondary traumatization" has been used to describe the finding that
individuals living in close proximity to victims of violent trauma can themselves
become indirect victims of that trauma (Rosenheck & Nathan, 1985, p. 538). We use the
term here in its broadest sense, to refer to "any transmission of distress from someone
who experienced a trauma to those around the traumatized individual" (Galovski &
Lyons, 2004, p. 478).

Most previous research on the families of Vietnam veterans relevant to the question
of secondary traumatization has been based on surveys conducted with a subsample
of male veterans from the National Vietnam Veterans Readjustment Study (NVVRS)
whose wives or domestic partners were also surveyed (Kulka et al., 1990). Because most
of the partners were wives, we henceforth refer to the veterans' wives or partners simply
as their wives. These studies investigated a number of important variables in relation to
the behavioral problems of the veterans' children, as reported by the wives (Jordan et al.,
1992; Kulka et al., 1990; Rosenheck & Fontana, 1998). They found that the children's
behavioral problems, as reported by the wife on the Child Behavior Checklist (CBCL;
Achenbach, 1991), were positively associated with four variables: first, the wife's own

psychological distress, as reported by her on the Psychiatric Epidemiology Research Interview (PERI) Demoralization Scale (Dohrenwend et al., 1980); second, the veteran's self-reported involvement in, or witnessing of, harm to civilians and prisoners (Rosenheck & Fontana, 1998); third, the veteran's self-reported combat experiences; and, especially, fourth, the veteran's own PTSD—the most direct measure of primary traumatization of the veteran himself.

PTSD in these studies was measured by the Mississippi Scale for Combat-Related PTSD (M-PTSD), a checklist of self-reported symptoms (Keane, Caddell, & Taylor, 1988). Checklists such as the M-PTSD are used for the self-reporting of current symptoms but are not intended to track their prior onset. This is a limitation in that factors associated with onset can be quite different from factors affecting course (e.g., Schnurr, Lunney, & Sengupta, 2004). A more serious problem is that the M-PTSD checklist may measure non-specific distress rather than PTSD (Lauterbach, King, & King, 1997; see also Chapter 4).

As elsewhere in this monograph, therefore, we use rigorous diagnoses of war-related PTSD onsets and chronic current war-related PTSD made by professional clinical interviewers of veterans in a subsample of the NVVRS. These diagnoses, along with clinical diagnoses of alcoholism with onset during or after the veterans' service in Vietnam and diagnoses of psychiatric disorders with onset before Vietnam, allow us to improve on earlier studies. We single out alcoholism (including both abuse and dependence) because it is highly likely to be disruptive of family life (e.g., Savarese et al., 2001) and less likely than other frequently occurring disorders, such as depression, to be comorbid with PTSD in Vietnam veterans (Dohrenwend et al., 2013).

We also investigate the roles of risk factors strongly associated with PTSD (see Chapters 3 and 5; and Dohrenwend et al., 2013). The first of these is pre-war vulnerability load, including history of pre-war psychiatric disorder. If fathers' PTSD is not associated with children's problems independently of pre-war vulnerability, that finding would rule out an interpretation that the problems are attributable to war-related PTSD. We examine the roles of potentially traumatic war experience for a different reason. An association of these experiences with the children's problems, even when PTSD is taken into account, would suggest that secondary traumatization, if any, may have occurred in some way other than through the father's PTSD. Finally, we test simultaneously father's PTSD and alcoholism to determine if either is independently associated with children's problems.

We investigate the roles of these factors as each may have affected the internalizing (e.g., anxious or depressive) and externalizing (e.g., aggressive) behaviors of the children, as measured by the CBCL, or the wife's psychological distress. We investigate in turn the effects the wife's distress may have on the couple's children.

In general, males and females have been found to differ in the nature and prevalence of their psychiatric disorders (e.g., Dohrenwend & Dohrenwend, 1976). And a national survey found that externalizing scores of boys referred for mental health services were relatively higher than their internalizing scores; for referred girls, internalizing scores were relatively higher than externalizing scores (Achenbach, et al., 1991, p. 30). Since girls and boys tend to differ in the nature of their behavior problems, we expected secondary traumatization of girls to be indicated more by internalizing symptoms, and the impact on boys to be more evident in externalizing symptoms.

METHOD
Participants and Procedure

Two overlapping subsamples were drawn by Kulka et al. (1988) from the larger 1,200-member NVVRS sample of male Theater veterans. One subsample received psychiatric examinations and were given clinical diagnoses ($N = 260$). In the other, veterans' wives were interviewed ($N = 257$). The two subsamples overlapped considerably.

We focused on 115 male veterans who received psychiatric examinations, whose wives were interviewed, and with whom the veterans had at least one child aged 6–16. This subsample was drawn entirely from greater urban areas, whereas the other 142 families (without diagnosed veterans) came from rural as well as urban areas. There were no statistically significant differences in rates of CBCL internalizing or externalizing problems in the two samples. Only one difference, in boys' internalizing behavior, approached statistical significance ($p = .057$). The two samples could not be compared on variables that were based on, or incorporated, the psychiatric diagnoses—veteran PTSD, alcoholism, and vulnerability load. The two samples did not differ with statistical significance on any of the other independent variables used in our analysis—combat exposure, harm to civilians or prisoners, and wife demoralization.

Each wife in these 115 families provided responses on her own demoralization and completed a CBCL about her children. We analyze CBCL data from one child in the selected age range for each veteran. If he had more than one such child, we randomly chose one (52 girls, 63 boys). With one exception, all analyses used the full sample with no missing cases. (The exception was analyses using veterans' reports of harm to civilians or prisoners, for which data were missing for the fathers of two girls and two boys. Missing item scores were rare in the continuous scales and were handled by taking the mean of available Demoralization Scale items and prorating the CBCL scales.)

MEASURES
The Child Behavior Checklist (CBCL)

CBCL internalizing and externalizing symptoms (Achenbach, 1991; Achenbach & Ruffle, 2000) have been investigated in many large samples, including nationwide samples of the general population that provide age and gender norms. The CBCL provides "clinical" and "borderline" ("clinical range") cut-points based on deviations from age- and gender-specific population norms for boys and girls aged 6–11 and 12–18. We used the available 12–18 cut-offs for our 12–16-year-olds (Achenbach & Rescorla, 2001). Achenbach and his colleagues developed their cut-points using a sample of children in the United States who had not been referred for mental health problems.

Table 9.1 PROPORTIONS OF VETERANS' CHILDREN WHOSE
CBCL SCORES ARE IN THE CLINICAL RANGE ("CLINICAL" AND
"BORDERLINE")

	CBCL Internalizing		CBCL Externalizing		Internalizing or Externalizing	
	n	%	n	%	n	%
All children (n = 115)						
Clinical or above	15	7.8	13	5.1	19	8.3
Borderline or above	25	13.5	22	14.8	30	19.6
Girls (n = 52)						
Clinical or above	11	14.2	9	8.1	13	15.1
Borderline or above	15	24.8	12	16.5	17	25.6
Boys (n = 63)						
Clinical or above	4	2.8	4	2.8	6	3.1
Borderline or above	10	4.8	10	13.5	13	15.0

Note: Percentages are weighted to the population from which the male subsample was drawn. *N*'s are unweighted numbers. Achenbach reported rates of 18% and 17% for clinical-range internalizing and externalizing problems in a non-referred national sample of boys and girls (Achenbach, 1991, p. 102).

They tested the effectiveness of various cut-points for their ability to discriminate between referred and non-referred children. We dichotomized the continuous CBCL scales (internalizing mean $[M]$ = 6.35, standard deviation $[SD]$ = 6.24; externalizing M = 7.23, SD = 5.06) into clinical range (borderline plus clinical) versus all others in our analyses—a distinction that should help to clarify implications of our findings for treatment. Table 9.1 gives proportions of veterans' children whose CBCL scores are in the clinical range.

PTSD Diagnoses

As elsewhere, we used diagnoses made by doctoral-level clinicians using the Structured Clinical Interview for DSM-III-R (SCID) (Spitzer, Williams, & Gibbon, 1987). For each PTSD symptom, the SCID distinguished between "lifetime" (i.e., occurring during the veteran's lifetime) and "current" (present at any time during the six months prior to the examination). Compiling this information and applying DSM-III-R criteria, it then determined the presence or absence of lifetime or current PTSD and recorded the respondent's age at onset. We used additional information to establish whether a PTSD diagnosis was war-related (e.g., Dohrenwend et al., 2006). Our sample for this analysis included no veterans who had had onsets of PTSD that had occurred prior to their service in Vietnam. Twenty-one percent of veterans in the sample used here had war-related onsets. Eleven percent had war-related PTSD that was current at the time of the interview. Our analysis distinguishes current PTSD from "past" PTSD; that is, war-related PTSD that was not current at the time of the interview. Dating of multiple remissions and onsets was not possible. Because current PTSD had persisted until the time of the interview, we expected that it would be the more severe disorder and more strongly associated than past PTSD with problems in the veterans' children and wives.

Alcoholism (Abuse or Dependence)

The clinicians made similarly rigorous diagnoses of other disorders (Dohrenwend et al., 2006; Dohrenwend et al., 2013). We focused here on alcohol problems that had developed during or after the veteran's service in Vietnam. In the sample used here, 30% of veterans had alcoholism onsets during or after their service in Vietnam; 3.4% were diagnosed with such alcoholism at the time of the interview.

Demoralization in the Veterans' Wives

Following Jerome Frank (1961), we think of our measure of nonspecific distress as indicating demoralization in the NVVRS dataset. The Demoralization Scale, derived from the PERI (Dohrenwend, 1980), consists of 27 items on helplessness, hopelessness, depressed mood, dread and anxiety, low self-esteem, and psychophysiological disturbances. It yielded an internal consistency reliability of .95 in the sample of veterans' wives used here. Expressed as the mean of item scores, the scale has possible scores of 0–5, with $M = 2.01$, $SD = .640$. We use a standardized version here ($M = 0$, $SD = 1$).

Pre-Vietnam Vulnerability Factors

Previous research has consistently shown PTSD to be associated with vulnerability factors such as childhood trauma, childhood family problems, and a history of psychiatric disorder, as well as age, education, and belonging to a minority racial or ethnic group (e.g., Brewin, Andrews, & Valentine, 2000; Schnurr, Lunney, & Sengupta, 2004). As explained in Chapter 3, our vulnerability load measure consisted of a simple count of nine dichotomously scored vulnerability factors previously shown to be related to PTSD. It had scores ranging from 0–8 ($M = 3.82$, $SD = 1.34$).

Measure of Severity of Exposure to War-Zone Stressors

We used the Combat Exposure Severity Scale (CESS) described in Chapter 3, dichotomizing it at the 75th percentile in the full diagnosed subsample on the basis of an inflection point identified in that chapter (also in Dohrenwend et al., 2013). Based on this dichotomization, 26% percent of veterans in the sample used here experienced high combat exposure.

Participation in Harm to Civilians or Prisoners

We used the indicator of harm to civilians or prisoners described in Chapter 3. In the full, diagnosed subsample, this measure of harm is strongly associated with PTSD onset and current PTSD (Chapter 6; and Dohrenwend et al., 2013). In the sample used here, 16% of veterans reported participating in harming civilians or prisoners.

DATA ANALYSIS

We first compared rates of clinical-range internalizing and externalizing behavior problems in veterans' daughters and sons with rates in the U.S. general population. We then tested bivariate associations between veterans' PTSD and their children's behavior problems, as well as their wives' demoralization. Next, through a series of multivariate models, we tested whether veterans' PTSD showed a positive association with the children's internalizing and externalizing behaviors and the wives' distress that was independent of each of the possible risk factors for PTSD—namely, the veterans' vulnerability load, combat exposure, involvement in harming civilians or prisoners, current alcoholism with onset in or after Vietnam (and the wives' demoralization when children's problems were the dependent variable). Because of our small sample size ($n = 115$), we tested each risk factor separately rather than combining all in a single model. We use Benjamini and Hochberg's false-discovery-rate controlling procedure (Benjamini & Hochberg, 1995) and $\alpha = .05$ (two-tailed) to adjust for multiple tests. The CBCL scores in these analyses were dichotomized to indicate the clinical-range level, which included Achenbach's borderline and clinical categories. We used logistic regression when these dichotomous indicators of children's problems were the dependent variable. We used linear regression to test for possible independent effects of the veteran variables on wife demoralization, a continuous variable. Where veteran PTSD was found to be associated with wife demoralization, and wife demoralization (after controlling for PTSD) was associated with children's behavior problems, we fitted a mediation model testing the indirect effect of PTSD on children's problems by way of their mothers' demoralization.

Data in all analyses were weighted to reflect NVVRS sampling procedures and were further adjusted for non-response (Kulka et al., 1988, p. 21). Statistical tests in all analyses except the mediation models used the SPSS (Statistical Package for the Social Sciences) Complex Samples package for analyzing stratified and weighted data. For the mediation models, estimation and testing was done with Mplus 7.3, using linear regression to predict mothers' demoralization and probit regression to predict children's problems. Because of racial and ethnic differences in rates of PTSD (Dohrenwend et al., 2008), the veteran's racial and ethnic group was included as a control in all regression analyses. This categorical variable distinguishes blacks, Hispanics, and non-Hispanic whites; other groups did not occur in the sample used here.

Results

Table 9.1 shows, as expected, that girls have higher clinical-range proportions of internalizing than externalizing behavior, while boys show the opposite pattern.

Among all children combined, 13.5% met the borderline/clinical criterion on the internalizing scale, and 14.8% met it on the externalizing scale. These figures are lower than the 18% and 17% rates of clinical-range internalizing and externalizing problems, respectively, in Achenbach's non-referred national sample (Achenbach, 1991, p. 102).

We expected veterans' PTSD, especially if still current, to have more impact on internalizing than externalizing symptoms for girls, while showing the reverse for boys. It can be seen in Table 9.2, however, that veteran PTSD, whether past or current, shows

Table 9.2 LOGISTIC MODELS TESTING BIVARIATE ASSOCIATIONS BETWEEN WAR-RELATED PTSD IN VETERANS AND INTERNALIZING AND EXTERNALIZING CLINICAL RANGE PROBLEMS IN THEIR DAUGHTERS AND SONS

Independent Variables	CBCL Internalizing Problems		CBCL Externalizing Problems	
	OR	95% CI	OR	95% CI
Girls				
Past PTSD	.09	[.006, 1.20]	.14	[.009, 2.24]
Current PTSD	1.12	[.20, 6.27]	2.48	[.41, 14.81]
Boys				
Past PTSD	1.11	[.09, 13.57]	13.81	[.52, 367.01]
Current PTSD	20.31*	[2.45, 168.41]	6.70	[.74, 60.90]

Note: These analyses take into account the complex subsample design. Father's racial/ethnic group (white, black, Hispanic) is included in every model as a control variable. Children whose veteran fathers had past (but not current) PTSD are contrasted with those whose fathers never had PTSD ($N = 40$ girls, 44 boys). Children whose veteran fathers had current PTSD are contrasted with those whose fathers did not ($N = 52$ girls, 63 boys). OR = odds ratio; CI = confidence interval.

*$p \leq .01$.

Table 9.3 LINEAR REGRESSION MODELS TESTING
BIVARIATE ASSOCIATIONS BETWEEN WAR-RELATED PTSD
IN VETERANS AND DEMORALIZATION IN THEIR WIVES

Independent Variables	Wife Demoralization	
	β	95% CI
Past PTSD	–.229	[–.564, .105]
Current PTSD	.235*	[.049, .422]

Note: These analyses take into account the complex subsample design. Father's racial/
ethnic group (white, black, Hispanic) is included in each model as a control variable.
CI = confidence interval.

*$p \leq .05$

no statistically significant association with internalizing or externalizing clinical-range
symptoms in girls.

Among boys, in contrast, veterans' current PTSD showed a statistically significant
association with internalizing problems. Contrary to our expectation, there was no
evidence that veteran PTSD was more strongly associated in boys with externalizing
behavior problems than with internalizing behavior problems.

Table 9.3 focuses on wife demoralization as the dependent variable.

It shows that veterans' current PTSD, but not past PTSD, has a statistically significant positive association with wife demoralization. The absence of any statistically
significant association of past PTSD with problems in veterans' children or with demoralization in their wives is consistent with our expectation that associations with
current PTSD would be stronger. Because we found no statistically significant effects
of past PTSD, we excluded it from further analyses.

A question arose as to whether other war-related or pre-war risk factors for PTSD
could account for children's internalizing and externalizing behavior problems or for
wife demoralization. Table 9.4 shows the results for boys' behavior problems in a series of multivariate models in which risk factors were combined with PTSD one at
a time.

Model 1, also shown in Table 9.2, is repeated here for inclusion in Benjamini and
Hochberg's false-discovery-rate controlling procedure. In accord with that procedure, none of the known risk factors for PTSD (pre-war vulnerability, combat exposure, harm to civilians or prisoners) showed a statistically significant association with
boys' problems independent of current PTSD in the father. Therefore, we have no
evidence that veterans' war experiences adversely affected their sons in any way other

Table 9.4 LOGISTIC MODELS TESTING ASSOCIATIONS BETWEEN BOYS'
CLINICAL RANGE CBCL SCORES AND CURRENT WAR-RELATED PTSD IN THEIR
FATHERS, IN COMBINATION WITH OTHER PARENTAL VARIABLES

Independent Variables	CBCL Internalizing Problems		CBCL Externalizing Problems	
	OR	95% CI	OR	95% CI
Model 1.				
Current PTSD	**20.31**	[2.45, 168.41]	6.70	[.74, 60.90]
Model 2.				
Current PTSD	**10.11**	[2.06, 49.75]	3.00	[.12, 77.78]
Vulnerability	1.41	[.72, 2.78]	1.35	[.45, 4.10]
Model 3.				
Current PTSD	**11.99**	[1.94, 73.96]	6.47	[1.02, 40.84]
Combat Exposure	4.41	[.62, 31.15]	1.09	[.20, 5.93]
Model 4.				
Current PTSD	**37.90**	[2.35, 611.29]	2.44	[.08, 70.77]
Harm to Civ./Prisoners	.23	[.01, 4.81]	7.84	[.33, 188.02]
Model 5.				
Current PTSD	**22.03**	[3.05, 159.18]	6.39	[.70, 58.38]
Current Alcohol	5.02	[.06, 409.80]	0	—
Model 6.				
Current PTSD	13.96	[1.34, 144.98]	6.08	[.85, 43.60]
Wife Demoralized	3.61	[.64, 20.19]	1.21	[.49, 2.98]

Note: These analyses take into account the complex subsample design. $N = 115$ ($N = 111$ for Model 4). Father's racial/ethnic group (white, black, Hispanic) is included in every model as a control variable. Vulnerability is a simple count, ranging from 0–8. Wife demoralization is a continuous scale expressed in standard deviation units with mean = 0 (based on the combined sample of girls and boys). Bolded odds ratios (ORs) significant at $p \le .023$ (Benjamini-Hochberg alpha correction for 5 of 11 hypotheses). OR = odds ratio; CI = confidence interval.

than through PTSD in their fathers. Similarly, current alcoholism showed no statistically significant independent association, nor did demoralization in the boys' mothers. Conversely, the association of PTSD with internalizing problems remained large when controlled for each of these factors and was statistically significant in all but Model 6, where wife demoralization was controlled. In Model 6, PTSD lost statistical significance when we applied Benjamini and Hochberg's procedure: even then, barely falling short of the required level of significance ($p = .028$ vs. $p \le .027$ for six of 11 hypotheses). In contrast, wife demoralization showed no statistically significant association with or without this procedure.

Table 9.5 shows the results for girls.

Table 9.5 LOGISTIC MODELS TESTING ASSOCIATIONS BETWEEN GIRLS'
CLINICAL RANGE CBCL SCORES AND CURRENT WAR-RELATED PTSD IN THEIR
FATHERS, IN COMBINATION WITH OTHER PARENTAL VARIABLES

Independent Variables	CBCL Internalizing Problems		CBCL Externalizing Problems	
	OR	OR	OR	95% CI
Model 1.				
Current PTSD	1.12	[.20, 6.27]	2.48	[.41, 14.87]
Model 2.				
Current PTSD	1.64	[.23, 11.52]	7.24	[.47, 112.13]
Vulnerability	2.04	[.69, 6.08]	3.86	[1.19, 12.55]
Model 3.				
Current PTSD	1.15	[.21, 6.27]	2.63	[.43, 15.93]
Combat exposure	1.73	[.23, 12.97]	2.31	[.20, 27.33]
Model 4.				
Current PTSD	1.15	[.20, 6.57]	2.72	[.43, 17.05]
Harm to Civ./Prisoners	1.69	[.18, 15.83]	2.25	[.23, 22.08]
Model 5.				
Current PTSD	.92	[.14, 6.02]	1.46	[.20, 10.99]
Current Alcohol	3.03	[.08, 116.54]	17.22	[.66, 445.43]
Model 6.				
Current PTSD	.27	[.04, 1.82]	.36	[.04, 3.16]
Wife Demoralized	**2.67**	[1.51, 4.72]	**4.61**	[1.72, 12.34]

Note: These analyses take into account the complex subsample design. N = 115 (N = 111 for Model 4). Father's racial/ethnic group (white, black, Hispanic) is included in every model as a control variable. Vulnerability is a simple count, ranging from 0–8. Wife demoralization is a continuous scale expressed in standard deviation units (based on the combined sample of girls and boys). Bolded ORs significant at p ≤ .004 (Benjamini-Hochberg alpha correction for 1 of 11 hypotheses). OR = odds ratio; CI = confidence interval.

Again, Model 1 is repeated from Table 9.2. Demoralization in the girls' mothers showed statistically significant associations with both internalizing and externalizing behavior problems. None of the other associations tested was statistically significant.

Wife demoralization is the dependent variable in Table 9.6.

It shows a statistically significant association, independent of PTSD, between wife demoralization and current veteran alcoholism with onset in or after Vietnam. Pre-war vulnerability and war-zone veteran variables show no such independent effects. Model 1 (repeated from Table 9.3) shows a statistically significant association between PTSD in veterans and demoralization in their wives. That association remains statistically significant in all but Model 2, where vulnerability was controlled. However, further analysis reveals that among girls (but not boys), veterans' PTSD and their pre-war vulnerability load were independently associated with demoralization in their wives at statistically significant levels (β=.373, p = .000 and β=.398, p = .048 for PTSD and vulnerability, respectively).

Table 9.6 LINEAR REGRESSION MODELS TESTING ASSOCIATIONS
BETWEEN WIFE DEMORALIZATION AND VETERAN CURRENT WAR-RELATED
PTSD, IN COMBINATION WITH OTHER VETERAN VARIABLES

Independent Variables	Wife Demoralization	
	β	95% CI
Model 1.		
Current PTSD	**.235**	[.049, .422]
Model 2.		
Current PTSD	.172	[−.056, .400]
Vulnerability	.155	[−.109, .419]
Model 3.		
Current PTSD	**.250**	[.070, .430]
Combat Exposure	−.060	[−.213, .093]
Model 4.		
Current PTSD	**.259**	[.085, .433]
Harm to Civ./Prisoners	−.071	[−.289, .147]
Model 5.		
Current PTSD	**.210**	[.026, .395]
Current Alcohol	**.268**	[.146, .390]

Note: These analyses take into account the complex subsample design. $N = 115$ ($N = 111$ for Model 4). Father's racial/ethnic group (white, black, Hispanic) is included in every model as a control variable. β = standardized coefficient. Bolded β's significant at $p \leq .028$ (Benjamini-Hochberg alpha correction for 3 of 9 hypotheses). CI = confidence interval.

The association of wife demoralization with veteran PTSD and with behavior problems in girls suggested to us that veteran PTSD might have affected girls' problems indirectly by way of demoralization in their mothers. A test (in girls only) of that indirect effect found it statistically significant for both internalizing ($p = .018$) and externalizing ($p = .004$) problems.

SUMMARY AND CONCLUSIONS

We found evidence consistent with the proposition that these families of male Vietnam veterans suffered effects of secondary traumatization. These effects differed markedly, however, for the veterans' sons and daughters and for their wives.

Consistent with the literature, we expected that girls would have more internalizing than externalizing behavior problems and that boys would have the opposite. This was the case in our sample. Thus, it seemed reasonable to expect that secondary traumatization would be more likely to take the form of internalizing than externalizing behavior problems for girls and the opposite for boys. This was not the case.

In veterans' sons, internalizing behavior problems were associated with current PTSD in their fathers even when each of four additional established risk factors—pre-war vulnerability, combat exposure, harming of civilians or prisoners, and alcoholism—was controlled. The pattern was quite different for veterans' daughters, for whom both internalizing and externalizing behavior problems were associated with degree of demoralization of the veteran's wife. Wife demoralization was associated in turn with veterans' current PTSD and alcoholism. Tests (in girls) of the paths from PTSD to internalizing and externalizing behavior problems via wife demoralization confirmed an indirect association in each case and were consistent with the possibility of indirect secondary traumatization.

Why the effects of secondary traumatization are so different for boys and girls is an important question for further investigation. A limitation for further research on the families of veterans, however, is that the children in the NVVRS are now well into adulthood. New research needs, therefore, to focus on a new generation of veterans of more recent wars and their families—different wars and different times. It is also important to examine these relationships in traumatic exposure other than combat.

A further limitation of this research is that the small sample size and the rarity of some of the child outcomes contributed to wide confidence intervals. A larger sample would be likely to reduce the confidence intervals around findings for behavior problems with relatively rare incidence, and it might reveal additional associations that need attention. A larger sample would also permit more comprehensive statistical analyses. In addition, we relied on the SCID's broad distinction between lifetime (current plus past) and current war-related PTSD. Data on multiple onsets and remittances of PTSD were unavailable, but they would have given us a more detailed account of how the veterans' exposure affects their children's functioning.

Nevertheless, the sample used here made it possible to discover some intriguing possible causes of secondary traumatization associated with one of our most important wars. The secondary traumatization we found was of insufficient magnitude to transform the children of these Vietnam veterans into an unusually problematic group on the measures we had available. Children of the veterans did not show higher rates of serious internalizing and externalizing behavior problems than did children in a national sample of the general population. Secondary traumatization seems to have affected an unusually healthy group of children who remained at least as free of serious emotional and behavior problems as their age counterparts. In fact, the veterans' children differ from the national sample in a number of positive ways in addition to having fathers who served in Vietnam. Notably, their fathers had to pass physical and psychiatric screening to be inducted into the military. In addition, to be included in the study, the children had to be living in intact families that included a father and a mother. Absent the possible causes of secondary traumatization summarized here, their mental health might have exceeded by even more than it did the national norms set by the children in Achenbach's sample.

Nevertheless, the behavior problems we investigated are not trivial. We focused on problems in the clinical range, which implies that treatment considerations are in order. Our results suggest that treatment to ameliorate problems of secondary traumatization, especially in girls, should include giving attention to the possibility of demoralization in the veteran's spouse or partner as well as to the veteran's PTSD.

ACKNOWLEDGMENT

This chapter is based on the following article: Yager, T. J., Gerszberg, N., & Dohrenwend, B. P. (2016), Secondary traumatization in Vietnam veterans' families. *Journal of Traumatic Stress, 29,* 349–355. Publisher: International Society for Traumatic Stress Studies: Wiley InterScience.

REFERENCES

Achenbach, T. M. (1991). *Manual for the Child Behavior Checklist/4-18 and 1991 profile.* Burlington, VT: University of Vermont, Department of Psychiatry.

Achenbach, T. M., Howell, C. T., Quay, H. C., Conners, C. K., & Bates, J. E. (1991). National survey of problems and competencies among fourteen to sixteen-year-olds: Parents' reports for normative and clinical samples. *Monographs of the Society for Research in Child Development, 56,* 1–131. doi:10.2307/1166156

Achenbach, T. M., & Rescorla, L. (2001). *ASEBA school-age forms and profiles.* Burlington, VT: Aseba.

Achenbach, T. M., & Ruffle, T. M. (2000). The Child Behavior Checklist and related forms for assessing behavioral/emotional problems and competencies. *Pediatrics in Review, 21*(1), 265–271. doi:10.1542/pir.21-8-265

Benjamini, Y., & Hochberg, Y. (1995). Controlling the false discovery rate: A practical and powerful approach to multiple testing. *Journal of the Royal Statistical Society. Series B (Methodological), 57,* 289–300. doi:10.2307/2346101

Brewin, C. R., Andrews, B., & Valentine, J. D. (2000). Meta-analysis of risk factors for posttraumatic stress disorder in trauma-exposed adults. *Journal of Consulting and Clinical Psychology, 68,* 748–766. doi:10.1037//0022-006X.68.5.748

Coleman, P. (2006). *Flashback: Posttraumatic stress disorder, suicide and the lessons of war.* Boston, MA: Beacon Press.

Dohrenwend, B. P., & Dohrenwend, B. S. (1976). Sex differences and psychiatric disorders. *American Journal of Sociology, 81,* 1447–1454. doi:10.1086/226229

Dohrenwend, B. P., Shrout, P. E., Egri, G., & Mendelsohn, F. S. (1980). Non-specific psychological distress and other dimensions of psychopathology: Measures for use in the general population. *Archives of General Psychiatry, 37,* 1229–1236. doi:10.1001/archpsyc.1980.01780240027003

Dohrenwend, B. P., Turner, J. B., Turse, N. A., Adams, B. G., Koenen, K. C., & Marshall, R. (2006). The psychological risks of Vietnam for U.S. veterans: A revisit with new data and methods. *Science, 313,* 979–982. doi:10.1126/science.1128944

Dohrenwend, B. P., Turner, J. B., Turse, N. A., Lewis-Fernandez, R., & Yager, T. J. (2008). War-related posttraumatic stress disorder in black, Hispanic, and majority white veterans: The roles of exposure and vulnerability. *Journal of Traumatic Stress, 21,* 133–141. doi:1002/jts.20327

Dohrenwend, B. P., Yager, T. J., Wall, M. M., & Adams, B. G. (2013). The roles of combat exposure, personal vulnerability, and involvement in harm to civilians or prisoners in Vietnam war-related posttraumatic stress disorder. *Clinical Psychological Science, 1,* 223–238. doi:10.1177/2167702612469355

Frank, J. D. (1961). *Persuasion and healing: A comparative study of psychotherapy.* Baltimore, MD; London: Johns Hopkins University Press.

Galovski, T., & Lyons, J. A. (2004). Psychological sequelae of combat violence: A review of the impact of PTSD on the veteran's family and possible interventions. *Aggression and Violent Behavior, 9*, 477–501. doi:10.1016/S1359-1789(03)00045-4

Jordan, B. K., Marmar, C. R., Fairbank, J. A., Schlenger, W. E., Kulka, R. A., Hough, R. L. (1992), et al. Problems in families of male Vietnam veterans with posttraumatic stress disorder. *Journal of Consulting and Clinical Psychology. 60*, 916. doi:10.1037//0022-006X.60.6.916

Keane, T. M., Caddell, J. M., & Taylor, K. L. (1988). Mississippi Scale for Combat-Related Posttraumatic Stress Disorder: Three studies in reliability and validity. *Journal of Consulting and Clinical Psychology 56*, 85. doi:10.1037/0022-006X.56.1.85

Kulka, R. A., Schlenger, W. E., Fairbank, J. A., Hough, R. L., Jordan, B. K., . . . Marmar, C. R. (1988). *National Vietnam Veterans Readjustment Study (NVVRS): Description, current status, and initial PTSD prevalence estimates.* Washington, DC: Veterans Administration.

Kulka, R. A., Schlenger, W. E., Fairbank, J. A., Hough, R. L., Jordan, B. K., Marmar, C. R. et al. (1990). *Trauma and the Vietnam war generation: Report of findings from the National Vietnam Veterans Readjustment Study.* New York: Brunner/Mazel.

Lauterbach, D., Vrana, S., King, D., & King, L. (1997). Psychometric properties of the civilian version of the Mississippi PTSD scale. *Journal of Traumatic Stress, 10*, 499–513. doi:10.1002/jts.2490100313

Rosenheck, R., & Fontana, A. (1998). Transgenerational effects of abusive violence on the children of Vietnam combat veterans. *Journal of Traumatic Stress, 11*, 731–742. doi: 10.1023/A:1024445416821

Rosenheck, R., & Nathan, P. Secondary traumatization in children of Vietnam veterans. *Hospital and Community Psychiatry, 36*, 538–539. doi:10.1176.5.538

Savarese, V. W., Suvak, M. K., King, L. A., & King, D. W. (2001). Relationships among alcohol use, hyperarousal, and marital abuse and violence in Vietnam veterans. *Journal of Traumatic Stress, 14*, 717–732. doi:10.1023/A:1013038021175

Schnurr, P. P., Lunney, C. A., & Sengupta, A. (2004). Risk factors for the development versus maintenance of posttraumatic stress disorder. *Journal of Traumatic Stress, 17*, 85–95. doi:10.1023/B:JOTS.0000022614.21794.f4

Spitzer, R., Williams, J., & Gibbon, M. (1987). *Structured Clinical Interview for DSM-III-R, version NP-V.* New York: New York State Psychiatric Institute, Biometrics Research Department.

PART III

Veterans' Post-War Readjustment

CHAPTER 10

⌒⌒⌒

Some Psychological Effects of Changing Public Attitudes on U.S. Vietnam Veterans

BRUCE P. DOHRENWEND, ELEANOR MURPHY, THOMAS J. YAGER, AND STEPHANI L. HATCH

Returning vets did not experience homecoming as the sweet end to their ordeal they had imagined; the reality was far more painful. We who were their homes found it difficult to listen. They were alive but often their friends were not. The streets of their hometowns had changed. As the war ground on overseas, the war at home became an unavoidable fact of life in every community in the United States. . . . Vietnam veterans were called baby-killers by some and losers by others; it was not an easy time to claim veteran status with pride. (Coleman, 2006, at pp. 86–87)

President Barack Obama, speaking to a gathering of Vietnam veterans on a May 27, 2012, pilgrimage to the Vietnam Memorial Wall, observed,

You were often blamed for a war you did not start when you should have been commended for serving your country with valor. . . . You were sometimes blamed for the misdeeds of a few, when the honorable service of the many should have been praised. It was a national shame that should never have happened. (Baker, 2012, p. A16)

Toward the latter stages of the Vietnam war, following the 1968 Tet Offensive by the North Vietnamese Army and their Vietcong allies throughout South Vietnam, majority public opinion in the United States turned against the war. (See Chapter 1, section *War, Tet, 1968: Fighting on All Fronts, Nixon's War,* and *The Final Years,* for descriptions of growing anti-war sentiment and protests.)

As summarized in Figure 10.1, U.S. polls showed that while only about 25% of the public surveyed in August 1965 believed that the United States had made a mistake

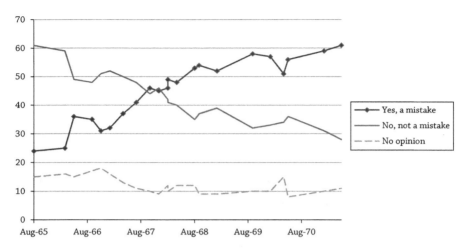

Figure 10.1 Distribution of public attitudes toward the Vietnam War from 1965 to 1971.
Note: Figures presented are from Hazel Erskine, "The Polls: Is War a Mistake?" *Public Opinion Quarterly 43* (Spring 1970): 141–142; and *Gallop Opinion Index,* numbers 56, 59, 61, 69, and 73.

in sending troops to Vietnam, about 60% thought so by August 1970. Some men also reported negative reactions of U.S. civilians to them as Vietnam veterans when they returned home.

It seemed possible to us that negative changes in public attitudes could have affected veterans' own attitudes, thereby undermining any positive motives veterans might have had about fighting this war. If so, increasingly negative attitudes on the part of the veterans who served during later, more unpopular periods of the war might have contributed to the development of adverse psychiatric outcomes.

As we reported in Chapter 4, involvement of U.S forces in combat, and often their involvement in related harm to civilians and prisoners, declined in later periods of the war when majority public attitudes were becoming unfavorable. We also found that rates of PTSD onset and current PTSD were high among veterans who served in high combat periods and low among those who served in low combat periods, especially the last period of the war—as one would expect, given the primary role of severity of combat exposure in the onset of the PTSD symptom syndrome.

In contrast, however, as discussed in Chapter 4, non-specific psychological distress at the time of the interview, similar in content to Jerome Frank's concept of demoralization (Frank, 1961; Dohrenwend et al, 1980), did not parallel variations in the level of combat depending on the period of the war when the veteran served. Like PTSD, demoralization is positively associated with severity of combat exposure; unlike PTSD, demoralization is also positively associated with a wide variety of stressful events and situations that would not qualify as Criterion A exposures. It is demoralization, therefore, that may have been most affected by the stress of changing public attitudes independently of combat exposure. This chapter is an account of our investigation of this possibility.

In this account, we examine relations among demoralization, period of the war, and the veterans' attitudes toward the war and the role of other possibly relevant variables.

CHANGING PUBLIC AND VETERAN ATTITUDES AND TIME OF WAR ENTRY

The full sample of male Theater veterans were retrospectively asked about their attitudes toward the war at the time of their entry into Vietnam and at the time of their exit, usually about a year later. Specifically, they were asked, "At the time when you first went to Vietnam [and also, "When you left the Vietnam Theater . . ."], how much were you opposed to or in favor of U.S. involvement in Vietnam—*extremely opposed, fairly opposed, somewhat opposed, neutral, somewhat in favor, fairly in favor,* or *extremely in favor?*" To overcome the problem of small sample sizes in these seven response categories, we collapsed them into three. We grouped the three opposed categories simply as "Opposed"; the fourth category remained "Neutral"; and we grouped the three favorable categories as "In favor."

Figure 10.2 shows that early in the war the veterans' attitudes started out more favorable than the public attitudes shown in Figure 10.1. Nevertheless, the increased opposition among veterans who served later in the war parallels the increased public opposition shown in Figure 10.1.

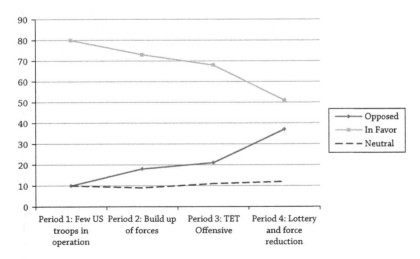

Figure 10.2 Distribution of Vietnam veterans who were in favor of, neutral toward, or opposed to the war at periods of war entry.

Note: Figures represent weighted percentages of veterans within each war entry period who reported that they were opposed to, in favor of, or neutral toward the war at time of their entry into the war. Period 1, $n = 89$; period 2, $n = 485$; period 3, $n = 369$; period 4, $n = 219$.

Wald χ^2 (6, 1162) = 26.53, $p < .0001$.

Table 10.1 CHANGE IN ATTITUDES TOWARD THE VIETNAM WAR FROM TIME
OF ENTRY TO EXIT

Attitudes at Time of Entry	Attitudes at Time of Exit		
	In Favor (*n* = 508)	Neutral (*n* = 68)	Opposed (*n* = 586)
In Favor (*n* = 747)	443 (63%)	18 (1%)	287 (36%)
Neutral (*n* = 131)	30 (27%)	44 (29%)	57 (43%)
Opposed (*n* = 283)	35 (13%)	6 (2%)	242 (86%)

Note: Percentages represent weighted estimates of those who were in favor of, neutral toward, or opposed to the war at time of entry. *N*'s are unweighted full sample numbers.

Since we had a measure of veterans' attitudes at exit as well as entrance, it was possible to examine stability and change within each veteran's tour of duty in Vietnam, usually about a year.

Table 10.1 shows the distribution of veterans among the nine possible combinations of entrance and exit attitudes. The modal group of veterans favored the war when they arrived in Vietnam and had not changed that attitude when they left. Among those who did change their attitudes from entrance to exit, however, there was a general trend toward opposing the war. Among the initially favorable, 36% became opposed, while among the initially opposed, only 13% became favorable. Likewise, more of the initially neutral became opposed (43%) than became favorable (27%). A substantial group of veterans were opposed to the war when they went to Vietnam and remained opposed when they left. These men may have been susceptible to demoralization resulting from the stress of having to fight a war in which they did not believe. However, we would expect those who changed from favorable upon entrance to unfavorable on exit to be especially demoralized because of possible feelings of betrayal.

DEMORALIZATION AND VETERAN ATTITUDES AT ENTRY AND AT EXIT

Table 10.2 shows rates of high demoralization among veterans who reported either favoring or opposing the war when they arrived in Vietnam and either favoring or opposing it when they left.

At entry, the relationship between demoralization and attitude is weak at best. The rate of high demoralization is only two percentage points higher among those who were opposed at entry (44%) than among those who were in favor (42%); and the rate among those who were neutral is higher (47%) than in either of these groups. On the other hand, at exit, demoralization is strongly related to attitude. The rate at exit is 50% among those who were opposed, versus only 36% among those who were in favor. The "neutrals" fall between these two values (41%), although closer to those who were in favor.

Table 10.2 RATES OF HIGH
DEMORALIZATION BY ATTITUDE
TOWARD THE WAR AT ENTRY AND
AT EXIT

Rate of High Demoralization

	At Entry	At Exit
In Favor	42% (748)	36% (508)
Neutral	47% (131)`	41% (68)
Opposed	44% (283)	50% (586)

Note: Percentages are weighted to the population from
which the full sample was drawn. Unweighted sample *n*'s
are in parentheses.

We used logistic regression models to test these relationships. Table 10.3 shows
models estimating the effects of attitude at entry and attitude at exit on high demoralization. We chose those who favored the war in each case as the reference group because,
as the modal group, they represent the norm.

Opposition at exit shows a substantial and statistically significant effect. All other
effects shown in Table 10.3 are not statistically significant. The fact that demoralization
is strongly associated with opposition at exit but not at entrance suggests that a change
of attitude during the veteran's tour of duty (as indirectly indicated in Table 10.2) might
have had a part in giving rise to demoralization.

Table 10.3 LOGISTIC REGRESSION MODELS
TESTING THE EFFECTS OF ENTRY AND EXIT
ATTITUDES ON HIGH DEMORALIZATION

	O.R.	(p)
Attitude at Entry		
In Favor	--Ref. Group--	
Neutral	1.22	(.45)
Opposed	1.08	(.67)
Attitude at Exit		
In Favor	--Ref. Group--	
Neutral	1.22	(.60)
Opposed	1.79	(.000)

Note: These analyses take into account the complex sample design.

DEMORALIZATION AND ATTITUDE CHANGE

We next examined the relationship between demoralization and attitude change.

Table 10.4 shows rates of high demoralization in each of the nine groups defined by attitudes at entry and at exit—in other words, for each of the nine attitude histories elicited from veterans. As we expected, those whose attitude changed from favorable to opposed exhibited a somewhat higher demoralization rate than those who were initially opposed or neutral. This modest elevation represents the effect of having become opposed during the veteran's tour of duty over and above the general effect of opposition at exit. However, as noted in the table, the difference between the rate for those opposed at exit who were initially favorable and the rate for those who were opposed from the beginning is not statistically significant ($p = .27$). Our expectation for the group who became opposed while serving in Vietnam is in the predicted direction but not statistically significant.

VETERANS' ATTITUDES AND PERIODS OF THE WAR

Table 10.5 shows the types of attitude stability and change in the different periods of the war. It was period 4, when public attitudes were most negative, that had the smallest proportion of veterans who remained favorable and the largest proportion of veterans who remained opposed during their tours. This last cohort had roughly as high a proportion of men who changed from favorable to opposed as the two high combat cohorts preceding it.

Table 10.4 RATE OF HIGH DEMORALIZATION FOR EACH OF NINE GROUPS DEFINED BY ATTITUDES AT ENTRY AND AT EXIT; CHANGE IN ATTITUDES TOWARD THE VIETNAM WAR FROM TIME OF ENTRY TO EXIT

Attitudes at Time of Entry	Attitudes at Time of Exit		
	In Favor ($n = 508$)	Neutral ($n = 68$)	Opposed ($n = 586$)
In Favor ($n = 747$)	35.4% (443)	63.5% (18)	53.4% (287)
Neutral ($n = 131$)	57.7% (30)	34.8% (44)	48.5% (57)
Opposed ($n = 283$)	25.3% (35)	45.8% (6)	46.8% (242)

$p = .008$ (linear regression with each of the 9 categories represented by a dummy variable)

Note: Percentages are weighted to the population from which the full sample was drawn. Unweighted sample n's are in parentheses.

The rates of high demoralization for the favor-to-opposed group (53.4%) and the opposed-to-opposed group (46.8%) do not differ significantly ($p = .27$). When this table is generated by a saturated regression model—i.e., one including main effects and the maximum possible number of interaction terms—the overall interaction between attitude at entry (3 categories) and attitude at exit (3 categories) is not statistically significant. ($p = .23$ in a saturated logistic model; $p = .21$ in a saturated linear model).

Table 10.5 DISTRIBUTION OF MAJOR ATTITUDE GROUPS ACCORDING TO PERIOD OF WAR ENTRY

Attitude Group	Vietnam War Entry Period			
	Period 1: Entry on/before July 27, 1965	Period 2: Entry from July 28, 1965, to Jan. 29, 1968	Period 3: Entry from Jan. 30, 1968, to Nov. 30, 1969	Period 4: Entry on/after Dec. 1, 1969
Opposed to opposed	9.2% (8)	14.8% (79)	17.8% (83)	32.7% (72)
Favor to favor	67.7% (57)	47.8% (201)	40.6% (125)	27.2% (60)
Opposed to favor	1.0% (3)	2.8% (14)	2.9% (12)	3.6% (6)
Favor to opposed	12.4% (11)	24.3% (130)	26.9% (94)	23.0% (52)
Neutral at entry or exit	9.6% (10)	10.3% (61)	11.9% (55)	13.5% (29)
TOTAL	100.0% (89)	100.0% (485)	100.0% (369)	100.0% (219).

$p = .000$ (Pearson chi-square).

Note: Percentages are weighted to the population from which the full sample was drawn. Unweighted sample n's are in parentheses.

DEMORALIZATION AND PERIODS OF THE WAR

Table 10.6 shows that demoralization was not lower in periods 1 and 4 than in the much higher-combat periods 2 and 3. As noted at the outset, this profile is very different from the one we saw in Chapter 4 for rates of war-related PTSD, both onset and current, which were much higher in periods 2 and 3 (see Figure 4.4 in Chapter 4). This suggested to us that factors more strongly related to demoralization than severity of combat exposure

Table 10.6 RATE OF HIGH DEMORALIZATION ACCORDING TO PERIOD OF WAR ENTRY

	Vietnam War Entry Period			
	Period 1: Entry on/ before July 27, 1965	Period 2: Entry from July 28, 1965, to Jan. 29, 1968	Period 3: Entry from Jan. 30, 1968, to Nov. 30, 1969	Period 4: Entry on/ after Dec. 1, 1969
Rate of High Demoralization	54.6% (89)	38.5% (485)	44.5% (369)	45.0% (219)

$p = .131$ (linear regression with a dummy variable representing each period).

Note: Percentages are weighted to the population from which the full sample was drawn. Unweighted sample n's are in parentheses.

might be involved in demoralization of veterans serving in the low-exposure periods 1 and 4. The high rates of negative attitudes in period 4 (see Table 10.2) are a plausible possibility. However, the substantial rate of demoralization in period 1, where veterans' attitudes were more positive than those of the veterans in any of the other three periods (see Table 10.2), is puzzling. We will return to this surprising result in the concluding section of this chapter.

OTHER POSSIBLY RELEVANT RISK FACTORS FOR DEMORALIZATION

We next considered variables other than attitudes toward the war that might be related to demoralization. If any of these variables were, like negative attitudes, elevated in period 4, it is they rather than, or together with, negative attitudes, that could be responsible for the fact that the rate of demoralization was as high in low-combat period 4 as in high-combat periods 2 and 3. In addition to attitudes toward the war, severity of combat, and involvement in harm to civilians or prisoners, we investigated whether any of the following variables were possible risk factors: racial or ethnic background, pre-Vietnam vulnerability load (including a separate analysis of psychiatric disorders in the diagnosed subsample), mode of entry into the military (drafted, enlisted to avoid the draft, enlisted voluntarily), branch of service (Army, Marines, Navy, and Air Force), severity of disciplinary actions, unit cohesion, and perception of negative homecoming reactions.

VARIABLES NOT DESCRIBED PREVIOUSLY

Most of these variables, like combat exposure (see Chapters 2 and 3), have been described previously. Two that have not are unit cohesion and perception of negative homecoming.

Unit Cohesion

Morale among the soldiers has been reported to have paralleled the decline in positive public attitudes toward the war in the latter stages of the war (Bates et al., 1998; Appy, 1993; Cortright, 2005). (See Chapter 1, section War, Nixon's War, which describes rising disillusionment, indiscipline, and low morale with the decline of U.S. troop strength in Vietnam.) We focused on the five items in the NVVRS that best assessed the respondent's perception of the cohesion of his unit as a measure of morale. These items dealt with issues of perceived competence of unit heads, and trust, closeness, and understanding among unit members. An example of such an item was, "How often did you feel that members of your unit understood you and your problems while in (or around) Vietnam?"

We initially scored each item on a Likert scale from 1–5, with 1 indicating most perceived competence, trust, closeness, or understanding, and 5 indicating the lowest perception of these attributes. We summed the five items to make a scale with a reliability index as measured by Cronbach's alpha of .74. To facilitate interpretability, we recoded and reverse-scored the items, with 0 indicating the least perceived competence, closeness, trust, or understanding, and 4 indicating the highest rating of these attributes. Consequently, scores on our unit cohesion scale could range from 0–20, with higher scores indicating greater perceived unit cohesion.

Negative Homecoming

A dichotomously scored "yes–no" item in the NVVRS that assessed a negative perception of homecoming reads as follows:

> It has been reported that some veterans experienced negative or even hostile events after returning from Vietnam. Did you ever experience any events like these after you returned from the Vietnam arena? (For example, some veterans were spit at, called "baby-killers," were challenged to fights in bars, or found that some friends or relatives would not talk to them).

Table 10.7 shows that all but two of these variables are strongly associated with demoralization at the .05 level of statistical significance or better. The two exceptions are branch of service and mode of entry, which show little relationship to demoralization. We therefore omitted these variables from our analysis of additional risk factors.

Table 10.7 BIVARIATE RELATIONSHIPS BETWEEN HIGH DEMORALIZATION AND INDEPENDENT VARIABLES THAT ARE CANDIDATES FOR INCLUSION IN A LOGISTIC REGRESSION MODEL: DEPENDENT VARIABLE IS HIGH DEMORALIZATION

Independent Variable	O.R.	(p)
Racial/Ethnic Group		
White	----ref. group----	
Black	1.60	(.001)
Hispanic	2.24	(.000)
Overall significance	---	(.000)
*Vulnerability Load**	1.35	(.000)
High Combat Exposure	1.97	(.000)
Harmed Civilians/Prisoners	2.35	(.000)

(continued)

Table 10.7   CONTINUED

Independent Variable	O.R.	(p)
Attitude Group		
Opposed to opposed	1.61	(.03)
Favor to favor	----ref. group----	
Neutral to neutral	.97	(.95)
Neutral to opposed	1.72	(.17)
Neutral to favor	2.49	(.06)
Opposed to favor	.62	(.40)
Favor to opposed	2.10	(.000)
Opposed to Neutral	1.54	(.69)
Favor to neutral	3.18	(.16)
Overall significance	---	(.013)
Mode of Entry to Military		
Drafted	1.02	(.91)
Enlisted but not voluntarily	1.37	(.22)
Enlisted voluntarily	---ref. group---	
Overall significance	---	(.46)
Branch of Service		
Army	---ref. group---	
Marines	1.46	(.14)
Navy	1.19	(.41)
Air Force	.89	(.60)
Overall Significance	---	(.34)
Disciplinary Action	1.88	(.000)
*Unit Cohesion**	.68	(.000)
Negative Homecoming	1.68	(.002)

Note: These analyses take into account the complex full sample design.

*Vulnerability load is a count of vulnerabilities; the odds ratio (O.R.) is the increase in odds of high demoralization for each additional vulnerability. Unit cohesion is a continuous scale, which has been standardized (expressed in standard deviation units). All other variables are dichotomous.

RISK FACTORS ELEVATED IN PERIOD 4

We have seen that severity of combat exposure and involvement in harm to civilians and prisoners are low in period 4 compared to their highs in periods 2 and 3. We have speculated that elevations in negative attitudes toward the war in period 4, paralleling increasingly negative attitudes in the United States, might be taking the place of combat and harm to keep the rates of demoralization as high in period 4 as in periods 2 and 3. We therefore considered whether there were elevations of other risk factors in period 4 that were more important than, or that may have acted together with, negative attitudes to raise the rate of high demoralization in period 4.

Table 10.8 MEANS AND PROPORTIONS OF SELECTED VARIABLES BY PERIOD
OF THE WAR

	Period 1	Period 2	Period 3	Period 4	Overall Significance
Racial/Ethnic Group					
White	80.1%	83.4%	83.6%	81.2%	
Black	12.9%	11.8%	10.3%	13.0%	
Hispanic	7.0%	4.8%	6.1%	5.8%	
TOTAL	100.0%	100.0%	100.0%	100.0%	(.68)
Vulnerability Load (number of	3.11	2.97	2.69	2.92	(.02)
vulnerabilities)					
*Pre-Vietnam Psych. Disorder**	1.6%	9.7%	14.0%	5.1%	(.39)
*Conduct Disorder**	1.6%	5.3%	6.2%	3.1%	(.77)
(childhood)					
*Any Other Disorder**	0.7%	6.1%	10.5%	2.0%	(.11)
High Combat Exposure	12.9%	27.6%	33.0%	9.8%	(.000)
Harmed Civilians/Prisoners	12.9%	15.1%	12.5%	6.9%	(.042)
Disciplinary Actions	28.5%	25.3%	21.2%	32.0%	(.17)
Unit Cohesion (Ranges from	15.5	14.5	13.8	13.5	(.000)
1–20, SD = 3.37)					
Opposed to War at Exit:	22.2%	43.8%	49.3%	61.1%	(.000)
Opposed to opposed	9.2%	14.8%	17.8%	32.7%	(.000)
Favor to opposed	12.4%	24.3%	26.9%	23.0%	(.047)
Negative Homecoming	34.1%	38.1%	33.4%	40.2%	(.55)

Note: Percentages are weighted to the populations from which the full sample and subsample (for psychiatric disorders) were drawn.

Significance test for racial/ethnic group is Pearson's chi-square. All other p-values are for comparisons of means and proportions. SD = standard deviation.

*Diagnosed subsample.

Table 10.8 shows our finding that only unit cohesion varied significantly with period of the war and was lowest in period 4. It was, however, only marginally lower than in the immediately preceding high-combat period. From early period 1 to later periods 2, 3, and 4, the mean scores went from a unit cohesion high of 15.5 in period 1 to progressively lower scores of 14.5 in period 2, 13.8 in period 3, and 13.5 in period 4. While statistically significant (Wald $F = 6.31, p < .001$), these differences on the 20-point scale do not suggest the kind of major overall decline in morale portrayed in anecdotal accounts (see Chapter 1, section War, *Nixon's War* and *The Final Years*). The high unit cohesion score in period 1 tends to compound rather than resolve the puzzle of the high rate of demoralization in period 1.

Over a third (37%) of the veterans reported that they had encountered a hostile reception upon their return in response to the question described, and we thought that such experiences would have increased as public attitudes became less favorable. (See Chapter 1, section Aftermath, *The Human Cost*, for a full discussion of treatment of returning veterans.)

Surprisingly, however, having a perception of negative homecoming was not significantly related to time of war entry ($p = .55$) or exit ($p = .47$). This finding calls into question the direction of the relationship between the veterans' reports of negative homecoming reactions and attitude change.

SUMMARY AND CONCLUSIONS

As reported in Chapter 4, we found that demoralization, unlike diagnosed PTSD, did not vary with the intensity of combat over the course of the war. It seemed possible, therefore, that increasingly negative U.S. public attitudes toward the war and hostile reactions to returning veterans might have adversely affected the attitudes of the veterans fighting it. Their negative attitudes, in turn, might have increased their risk of nonspecific distress or demoralization at the same time that the risk of demoralization due to combat experiences was declining toward the end of the war. To examine this possibility, we investigated, first, the relationship of changing public attitudes toward the Vietnam war to the attitudes of veterans who began serving in Vietnam in earlier popular and later unpopular periods of the war. Second, we investigated the relationship of the veterans' attitudes toward the war to their likelihood of developing demoralization.

We found, as expected, that later cohorts of U.S. veterans had less favorable attitudes than earlier cohorts. This contrast in veterans' attitudes, although less pronounced, paralleled changes in public attitudes over the course of the war. Furthermore, we found, as hypothesized, that negative attitudes at entrance and exit and negative changes in the veterans' favorable attitudes from entrance to exit were related to the period of the war in which they served and were associated with demoralization. Moreover, negative attitudes, unlike other strong risk factors for demoralization, were elevated in period 4, as was lesser unit cohesion. These results are consistent with the hypothesis that the elevation of negative attitudes in period 4 replaced more severe combat exposure in periods 2 and 3 in producing an equivalent rate of demoralization.

Negative perception of homecoming, surprisingly, did not vary with period of the war. This makes reverse causation a more plausible possibility with the variable of perception of negative homecoming than with unit cohesion—though the problem of possible reverse causation cannot be dismissed for unit cohesion.

It remains a puzzle to us why the rate of demoralization is at least as high in period 1 as in the other three periods. Period 1 was one of limited U.S. engagement. We have no data on public opinion about the war in that period, but we do know that veterans who served then reported more favorable attitudes toward the war when they arrived in Vietnam (80%, Figure 10.2) than veterans who served in any other period. Most of these veterans remained favorable. The small minority (12.4%, Table 10.5) who changed from favorable to unfavorable may have done so for reasons that were atypical and unaffected by changing public attitudes.

We can speculate that once they changed their attitudes, they may have experienced increased isolation and cognitive dissonance as a result of having opinions that differed from those of the large majority of their fellow soldiers, who were still very positive about the war. Possibly these men's change of attitude had something to do with their personal involvement in harm to prisoners and civilians, which had a rate at least as high in period 1 as in the high-combat periods 2 and 3. Given the strong association between severity of combat exposure and involvement in harm to civilians and prisoners, this high rate of harm in period 1 is also a puzzle.

The veterans' attitudes toward the war at entrance and exit were both measured at one point in time only, and this point was long after their service in Vietnam. As with any retrospective report, there is the possibility that memory distortions played a role in the findings. This distortion would be especially serious if demoralization influenced recalled attitudes toward the war, rather than vice versa. The relationship of our record-based data on veterans' period of war service to their positive and negative attitudes shows, however, that retrospective bias cannot be the only factor responsible for our findings. The fact that declining favorable and increasing negative attitudes of the veterans' attitudes are related to time of war entry suggests that factors other than demoralization influenced their attitudes. It is plausible that increasingly negative public attitudes were among these factors.

We conclude that the main results strongly suggest that changing public attitudes had a substantial effect on veterans' attitudes, unit cohesion, and demoralization in the U.S. armed forces toward the end of the war.

REFERENCES

Appy, C. (1993). *Working-class war: American combat soldiers and Vietnam.* Chapel Hill, NC: University of North Carolina Press.

Baker, P. (2012, May 27). Obama Begins Commemoration of Vietnam Era, *The New York Times,* p. A16).

Bates, Lichty, Miles, Spector and Young (Eds.). (1998). Chronology 1945–1995. *Reporting Vietnam. Part I: American Journalism 1959–1969.* New York, NY: Literary Classics of the United States, Inc. (pp. 775–803).

Coleman, P. (2006). *Flashback: Posttraumatic stress disorder, suicide and the lessons of war.* Boston, MA: Beacon Press.

Cortright, D. (2005). *Soldiers in revolt: GI resistance during the Vietnam war.* Chicago, IL: Haymarket Books.

Dohrenwend, B. P., Shrout, P. E., Egri, G., & Mendelsohn, F. S. (1980). Measures of non-specific psychological distress and other dimensions of psychopathology in the general population. *Archives of General Psychiatry, 37,* 1229–1236.

Erskine, H. (1970). The polls: Is war a mistake? *Public Opinion Quarterly (Spring 1970), 34*(1), 141–142.

Frank, J. D. (Ed.). (1961). *Persuasion and healing: A comparative study of psychotherapy* (1st ed.). Baltimore, MD: The Johns Hopkins University Press.

Gallup Opinion Index. (1969–1971). Numbers 56, 59, 61, 69, and 73. The following question was asked annually, with responses tabulated in the editions cited: "In view of the developments since we entered the fighting in Vietnam, do you think the U.S. made a mistake in sending troops to fight in Vietnam?"

CHAPTER 11

⌀⌀

Veterans' Appraisals of the Impact of the War on Their Lives 10-Plus Years After the War Ended

BRUCE P. DOHRENWEND, THOMAS J. YAGER, YUVAL
NERIA, J. BLAKE TURNER, NICK TURSE, RANDALL
MARSHALL, ROBERTO LEWIS-FERNÁNDEZ, AND
KARESTAN C. KOENEN

Vietnam changed me, in significant ways, for the better. It is a surpassing irony that war, for all its horror, provides the combatant with every conceivable human experience. . . . Such an experience is transforming. And we can be much the better for it. (McCain & Salter, 1999, p. 347)

Research on the psychological consequences of military service during wartime has been conducted for the most part from a pathogenic perspective. Despite calls for a broader vision (e.g., Elder & Clipp, 1989), this narrower focus has been especially true of research on U.S. veterans of the war in Vietnam.

The emphasis on negative outcomes increased with growing interest in the relatively new diagnosis of PTSD, a classification that coincided with, and provided impetus to, the study of Vietnam veterans (Kulka et al., 1990). Nevertheless, studies of combat veterans of previous wars (e.g., Elder & Clipp, 1989) and studies of persons who have encountered various other types of traumatic events (e.g., Tedeschi, Park, & Calhoun, 1998) have found that some exposed persons report positive changes and significant benefits from their experiences. What do these positive reports represent, and how are they related to adaptive and maladaptive outcomes?

Lazarus and Folkman (1984) have distinguished between "primary appraisals" and "secondary appraisals," both of which occur during or immediately after the event.

Primary appraisals involve judgments about whether the individual is in jeopardy, whereas secondary appraisals involve judgments about the options and resources available to the individual in responding to the event. Janoff-Bulman (1992) has described a third type of appraisal, which consists of the ongoing evaluation, sometimes over many years, of the impact of an experience after it has occurred. We call these tertiary appraisals.

As Janoff-Bulman and Berg (1998) point out, what we are calling positive and negative tertiary appraisals often coexist for a person who has been exposed to traumatic events. When tertiary appraisals are mainly negative, they are hypothesized to contribute to maladaptive outcomes:

> For survivors who have painfully experienced disillusionment, the malevolence and meaninglessness of the universe is acknowledged in the new assumptive world. If these negative views are wholly embraced and therefore overwhelm the survivor's new assumptive world, the result will be profound anxiety and despair. (Janoff-Bulman & Berg, 1998, p. 42)

When tertiary appraisals are mainly positive with reference to life-threatening and other potentially traumatic events, Janoff-Bulman hypothesizes that these "creative reformulations" are adaptive "cognitive strategies that ultimately contribute to the difficult process of rebuilding the victim's inner world" (Janoff-Bulman, 1992, pp. 116–117). Such strategies provide "a new 'valuation' or reevaluation of living. . . . Typically, this involves a newfound appreciation of their lives, and a consequent reordering of priorities" (Janoff-Bulman & Berg, 1998, p. 42). It is a developing balance in favor of the positive in the content of tertiary appraisals that theoretically contributes to healthy adaptation.

Few studies have investigated tertiary appraisals in the lives of war veterans. One of the best-designed was conducted in 1976 shortly after the end of the Vietnam war. It compared U.S. Air Force pilots and navigators who had been held captive in Vietnam with carefully chosen Air Force controls (Sledge, Boydstun, & Rahe, 1980). Prior to conducting this study, Sledge and his colleagues had participated in examinations given to all repatriated prisoners of war (POWs). The researchers were impressed by the veterans' reports of positive personal benefits from their captivity and felt that these appraisals served two very different functions for different veterans:

> For some POWs, the sense of having been changed favorably by captivity is clearly a defensive maneuver aimed at denying a deeper sense of having been impaired, both physically (some do have enduring disabilities) and psychologically (in terms of mental functioning) (Sledge, Boydstun, & Rahe, 1980, pp. 430–431).

In contrast,

> [O]ther POWs . . . have approached their lives with a new set of values concerning work, family, and relationships with others, and insist that they are wiser, more content, and

know themselves and their environment better. They responded to the challenge of captivity as an opportunity to experience their human limits, and they defined their abilities
and limitations more sharply than most people ever will. (Sledge, Boydstun, & Rahe,
1980, pp. 430–431)

The latter appear to be examples of creative reformulations previously described by
Janoff-Bulman (1992) and Janoff-Bulman and Berg (1998).

In their questionnaire follow-up of these veterans in 1976 while the pilots and
navigators were still in military service, Sledge, Boydstun, and Rahe found that the former
POWs, especially those treated more harshly over longer periods of imprisonment, reported more positive tertiary appraisals of the personal impact of their experiences than
controls did; for example, more optimism, insight, and ability to distinguish between
the important and the trivial. They interpreted this dose–response relationship between
severity of exposure and positive appraisals as evidence of "an adaptive attempt to make
the most of an extraordinarily stressful situation" rather than as either a "defensive ra-
tionalization or an actual fact" (Sledge, Boydstun, & Rahe, 1980, p. 443).

This interpretation by Sledge and his colleagues is consistent with Janoff-Bulman's
(1992) hypothesis that positive tertiary appraisals function as reformulations that contribute to adaptive outcomes. It is also possible, however, that positive tertiary appraisals
are after-the-fact affirmations of prior and current adaptive outcomes rather than antecedent contributors to such outcomes, as Sledge, Boydstun, and Rahe and others
(e.g., Frazier, Conlon, & Glaser, 2001) have pointed out. Nor does this exhaust the
possibilities. For some veterans, as Sledge et al. suggested, defensive denial associated
with serious psychological problems may be involved. Unfortunately, Sledge, Boydstun,
and Rahe did not investigate the relationship of the positive tertiary appraisals to actual adaptive and maladaptive outcomes. They could not, therefore, test the extent to
which the positive tertiary appraisals represented affirmation, reformulation, or defensive denial.

Solomon et al. (1999) conducted a study of repatriated Israeli soldiers who were
captured by the Egyptians and Syrians during the Yom Kippur War in 1973. Unlike the
prior study by Sledge, Boydstun, and Rahe (1980) on which it was modeled, the Israeli
study included a measure of PTSD symptoms (Solomon et al., 1999). Within both the
Israeli POWs and combat controls, only the negative tertiary appraisals were associated
with elevated PTSD symptoms. In their research with veterans mainly from World War
II and the Korean War, Aldwin, Levenson, and Spiro (1994) also found that negative,
but not positive, tertiary appraisals were correlated with elevated PTSD symptoms controlling on self-reported severity of combat exposure, as did Fontana and Rosenheck
(1998) in research with Vietnam veterans. This finding is not limited to studies of veterans exposed to wartime stressors. Frazier, Conlon, and Glaser (2001), for example,
got similar results in their research with victims of sexual assault.

Findings to date on the relationship between positive appraisals and symptoms of
PTSD or other types of psychological distress, however, are less consistent than those
for negative tertiary appraisals. In the research with samples of war veterans, Aldwin,
Levenson, and Spiro (1994) found that positive tertiary appraisals were associated with

lower rates of PTSD symptoms. Solomon et al. (1999), however, found no relationship between such positive appraisals and PTSD symptoms in either their POW or combat control samples. Frazier, Conlon, and Glazer (2001) cited five studies of various types of severe but nonmilitary stressors in which positive appraisals were unrelated to distress, three such studies in which positive appraisals were negatively correlated with distress, and one in which positive appraisals were positively correlated with distress. In view of these inconsistencies, it seems possible that, in some circumstances, positive tertiary appraisals are neither reformulations that contribute to adaptive outcomes nor after-the-fact affirmations of adaptive outcomes. Rather, consistent with the observation by Sledge, Boydstun, and Rahe (1980) previously discussed, and the research of Shedler, Mayman, and Manis (1993) on the "illusion of mental health," it seems possible that, for some individuals, positive appraisals represent defensive denial related to maladaptive outcomes.

In sum, although both theory and research results to date suggest that mainly negative tertiary appraisals are associated with maladaptive outcomes, the picture is more complicated when tertiary appraisals are mainly positive. This may be because positive tertiary appraisals can represent three very different processes: *Reformulation* that involves recasting the meaning of a difficult experience in a positive light; *affirmation* that consists of acknowledging a positive adaptation to a difficult experience; and *defensive denial* of negative features and effects of a difficult experience as a pathological maneuver. Two of these—after-the-fact affirmation and reformulation—associate mainly positive appraisals with adaptive outcomes. In contrast, the third—defensive denial—associates mainly positive appraisals with maladaptive outcomes.

MEASURES OF TERTIARY APPRAISALS AND SOME RESULTS FROM OUR PREVIOUS INVESTIGATION

In a previously reported investigation, we used interview data from the full NVVRS Theater sample and data from military records and historical accounts to investigate appraisals by these Theater veterans of the effects of their service in Vietnam on their present lives (Dohrenwend et al., 2004).

Unlike primary and secondary appraisals that occur in the midst of a dangerous situation, tertiary appraisals begin after the immediate danger is over—in the present case, presumably after the end of the veteran's tour in Vietnam. As described by Janoff-Bulman (1992), tertiary appraisals are ongoing processes that can continue for years. In this study, tertiary appraisals were measured at the time of the NVVRS interviews conducted with the veterans 11–12 years after the end of the war. We developed measures of valence and salience from the NVVRS survey interview, called the National Survey of the Vietnam Generation (NSVG), conducted with the full sample of Theater veterans.

VALENCE

We measured valence by two questions from the NSVG about whether the effects of military service and the war were positive or negative. The first question was, "Overall, do you feel that you personally benefited in the long run or were set back in the long run by having been involved in the Vietnam War?" with the fixed alternative response categories of *personally benefited, set back,* or *no impact* (if this answer was volunteered). The second question was, "What effect has military service had on your life?" with fixed alternative response categories of *entirely positive, mainly positive, equally positive and negative, mostly negative,* and *entirely negative.*

These two items are inter-correlated (.43). However, there are ambiguities in the response category "no impact," which mixes salience with valence in the first item, and the category of "equally positive and negative," which may do the same in the second item. To deal with these ambiguities, we defined positive valence and negative valence as follows.

Positive valence was indicated by either of the following combinations of responses: (a) *personally benefited* on the first item, which most specifically referred to experiences in Vietnam; or (b) *no impact* on the first item and *entirely positive* or *mainly positive* on the second, which referred more generally to their military service. Negative valence was defined either by (a) *set back* on the first item; or by (b) *no impact* on the first item and *mostly negative* or *entirely negative* on the second item. We removed the 59 respondents who could not be classified because of their "no impact" or "equally positive and negative" responses.

Strikingly, of the 1,089 remaining male veterans in the NVVRS sample, 70.9% gave positive tertiary appraisals of the impact of the war on their present lives. This figure was almost identical for veterans who served in Vietnam before the Tet Offensive, when the war was relatively popular in the United States, and after the Tet Offensive, when the popularity of the war started to decline. Most of the veterans (75.5%) who enlisted voluntarily gave positive tertiary appraisals, but so, also, did a substantial majority (64.0%) who were drafted or enlisted to avoid the draft (Dohrenwend et al., 2004).

The question arises as to whether military service per se would be judged by veterans to have such positive effects on their civilian lives. Fortunately, the NVVRS included a sample of Era veterans who served during the period of the Vietnam War but not in Vietnam. These Era veterans were asked one of the two questions we used to measure valence in the Vietnam veteran sample: "What effect has military service had on your life?" Of the veterans who served in the Vietnam war-zone, 58.2% replied "entirely positive" or "mainly positive," in contrast with 49.5% of the Era veterans who served elsewhere ($p < .05$) (Dohrenwend et al., 2004).

Qualitative Illustrations

The NSVG interview also included three open-ended questions about the content of the appraisals. The first, asked prior to the closed questions, was, "In what ways has the Vietnam war affected your everyday life?" The next two followed the closed questions on whether effects were mainly positive or negative: "First, what were some of the *positive* things that you gained from your Vietnam experience?" and "What were some of the *negative* things?" Responses were recorded verbatim.

In addition to these questions in the NSVG, the subsample of 254 male Theater veterans who were given diagnostic interviews were asked in the introductory section to the questions about PTSD, "Overall, what do you think has been the impact of your military experience since that time?" The clinician was instructed as follows: "Record details on the facing page. If R [respondent] does not mention, probe for both perceived positive and perceived negative effects, and for various aspects of adjustment—family, work, school, etc." These diagnostic interviews were tape-recorded.

Because of this additional detail from the clinical interviews, the most complete qualitative data on the content of positive and negative appraisals are available only on the small, diagnosed subsample. Examples of the positive things gained were, "growing up," "understanding others," "being able to deal with matters as they came up," and having become a "better person." Examples of the negative things were, "people back home not really understanding," accusations that lives were lost "for political reasons," returning to the United States and "just being put on the street," and psychiatric problems, such as drug use.

Salience

We measured salience by two items from the NSVG that asked about the current importance of the Vietnam War in the veteran's life. The first and most direct, in terms of present impact, asked, "How much would you say the Vietnam War has affected your everyday life? *A great deal, a fair amount, hardly at all, not at all?*" The second item asked how closely the following statement described the veteran: "Being in the Vietnam War was the biggest event in my life up until now: *Very closely, somewhat closely, not too closely, not at all?*" These two items were only modestly correlated (.24), so we gave priority to the first, more direct item assessing effect on everyday life. Accordingly, high salience was operationalized as (a) a response to the first question that Vietnam had "a great deal" of effect on the veteran's everyday life; *or* (b) a response of "a fair amount" of effect on the first question *and* a response of either "very" or "somewhat" on the second question about how closely the statement about Vietnam as the biggest event in life up to now described the veteran. Low salience was indicated by all other responses to the two questions. An estimated 41.7% of the male veterans in the larger sample gave high-salience appraisals of the impact of their service in Vietnam on their present lives (Dohrenwend et al., 2004).

Valence and Salience Typology

We combined the valence and salience measures into four types of tertiary appraisal. These types, and the estimated percentage of the full sample of veterans in each, were as follows: Positive/high salience (23.2%); positive/low salience (47.7%); negative/high salience (18.5%); and negative/low salience (10.6%). By far the largest group, almost half the veterans, were in the mainly positive/low salience type.

ADAPTIVE AND MALADAPTIVE WARTIME AND POST-WAR ROLE FUNCTIONING

Wartime Functioning

We used two indicators of wartime role functioning according to military standards, both of which were taken from the service records (DD-214s) of the sampled veterans. The first was whether the veteran had received a medal for superior performance during his service in Vietnam. We excluded from the category of performance medals those that were either universally awarded (i.e., the Vietnam Service Medal) or nearly universally awarded (i.e., the Vietnam Combat Medal). We also excluded Combat Infantry Badges and Purple Hearts, neither of which is explicitly tied to superior performance. We included all medals that acknowledged meritorious action—whether that action involved valor or other kinds of superior military service—in the category of performance medals.

The second indicator of wartime role functioning was whether the veteran's record contained a disciplinary action. We included any formal action—Article 15s (involving formal but non-judicial punishment) and/or any kind of court martial. Like the previous measures of combat exposure, these record-based measures of role performance during military service are independent of self-reported recall and antecedent to tertiary appraisals, current PTSD, and post-war role functioning. In general, these measures of less adequate role performance in Vietnam were most elevated in those who made negative/high salience appraisals and lowest in those who made positive/low salience appraisals (Dohrenwend et al., 2004).

Post-War Functioning

Results for the sample as a whole show that 84% of the male Theater veterans in this study had never been married before going Vietnam, and, as most had not advanced in their educational or occupational careers, we used their current statuses on these three variables (i.e., marital status, education, and career attainment levels) as indicators of post-war functioning. Veterans currently married who had never separated or divorced were compared with veterans who had divorced or separated, regardless of their current status, and with those who never married. We also assessed the relationships of level of educational attainment and occupational attainment (Stevens & Cho, 1985) to veterans' tertiary appraisals and to PTSD. The education categories we used were college graduate or more, high school graduate, and less than high school graduate. Occupation was grouped into high versus low socioeconomic status by use of a cut-point of 30 on Duncan's (1961) measure, calibrated to the 1980 Census Occupational Scheme by Stevens and Cho (1985). This cut-point yielded as closely as we found possible an even split of the male Theater sample (40.2% low and 59.8% high).

We evaluated their assessments of the importance (salience) of their experiences in Vietnam and whether they saw the effects of these experiences as mainly positive or mainly negative (valence). In formulating hypotheses about the relationship of the resulting four types of tertiary appraisals (positive/high salience, positive/low salience, negative/high salience, and negative/low salience) to current PTSD and post-war social functioning, we initially assumed that high salience, as a measure of intensity, increases whatever association is found between the valence of tertiary appraisals and the outcomes. As negative outcomes increase with the severity of war-zone stressors veterans experienced, we took into account exposure as measured with our record-based MHM in testing hypotheses about the role of tertiary appraisals.

MAIN RESULTS FROM OUR PREVIOUS RESEARCH

In this previous research, our main outcome variable was the Mississippi Scale of self-report items that was included in the NVVRS as a measure designed to screen for the presence of current PTSD (M-PTSD). (See Chapter 2 and the following sections for more detail on this measure.) We also used performance medals and disciplinary actions to measure adaptive and maladaptive functioning during the veteran's time in Vietnam. We measured post-war functioning by educational attainment, occupational attainment, and marital status.

With the M-PTSD and these other measures of outcome, we found that positive tertiary appraisals were associated with affirmations of successful wartime and post-war adaptation rather than defensive denials related to maladaptive outcomes. While we could not test it directly, it seemed possible that positive reformulation was also involved. Contrary to our hypothesis, however, positive/low salience appraisals were more likely than positive/high salience appraisals to be associated with positive outcomes, including the absence of current PTSD as measured by the M-PTSD.

However, we now had the same concerns about what this symptom scale was measuring that we had about the NVVRS Projected Probability algorithm (see Chapter 4). Also, as in previous chapters, we wanted to be able to distinguish between the onset of war-related PTSD and its adverse course, represented by current war-related PTSD. This distinction is especially important not only for reasons mentioned previously, but also because onset is antecedent to current functioning, while current PTSD, however measured, could be either the cause or the consequence of such functioning. For these several compelling reasons, therefore, for the additional analyses, we now focused on the clinical diagnoses in the much smaller subsample of veterans on whom such diagnoses were obtained.

FURTHER ANALYSES WITH CLINICAL DIAGNOSES
OF PTSD IN SUBSAMPLE VETERANS

In these further analyses, we expanded our previous research, this time using diagnoses of war-related PTSD onset and current PTSD, rather than current PTSD only, as measured less adequately by M-PTSD. We also used more comprehensive controls of relevant variables, including the addition of the veteran's involvement in harm to civilians or prisoners, pre-war vulnerability load, and his attitudes toward the war. These further analyses were confined to the much smaller subsample of male veterans who received psychiatric examinations by experienced clinicians.

Influence of PTSD Onset and Current PTSD
on Tertiary Appraisals

We found that both PTSD onsets and current PTSD were strongly associated with veterans' tertiary appraisals of the effects of the Vietnam war on their current lives.

The elevated rates of positive tertiary appraisals seen in Table 11.1 for those with no war-related PTSD are consistent with the results of the earlier study in suggesting that positive tertiary appraisals are associated with affirmations of successful wartime and post-war adaptation rather than defensive denials related to maladaptive outcomes. The sharpest difference is again between the relationship of PTSD to positive/low salience and negative/high salience appraisals. For example, almost two-thirds of the veterans with no war-related PTSD made positive/low salience appraisals of the effect of the war on their present lives; in contrast, almost two-thirds of those with current PTSD

Table 11.1 TERTIARY APPRAISAL TYPES FOR VETERANS
WITH NO PTSD ONSET, WITH PTSD ONSETS, AND
WITH CURRENT PTSD

War-related PTSD	Positive/ High Salience	Positive/ Low Salience	Negative/ Low Salience	Negative/ High Salience	Total
None	21.2%	63.6%	9.6%	5.5%	100%
	41	70	16	19	146
All onsets	21.5%	21.5%	8.8%	48.2%	100%
	27	10	9	38	84
Current	17.2%	7.6%	10.8%	64.4%	100%
	15	4	7	30	56

Note: Percentages are weighted to the population from which the subsample was drawn. *N*'s are unweighted subsample numbers.
All onsets vs. none: Pearson's chi-square *p* = .000.

Current vs. not current (not shown): Pearson's chi-square *p* = .000.

made negative/high salience appraisals. The association of current PTSD and tertiary appraisals seems especially strong, suggesting that persons with onsets that had remitted were less likely to make negative/high salience appraisals.

Other Factors That May Have Influenced Tertiary Appraisals

We also investigated several important factors that are positively associated with war-related PTSD for their possible influence on the veterans' appraisals of the impact of the war on their present lives. These are pre-Vietnam personal vulnerability load; severity of combat exposure; involvement in harm to civilians or prisoners, described in Chapters 5 and 6; changes in the veterans' attitudes toward the war, described in Chapter 10; and, finally, religious affiliation, a factor newly introduced here.

Table 11.2 shows that the first three clearly antecedent factors—that is, pre-Vietnam vulnerability load, severity of combat exposure, and personal involvement in harm to civilians or prisoners—are all strongly associated with tertiary appraisals. The contrast,

Table 11.2 TERTIARY APPRAISAL TYPES BY COMBAT EXPOSURE, PARTICIPATION IN HARM TO CIVILIANS OR PRISONERS, AND PRE-WAR VULNERABILITY

	Positive/ High Salience	Positive/ Low Salience	Negative/ Low Salience	Negative/ High Salience	Total
Combat exposure					
Below 75th percentile	18.9%	64.6%	5.6%	10.8%	100%
	39	60	11	25	135
75th percentile	27.9%	24.5%	20.2%	27.3%	100%
or above	29	20	14	32	95
Participation in harm					
Did not participate	22.3%	56.4%	9.7%	11.6%	100%
	56	70	20	32	178
Participated	15.9%	37.7%	8.7%	37.7%	100%
	10	8	4	24	46
Pre-war vulnerability load					
Mean vulnerability count	4.1	3.3	3.7	4.2	

Note: Percentages are weighted to the population from which the subsample was drawn. N's are unweighted subsample numbers.

Combat exposure: Pearson's chi-square $p = .000$.

Participation in harm: Pearson's chi-square $p = .014$.

Vulnerability count: Overall difference of means $p = .003$.

Our measure of combat exposure is the Combat Exposure Severity Scale (CESS). The vulnerability count has a maximum possible score of 9. Actual counts in this sample range from 0–8.

Table 11.3 TERTIARY APPRAISAL TYPES BY ATTITUDE CHANGE

Attitude Change	Positive/ high Salience	Positive/ Low Salience	Negative/ Low Salience	Negative/ High Salience	Total
Opposed to opposed	16.3%	54.0%	15.2%	14.5%	100%
	11	13	8	12	44
Favor to favor	27.2%	54.9%	4.8%	13.0%	100%
	32	37	6	19	94
Favor to opposed	20.3%	50.4%	8.9%	20.4%	100%
	17	18	8	18	61
All others	17.9%	52.5%	16.4%	13.1%	100%
	11	11	3	9	34

Note: Percentages are weighted to the population from which the subsample was drawn. *N*'s are unweighted subsample numbers.

Table as whole: Pearson's chi-square *p* = .82.

as with PTSD onset as a possible antecedent influence, is especially sharp between rates of positive/low salience and negative/high salience appraisers in each of these factors.

In contrast with the factors investigated, the veterans' reports of their attitudes towards the war when they went to Vietnam and when they left Vietnam are unrelated, as we can see in Table 11.3, to their tertiary appraisals of the effects of the war on their current lives.

Religious Affiliation

We did not investigate the role of the veterans' religious affiliation previously, but it seemed reasonable that such affiliation might be related to both PTSD, especially current PTSD, and to tertiary appraisals. Although religious affiliation is a possible contributor to, or indicator of, a veteran's social integration into his home community, research reviewed by Douthat (2014) suggests that only very strong religious affiliation would contribute in this way.

Fortunately, we have reports of the veteran's current religious affiliations (e.g., Catholic, Protestant, etc.), of the frequency of their usual attendance at religious services, and of their attendance in the preceding month. We, therefore, constructed our measures from these three relevant questions from the NSVG:

- Other than for weddings or funerals, have you attended services at a church or other place of worship since you were 18 years old? *No/Yes*
- [If yes] How often have you attended a religious service during the <u>past</u> <u>month</u>? *Every day, more than once a week, once a week, 2 or 3 times, once, or not at all?*

- How often do you <u>usually</u> attend religious services (attend church or other religious meetings)? *More than once a week, once a week, two or three times a month, once a month, a few times a year, or less than once a year?* [Responses of *never* were also recorded.]

As would be expected, frequency of usual attendance and frequency of attendance in the preceding month were highly correlated ($r = .80$, assuming equal distances between successive response categories). We gave preference to "usual" attendance in the analyses. The reason was that frequency of attendance in the preceding month is likely to be more variable and, therefore, less characteristic than "usual" attendance.

The great majority, four-fifths, of the veterans were either Protestant (49%) or Catholic (31%). We thought more Catholics than Protestants would report attending church once a week or more, because weekly mass is obligatory for Catholics. Had this been the case, we anticipated setting different cut-points to define frequent attendance for each denomination. However, this proved unnecessary. As Table 11.4 shows, Catholics and Protestants differed little in the proportions who attended religious services once a week or more. We, therefore, measured strong versus progressively weaker religious affiliation, as shown in Table 11.4, for all respondents regardless of particular denomination. We called this measure *religious affiliation*—a name meant to suggest not only the concrete behavior described by the items, but also possible broader aspects of religiosity such as adherence to the beliefs of one's religious group.

Table 11.5 shows that the main difference in rates of PTSD onset and current PTSD was between the veterans who usually attended religious services once a week or more

Table 11.4 USUAL FREQUENCY OF ATTENDANCE
AT RELIGIOUS SERVICES BY PROTESTANTS AND CATHOLICS

	Protestants		Catholics	
	%	(n)	%	(n)
More than once a week	15.5	(16)	0.7	(1)
Once a week	14.4	(18)	33.5	(21)
2–3 times a month	7.3	(14)	4.6	(11)
Once a month	4.6	(10)	2.9	(6)
A few times a year	29.7	(26)	30.0	(20)
Less than once a year	15.4	(16)	10.0	(7)
Never	13.1	(16)	18.3	(16)
TOTAL	100.0	(116)	100.0	(82)

Note: Percentages are weighted to represent the population. *N*'s are unweighted sample *n*'s.

Members of other major religious groups are too few to tabulate (Jewish $n = 2$; Black Muslim $n = 1$; Other $n = 5$). An additional 40 veterans said they had no religious preference.

Table 11.5 RATES OF PTSD ONSET AND CURRENT PTSD BY LEVEL
OF RELIGIOUS AFFILIATION

Religious Affiliation	PTSD Onset	Current PTSD	N
Attends services once a week or more often	12.3%	2.2%	62
Attends services 1–3 times a month	25.8%	16.8%	41
Attends services less often than once a month	22.8%	11.4%	82
Has a religious preference but never attends services	37.2%	19.4%	32
No religious preference and never attends services	22.9%	20.5%	29
TOTAL	21.7%	11.0%	246

Note: Percentages are weighted to reflect the population. N's are unweighted sample n's.
Rate of PTSD onset:
Religious services once a week or more: 12.3%.
Religious services less than once a week: 25.6%.
Difference of means: $p = .040$.
Rate of current PTSD:
Religious services once a week or more: 2.2%.
Religious services less than once a week: 14.7%.
Difference of means: $p = .000$.

and those who attended less than once a week. If we assume that stronger or weaker religious affiliation was characteristic of the veterans before as well as after their service in Vietnam, it seems possible that strong affiliation protected against the onset of war-related PTSD, as research with civilian samples shows that such affiliation does against the negative impact of divorce among Protestants (Douthat, 2014).

However, as Table 11.6 shows, there was no relationship between strength of religious affiliation and tertiary appraisals of the effect of the war on the current lives of the veterans. Like the veterans' changes in attitudes toward the war, therefore, strength of religious affiliation, while of interest for its relationship to low rates of PTSD, cannot help us explain the sources of differences in the veterans' appraisals of the effects of the war on their current lives. Rather, the main sources of the differences in tertiary appraisals appear to be their pre-Vietnam vulnerability loads, severity of combat exposure, involvement in harm to prisoners and civilians, and whether or not they developed war-related PTSD.

However, these four factors are not only correlated with tertiary appraisals, they are also correlated with each other (see Chapter 4). The question arises, therefore, as to which of these factors made independent contributions to differences in the veterans' tertiary appraisals of the impact of the war on their current lives. Before we answer this question, it is important to point out that our analyses so far have ignored possible differences in tertiary appraisals made by the main racial/ethnic subgroups in the male veteran population.

Table 11.6 TERTIARY APPRAISAL TYPES BY FREQUENCY OF ATTENDANCE AT RELIGIOUS SERVICES

Religious Service Attendance	Positive/ High Salience	Positive/ Low Salience	Negative/ Low Salience	Negative/ High Salience	Total
Less than once a week	20.2%	55.1%	8.7%	16.0%	100%
	48	58	20	44	170
Once a week or more	24.1%	52.9%	9.9%	13.2%	100%
	20	22	4	12	58

Note: Percentages are weighted to the population from which the subsample was drawn. N's are unweighted subsample numbers.
Table as a whole: Pearson's chi-square $p = .95$.

Table 11.7 shows that there are differences among these racial/ethnic subgroups, and the differences are most striking between positive/high salience and positive/low salience appraisals. There is little in the way of racial/ethnic difference in the negative/high salience or negative/low salience types. In Table 11.8, we examine the independence of the four factors discussed that show strong bivariate relationships to tertiary appraisals, with statistical controls on racial/ethnic background to ensure that any impacts are independent of the racial/ethnic difference as well.

Table 11.7 TERTIARY APPRAISAL TYPES BY RACIAL/ETHNIC GROUP

	Positive/ High Salience	Positive/ Low Salience	Negative/ Low Salience	Negative/ High Salience	Total
Majority white	16.3%	61.3%	8.7%	13.8%	100%
	14	46	7	17	84
Black	43.2%**	22.9%***	14.2%	19.6%	100%
	24	13	10	20	67
Hispanic	31.5%*	39.0%*	8.5%	21.0%	100%
	30	21	8	20	79

Note: Percentages are weighted to the population from which the subsample was drawn. N's are unweighted subsample numbers.
Table as a whole: $p = .000$ (Pearson chi-square).
* Trend towards difference from whites ($p \leq .10$).
** Significantly different from whites ($p \leq .01$).
*** Significantly different from whites ($p \leq .001$).

TESTS OF INDEPENDENCE

Table 11.8 summarizes the results of a series of logistic regression analyses designed to answer the question about which of the factors—vulnerability load, severity of combat exposure, involvement in harm to prisoners or civilians, and war-related PTSD—remained associated with tertiary appraisals, with the other factors and racial/ethnic background statistically controlled. In these comparisons, the reference category consists of the modal group of positive/low salience veterans who had the lowest rates of PTSD onset and current PTSD.

The most striking finding is that PTSD onset and current PTSD were the *only* factors that were independently related to elevations of negative/high salience appraisals of the impact of the war on the present lives of the veterans with the other factors controlled. In contrast, severity of combat exposure showed associations with elevated positive/high salience appraisals and negative/low salience appraisals. It is also noteworthy that involvement in harm to civilians and prisoners not only showed no independent elevation in negative/high salience appraisal, but was also less likely to be associated with positive/high salience appraisals and negative/low salience appraisals. Vulnerability load showed little independent association with any of the types of appraisals, possibly excepting a trend toward elevation of the positive/high salience appraisal type.

Table 11.8 LOGISTIC MULTIPLE REGRESSION MODELS PREDICTING TERTIARY APPRAISAL TYPES FROM FIVE INDEPENDENT VARIABLES

	Positive/ High Salience	Positive/ Low Salience (ref. group)	Negative/ Low Salience	Negative/ High Salience
Independent variables	O.R.(p)	O.R. (p)	O.R. (p)	O.R. (p)
Vulnerability load*	1.610 (.097)	1	1.139 (.73)	1.073 (.83)
Combat exposure**	3.308 (.054)	1	10.290 (.01)	1.557 (.54)
Harmed civilians/ prisoners	.262 (.046)	1	. 346 (.43)	.998 (.998)
PTSD onset	1.443 (.62)	1	1.357 (.83)	9.937 (.01)
Current PTSD	1.484 (.70)	1	1.967 (.66)	7.324 (.06)

Note: These analyses take into account the complex sample design.

Each variable is tested with the other independent variables statistically controlled; racial/ethnic groups are controlled in all models. The odds ratio (O.R.) of the reference group is 1 by definition.

* Standardized continuous variable.

** Dichotomized at 75th percentile.

SUMMARY AND CONCLUSIONS

Before the war in Vietnam ended without a victory by U.S. forces, it came to be opposed by the majority of U.S. citizens. Parallel to this change in public attitudes, the attitudes of the veterans who served later in the war were far less favorable than the attitudes of those who served earlier—as we saw in Chapter 10. Against this background, it is striking to find that, when the data were collected by the NVVRS more than 10 years after the war, a large majority of the U.S. male veterans who served in Vietnam perceived the impact of their wartime experiences on their present lives as mainly positive. With regard to salience, moreover, over 40% of the Theater veterans felt that the war's influence was still highly important in their lives.

These Theater veterans were more positive than veterans who served in the military at the same time but not in Vietnam. It did not matter whether the Vietnam veterans served before or after the Tet Offensive, when the war became increasingly unpopular, or whether or not they enlisted voluntarily. These results held regardless of whether the veterans were frequent church attenders.

We conclude that these appraisals had more to do with the individual experiences of the veterans in Vietnam than with the wider context of why the United States and these individuals themselves went to Vietnam in the first place. Additional evidence of the importance of individual experiences is the strong associations of severity of combat exposure, involvement in harm to civilians or prisoners, and PTSD onset with negative tertiary appraisals—contrasted with the lack of association of negative tertiary appraisals with changes in veterans' attitudes toward the war.

Especially striking, and consistent with our expectations, are the dramatically high rates of negative/high salience appraisers among those with PTSD onset and current PTSD. We expected that the greatest contrast with this group of negative/high salience appraisers would be the positive/high salience appraisers. The rationale for this hypothesis was that salience, a measure of intensity, would increase whatever association was being predicted between the valence of tertiary appraisals and adaptive as well as maladaptive functioning. This was not the case. It was the positive/low salience appraisers who were most under-represented in the veterans who developed war-related PTSD.

Positive appraisers tended to be more likely to receive medals for superior performance in Vietnam, be married at follow-up, and have stronger educational and occupational attainments than negative appraisers, especially negative/high salience appraisers. Taken together, these results are inconsistent with positive appraisals as defensive denials masking high rates of maladaptive behavior. They are consistent with the affirmation hypothesis that positive appraisals reflect positive functioning. There is no direct evidence for the positive reformulation hypothesis, but reformulation is probably not mutually exclusive with affirmation. Affirmation of positive experiences may change the balance between positive and negative appraisals, making them mainly positive. The fact that low salience appraisals, both positive and negative, show less association with

PTSD than high salience appraisals suggests that positive reformulation may have taken place as important and satisfying post-Vietnam activities related to family, education, and work supplied new, or newly reaffirmed, positive meanings that supplanted in importance those veterans' war-zone experiences.

It is of interest that pre-Vietnam vulnerability load, despite its strong bivariate relationship with tertiary appraisals in Table 11.2, showed no independent association with negative/high salience appraisals. It is also of note that severity of combat exposure did not show an independent relationship with negative/high salience appraisals. It is possible that combat exposure contributed to negative/high salience appraisals only when it was accompanied by the onset of war-related PTSD. Harm to civilians and prisoners may have been a major factor in these negative/high salience appraisals (see Table 11.2) only when accompanied by both severe combat exposure and war-related PTSD.

ACKNOWLEDGMENTS

This chapter expands on the following article: Dohrenwend, B. P., Neria, Y., Turner, J. B., Turse, N., Marshall, R., Lewis-Fernández, R., and Koenen, K. (2004), Positive tertiary appraisals and posttraumatic stress disorder in U.S. male veterans of the war in Vietnam: The roles of positive affirmation, positive reformulation, and defensive denial. *The Journal of Consulting and Clinical Psychology*, 72(3), 417–433. Publisher: American Psychological Association.

REFERENCES

Aldwin, C. M., Levenson, M. R., & Spiro, A., III. (1994). Vulnerability and resilience to combat exposure: Can stress have lifelong effects? *Psychology and Aging, 9*, 34–44.

Dohrenwend, B. P., Neria, Y., Turner, J. B., Turse, N., Marshall, R., Lewis-Fernández, R., & Koenen, K. (2004). Positive tertiary appraisals and post-traumatic stress disorder in U.S. male veterans of the war in Vietnam: The roles of positive affirmation, positive reformulation, and defensive denial. *Journal of Consulting and Clinical Psychology, 72*, 417-433.

Douthat, R. (2014). The Christian penumbra. *New York Times*, Sunday Review, March 30, p. 11.

Duncan, O. D. (1961). A socioeconomic index for all occupations. In A. J. Reiss (Ed.), *Occupations and social status* (pp. 109–138). New York: Free Press.

Elder, G. H., & Clipp, E. C. (1989). Combat experience and emotional health: Impairment and resilience in later life. *Journal of Personality, 57*, 311–337.

Fontana, A., & Rosenheck, R. (1998). Psychological benefits and liabilities of traumatic exposure. *Journal of Traumatic Stress, 11*, 485–503.

Frazier, P., Conlon, A., & Glaser, T. (2001). Positive and negative life changes following sexual assault. *Journal of Consulting and Clinical Psychology, 69*, 1048–1055.

Janoff-Bulman, R. (1992). *Shattered assumptions: Toward a new psychology of trauma.* New York: Free Press.

Janoff-Bulman, R., & Berg, M. (1998). Disillusionment and the creation of value: From traumatic losses to existential gains. In J. H. Harvey (Ed.), *Perspectives on loss: A sourcebook* (pp. 35–47). Philadelphia, PA: Brunner/Mazel.

Kulka, R. A., Schlenger, W. E., Fairbank, J. A., Hough, R. L., Jordan, B. K., Marmar, C. R., et al. (1990). *Trauma and the Vietnam war generation: Report on the findings from the National Vietnam Veterans Readjustment Study.* New York: Brunner/Mazel.

Lazarus, R. S., & Folkman, S. (1984). *Stress, appraisal and coping.* New York: Springer.

McCain, J., & Salter, M. (1999). *Faith of my fathers.* Random House: New York.

Shedler, J., Mayman, M., & Manis, M. (1993). The illusion of mental health. *American Psychologist, 48,* 1117–1131.

Sledge, W. H., Boydstun, J. A. & Rahe, A. J. (1980). Self-concept changes related to war captivity. *Archives of General Psychiatry, 37,* 430–443.

Solomon, Z., Waysman, M., Neria, Y., Ohry, A., Schwarzwald, J., & Wiener, M. (1999). Positive and negative outcomes in the lives of Israeli former POWs. *Journal of Social and Clinical Psychology, 18,* 419–435.

Stevens, G., & Cho, J. H. (1985). Socioeconomic indexes and the new 1980 census occupational classification scheme. *Social Sciences Research, 14,* 142–168.

Tedeschi, R. G., Park, C. L., & Calhoun, L. G. (1998). *Post-traumatic growth: Positive changes in the aftermath of crisis.* Mahwah, NJ: Erlbaum.

CHAPTER 12

∽

Long-Term Impact of the War on Veterans' Lives Nearly 40 Years After the War Ended

BRUCE P. DOHRENWEND, THOMAS J. YAGER, AND
MELANIE M. WALL

Some few who came home from war struggled to recover the balance that the war had upset. But for most veterans, who came home whole in spirit if not body, the hard uses of life will seldom threaten their equanimity. (McCain & Salter, 1999, p. 347)

Haunted and haunting, human and inhuman, war remains with us and within us, impossible to forget but difficult to remember. (Nguyen, 2016, p. 19)

Between July 3, 2012, and May 13, 2013, a number of the original National Vietnam Veterans Readjustment Study (NVVRS) investigators undertook a follow-up study of the NVVRS sample of veterans, especially those who had served in the Vietnam theater of operations. The follow-up was called the National Vietnam Veterans Longitudinal Study (Longitudinal Study) and, like the NVVRS, it was mandated by Congress and conducted with funds from the Veterans Administration. The design and methods of the Longitudinal Study have been described in detail by Schlenger et al. (2015).

The Longitudinal Study was a more limited investigation than the original NVVRS, but it contained data that are very important to the questions we address in this monograph. For example, the Longitudinal Study conducted additional clinical examinations with a substantial portion of the subsample of veterans who received clinical examinations by experienced clinicians in the NVVRS. The Longitudinal Study also included the NVVRS questions that we used to measure the valence and salience of the veterans' tertiary appraisals of the impact of the war on their lives at the time of the

NVVRS (Chapter 11). We thus had the rare opportunity to investigate the long-term course of war-related PTSD onsets from the time when these veterans were young men in their late teens and early twenties to the time when most were in their sixties. This enabled us to assess the continuing psychological effects of the war on the veterans over most of their adult lives.

Our key questions were:

1. Did the prevalence of war-related PTSD that was current at the time of the NVVRS in 1986–1987 increase, decrease, or remain the same by the time of the Longitudinal Study in 2012–2013?
2. Did the veterans' appraisals of the valence and/or salience of the impact of the war on their present lives change?
3. How well have the veterans readjusted after their experiences as young men in Vietnam?

We did not have Longitudinal Study data for the entire intensively studied sub-sample of NVVRS male Theater veterans on whom most of our analyses focused. It was important for purposes of generalizability, therefore, that we started our inquiry into these three questions by comparing the NVVRS veterans we did have to those we did not have in the Longitudinal Study data set.

THE LONGITUDINAL STUDY SAMPLE—ATTRITION IN THE NVVRS SAMPLE

The work in preceding chapters of this monograph centered on 248 male veterans who received clinical diagnostic examinations. As described earlier in Chapter 2, these veterans are quite representative of the urban portion of the 1,200 male veterans in the Theater sample. Of these 248 veterans, 111 were successfully included in the Longitudinal Study. The remainder consisted of two groups: (a) those who died in the interval between the two surveys ($n = 66$); and (b) non-responders among the living; that is, those who could not be located and those who refused to participate, including those who were not available after numerous contacts ($n = 71$).

Table 12.1 shows the distribution of important demographic, risk factor, and psychiatric variables in each of the three Longitudinal Study groups—responders, those living but non-responsive, and those who had died in the interval between the two surveys.

The dead did not differ with statistical significance ($p \leq .05$) from the responders on any of the variables shown in Table 12.1. Living non-responders, however, showed statistically significant differences from responders on three variables; they were younger when they arrived in Vietnam, their vulnerability load was greater, and their rate of alcoholism with onset in or after Vietnam was much higher (40.0% vs. 15.5%). The rate of such alcoholism among the dead was also higher (35.8% vs. 15.5%) but not statistically significant.

In the context of the current focus on suicide in the military, it is interesting that none of the veterans in this sample were identified as having died from suicide, and just

Table 12.1 DISTRIBUTION OF RISK FACTORS AND PSYCHIATRIC VARIABLES AMONG LONGITUDINAL STUDY RESPONDERS, NON-RESPONDERS, AND NVVRS VETERANS WHO DIED BEFORE THE LONGITUDINAL STUDY

	Alive at time of Longitudinal Study			Dead	Total Alive and Dead
Variable	Responders % (n)	Non-responders % (n)	Total % (n)	% (n)	% (n)
Sample	100.0 (111)	100.0 (71)	100.0 (182)	100.0 (66)	100.0 (248)
Racial/Ethnic Background					
White	85.0 (51)	72.2 (22)	80.9 (73)	76.9 (21)	79.8 (94)
Black	9.9 (24)	15.1 (17)	11.5 (41)	18.5 (29)	13.4 (70)
Hispanic	5.2 (36)	12.7 (32)	7.6 (68)	4.6 (16)	6.8 (84)
Vulnerability Load Mean count[a]	3.48 (111)	4.02 (71)*	3.66 (182)	3.48 (66)	3.61 (248)
Mean age when arrived in Vietnam	22.2 (108)	20.7 (71)*	21.7 (179)	23.9 (66)	22.3 (245)
Mean unit cohesion[b]	2.87 (107)	2.81 (71)	2.85 (178)	2.86 (66)	2.86 (244)
Combat Exposure					
Low	75.5 (66)	70.8 (42)	74.0 (108)	75.7 (39)	74.5 (147)
High	24.5 (45)	29.2 (29)	26.0 (74)	24.3 (27)	25.5 (101)
Took Part in Harm to Civilians or Prisoners					
No	89.6 (85)	77.3 (55)	85.5 (140)	89.9 (49)	86.7 (189)
Yes	10.4 (21)	22.7 (15)	14.5 (36)	10.1 (14)	13.3 (50)
PTSD Onset					
No	80.9 (76)	71.6 (40)	77.9 (116)	79.8 (44)	78.4 (160)
Yes	19.1 (35)	28.4 (31)	22.1 (66)	20.2 (22)	21.6 (88)
Current PTSD at Time of NVVRS					
No	90.9 (88)	87.2 (52)	89.7 (140)	87.3 (50)	89.1 (190)
Yes	9.1 (23)	12.8 (19)	10.3 (42)	12.7 (16)	10.9 (58)
Alcoholism with Onset In or After Vietnam					
No	84.5 (81)	60.0 (40)	76.7 (121)	64.2 (40)	73.2 (161)
Yes	15.5 (17)	40.0 (26)*	23.3 (43)	35.8 (22)	26.8 (65)
Major Depression with Onset In or After Vietnam					
No	82.2 (86)	82.0 (52)	82.1 (138)	86.7 (49)	83.3 (187)
Yes	17.8 (25)	18.0 (19)	17.9 (44)	13.3 (17)	16.7 (61)
Negative/High Salience					
No	85.2 (80)	87.0 (61)	85.8 (141)	88.4 (50)	86.5 (191)
Yes	14.8 (31)	13.0 (10)	14.2 (41)	11.6 (16)	13.5 (57)

Note: Percentages are weighted using the original NVVRS subsample weights. Unweighted sample *n*'s are in parentheses.

Total sample does not always equal 248, owing to missing data.

[a] Maximum possible vulnerability count is 9.

[b] Maximum possible unit cohesion score is 4.

*Differs significantly from value for responders ($p \leq .05$).

five were identified in the full sample (1,183) of male Theater veterans, for a weighted rate of 0.3%. Deaths attributed to non-natural causes were rare, with a weighted 3.0% due to injury or poisoning. Deaths due to identified natural causes amounted to 79.8% (40.2% due to cancer and 9.7% to heart disease). Surprisingly, given the high incidence among the dead of alcoholism onsets during and after their service in Vietnam, only one death (a weighted 1.0%) was attributed to chronic liver disease or cirrhosis. Deaths for which the cause was unknown accounted for 17.2% of the total. It is possible that some suicides may be included in this group.

Some notable differences were found among the Longitudinal Study groups that do not achieve statistical significance but that can nonetheless have an important effect on our analyses. While rates of severe combat exposure were quite similar in the three groups, rates of PTSD onset and current PTSD as diagnosed in the NVVRS were less similar, and non-responders had an elevated prevalence of participation in harm to civilians or prisoners compared with responders (22.7% versus 10.4%). Blacks were relatively under-represented among those who responded (9.9%) and over-represented among those who did not—that is, the non-responder group (15.1%) and those who had died (18.5%). Hispanics were over-represented in the non-responder group (12.7% compared with 5.2% in the responder group).

The differences between the living veterans who responded to the survey and those who did not respond limited our ability to generalize the results to the whole group of living veterans without further adjustment. The Longitudinal Study research team provided sampling weights for the diagnosed subsample, but those weights did not adequately adjust the subsample because they did not take into consideration important differences shown in Table 12.1. Therefore, we did not use them. Rather, we addressed this problem by creating a new set of weights by adjusting the original NVVRS weights so that the Longitudinal Study responders became representative of the entire population of living male Theater veterans represented by the original NVVRS subsample. The procedure for developing these weights is described in detail in Appendix A of this chapter.

DID CURRENT WAR-RELATED PTSD INCREASE, DECREASE, OR REMAIN THE SAME BETWEEN THE TIMES OF THE TWO SURVEYS?

Only one measure of PTSD-like symptoms was included in both the NVVRS and the follow-up Longitudinal Study (Marmar et al., 2015). This was the self-report Mississippi Scale (M-PTSD), a flawed measure, as we suggested in Chapter 4. Its main use for our purposes was what it showed about what Shrout et al. (2017) call "initial elevation bias" in subjective reports.

These investigators report that there was inflation of negative symptoms and moods in initial self-reports. This phenomenon casts doubt on the ability of follow-up interviews to provide valid assessment of whether symptoms decreased over time. The Shrout et al. studies conducted follow-up interviews over periods ranging from daily to every two months. In contrast, the Longitudinal Study conducted its study more than 25 years after the initial M-PTSD measurement. This study found a statistically significant, though modest, increase over more than two decades in the M-PTSD symptoms. This was, of course, the opposite of what would be predicted by the initial elevation bias hypothesis. This contrast between the M-PTSD data in the NVVLS and in the Longitudinal Study suggests that initial elevation bias either did not operate over long periods of time or, if it was present, it occurred on both the initial and subsequent measurements. In either case, the passage of time allowed a valid comparison of increase or decrease in what was being measured. Knowing this helped us interpret the results of our main analyses focusing on the clinical diagnoses, which also differed from self-reports in being scored by experienced psychologists and psychiatrists, in the NVVRS and the Longitudinal Study follow-up.

As we reported in Chapter 2, the estimates of war-related PTSD at the time of the NVVRS, conducted in the 1980s about 10–11 years after the war ended in 1975, used an instrument called the Structured Clinical Interview for Diagnosis (SCID) (Spitzer, Williams, & Gibbon, 1987). These diagnoses, which we have relied on throughout this monograph, were made according to the then-current DSM-III-R criteria, at a time when most of the veterans were in their early forties. In contrast, diagnoses in the Longitudinal Study, conducted over 25 years after the NVVRS, were made according to DSM-5, using a new diagnostic instrument called the Clinician-Administered PTSD Scale for DSM-5 (CAPS-5) (Weathers et al., 2013). Differences in both diagnostic methods and criteria posed a considerable problem for assessing whether rates of war-related PTSD in the Longitudinal Study remained the same, increased, or decreased in the intervening years.

Measures

Our focus in the following analyses was on changes between current PTSD in veterans participating in the NVVRS and in the Longitudinal Study. To deal with the problem of changing methods and diagnostic criteria between the two surveys, we constructed measures that allowed a more direct comparison between the NVVRS and Longitudinal Study rates of current PTSD than was possible using the SCID and CAPS diagnoses as they were originally made. We could do this because there is considerable overlap between the DSM-III-R criteria and the DSM-5 diagnostic criteria.

The diagnostic criteria of the Longitudinal Study's DSM-5 differed from those of the NVVRS's DSM-III-R criteria mainly in that DSM-5 added both more symptoms and a requirement of impairment in functioning. By omitting these new features from the DSM-5 diagnoses, therefore, we developed two useful measures. The first was a DSM-III-R version of CAPS to compare with a DSM-III-R version of SCID. For the second measure, we compared simple counts of DSM-III-R symptoms in the SCID and DSM-III-R symptoms in the CAPS. In order to count only symptoms that are included in both instruments, we omitted the symptom "foreshortened future," which occurred only in the SCID DSM-III-R diagnosis.

It should be noted that our attempt to create matching Longitudinal Study and NVVRS measures was not perfect. The CAPS's probing procedure for eliciting information about symptoms is more intensive than the SCID's, a difference that could either increase or decrease the number of PTSD diagnoses. As it turns out, however, the difference would be very small because the two measures are highly inter-correlated. The correlation is 99.2% between the two measures; the sensitivity of the SCID version as a predictor of the CAPS version of DSM-III-R PTSD using the items they have in common is 94.0% with a specificity of 99.5%.

Findings

Almost half of war-related PTSD onsets had remitted by the time of the NVVRS. This was true whether the diagnostic data came from the 111 responders available from the diagnosed subsample in the Longitudinal Study (see Table 12.1) or from the 248 members of the full NVVRS subsample (Chapter 2, Table 2.4). Was there further remission in the decades between the NVVRS and the Longitudinal Study?

Figure 12.1 shows levels of current PTSD according to the original diagnostic instruments and according to our new measures, both at the time of the NVVRS and

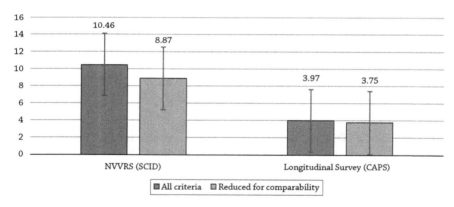

Figure 12.1 Rates of current PTSD (%) at the times of the NVVRS and the Longitudinal Study in male Theater veterans who were assessed in both interviews.

Note: The darker bars represent rates of current PTSD based on criteria that were current at the time of each survey (DSM-III-R for the NVVRS, DSM-5 for the Longitudinal Survey).

The lighter bars represent rates of current PTSD based on a reduced set of criteria in each survey that we selected to make them more comparable with criteria used in the other survey. Thus, "foreshortened future" is omitted from the SCID because it does not appear in CAPS, and the reduced version of CAPS attempts to simulate the SCID diagnosis by including only items that also occur in the SCID.

The vertical lines represent 95% confidence intervals around each rate.

Data are weighted to reflect the living NVVRS population at the time of the Longitudinal Study (see Appendix A, this chapter). Sample size is 111 for CAPS diagnosis and for both versions of the SCID diagnosis; 108 for the simulated SCID diagnosis due to three missing cases in Longitudinal Study symptom data.

Statistical significance of differences in proportions between the two interviews was tested using a sampling weighted version of McNemar's test—namely, testing whether the weighted proportion of discordant pairs across time that indicate an increase versus a decrease is different from 50% using the Rao-Scott (RS) Chi-square obtained from the PROC SURVEYFREQ procedure in the SAS statistical package. Three differences were tested: full SCID vs. full CAPS, full SCID vs. the reduced CAPS simulating SCID, and SCID omitting "foreshortened future" vs. the reduced CAPS simulating SCID. In all three cases, $p < .0001$.

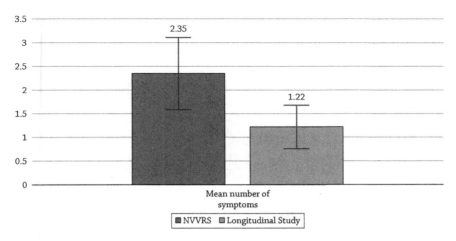

Figure 12.2 Mean numbers of symptoms common to DSM-III-R and DSM-5 that were current at the time of each survey.
Note: Vertical lines indicate 95% confidence intervals around mean numbers of symptoms.
Results are weighted as in Figure 12.1. Sample size is 111 for the NVVRS (darker bar), 108 for the Longitudinal Study (lighter bar) due to three missing cases in the symptom data.
Statistical significance of differences in means was tested using a paired t-test with PROC SURVEYMEANS: $p = .0041$.

the time of the Longitudinal Study. Figure 12.1 also shows that the rate of current PTSD according to DSM-5 (as measured by CAPS) was lower at the time of the Longitudinal Study than the rate according to DSM-III-R (as measured by SCID) at the time of the NVVRS. The diagnostic measures designed to be more comparable with each other showed a similar decline in PTSD between the two interviews. The prevalence of PTSD at the time of the NVVRS decreased by over half, from 10.46% or 8.87% (depending on which diagnostic measure is used) down to 3.97% or 3.75% at the time of the Longitudinal Study.

Figure 12.2 compares simple counts of PTSD symptoms at the times of the NVVRS and the Longitudinal Study. The comparison includes only symptoms assessed in both surveys (i.e., in both the SCID and CAPS). On average, the veterans had barely more than half as many symptoms in the second survey—1.22 versus 2.35. Thus, by all measures tested, the level of PTSD was considerably lower in the Longitudinal Study. As noted in Figures 12.1 and 12.2, these differences are statistically significant.

A few of those with DSM-III-R diagnoses at the time of the Longitudinal Study did not have current PTSD at the time of the earlier NVVRS. Table 12.2 shows that there were only three such cases in our sample—a weighted 2.6% of those not initially diagnosed with current PTSD, no matter which version of the SCID was used to make that diagnosis. These three men may have had recurrences in later life of disorders that had remitted at the time of the earlier assessment.

Table 12.2 also shows that only six men who had current PTSD at the original NVVRS interview had it at the time of the Longitudinal Study. These were the same

Table 12.2 RATES OF CURRENT PTSD AT THE LONGITUDINAL STUDY
INTERVIEW AS MEASURED BY THE SIMULATED SCID DIAGNOSIS, ACCORDING
TO TWO DIAGNOSTIC METHODS AT THE NVVRS INTERVIEW

Current PTSD in the NVVRS		Rates of current PTSD in the Longitudinal Study Using the Simulated SCID diagnosis
SCID diagnosis:	No	2.6% (3 of 85)
	Yes	13.1% (6* of 23)
SCID diagnosis omitting	No	2.6% (3 of 88)
"foreshortened future":	Yes	15.5% (6* of 20)

Note: Results are weighted to represent the living population at the time of the Longitudinal Study. Unweighted sample *n*'s are in parentheses. Sample size is 108.
*These are the same six men receiving both diagnoses.

six men regardless of which version of the SCID was used to make the initial diagnosis. When the data are weighted to represent the population, these six men represent only 1.4% of the veterans. This very low rate of persistent PTSD along with the decreased prevalence suggests that war-related PTSD, as manifested in this sample of male U.S. veterans of the war in Vietnam, was not a lifetime disorder for the large majority of those who developed it.

It is necessary, however, to qualify this conclusion on the basis of further analysis of the 14 responders whose PTSD had remitted (i.e., those who had onsets of war-related PTSD diagnosed at the time of the NVVRS, but for whom the disorder was no longer current at the time of the Longitudinal Study). Using appropriate weights, a little over a third (33.5%) were diagnosed with one of three other current disorders: alcohol abuse/dependence (19.1%), drug abuse/dependence (13.2%), and major depressive disorder (1.2%). The preponderance of alcoholism and substance use disorders suggests the possibility that some veterans with seemingly remitted PTSD were self-medicating.

Moreover, when we looked further at the group of veterans who remitted, we found that 77.8% still had one or more CAPS symptoms at the time of the Longitudinal Study, with 65% having two or more. This suggests that there was a long-standing residue of the disorder in most of those who no longer met full criteria for the diagnosis.

In Chapter 7, we reported that blacks and Hispanics had higher rates of PTSD onset (both 33%) than whites (18.7%). Hispanics at the time of the NVVRS had a higher rate of then-current PTSD (22.0%) than either blacks (16.8%) or whites (9%). Hispanics remained the group with the highest rate at the time of the Longitudinal Study (24.6% in Hispanics versus 3.7% in blacks and 2.0% in whites). The Longitudinal Study included a question that asked, "Did you receive any professional treatment for your reactions related to your war experiences in the last 12 months?" It is not surprising, given their higher rates of PTSD than whites at the time of the NVVRS, that blacks and Hispanics reported higher rates of current treatment than whites (4.7% for whites, 24.2 % for blacks, and 20.9% for Hispanics). It is striking, however, that while the rate of current PTSD became much lower for blacks (3.7% versus 16.8% earlier) and whites (2.0% versus 9.0% earlier), it remained high for Hispanics (24.6%). It is possible that professional treatment was less helpful to Hispanics. This is a matter that needs more investigation.

On balance, the weight of the evidence suggests that, except for Hispanics, there was a decline from initial onset in the rate of PTSD that was evident at the time of the NVVRS, and that that decline continued to the time of the Longitudinal Study. Would these results be different if we had Longitudinal Study data on war-related PTSD before the time of their deaths for those who died? We cannot be certain. However, as Table 12.1 shows, the dead had not differed from the Longitudinal Study responders in rates of current war-related PTSD at the time of the NVVRS—a strong predictor of whether the veteran would have current PTSD at the time of the Longitudinal Study.

The original NVVRS did not include male Theater veterans from largely rural areas in the diagnosed subsample. The Longitudinal Study added male veterans from the previously unrepresented areas and gave them diagnostic examinations. Despite these differences, this augmented sample found similar rates of current PTSD according to CAPS-5. In the augmented sample ($n = 275$), an estimated rate of 4.5% had DSM-5 diagnoses of current, war-related PTSD (Marmar et al., 2015) at the time of the Longitudinal Study. This compares with a rate of 4.0% with our smaller sample ($n = 111$), whose crucial advantage was that all members had baseline diagnostic and other important data from the original NVVRS.

DID THE VETERANS' APPRAISALS OF THE VALENCE AND SALIENCE OF THE IMPACT OF THE WAR ON THEIR PRESENT LIVES CHANGE BETWEEN THE TIMES OF THE TWO SURVEYS?

As we reported Chapter 11, the large majority of male veterans in the full Theater sample perceived the impact of the war on their lives at the time of the NVVRS survey to be mainly positive. In order to compare responses in the NVVRS and the Longitudinal Study in our much smaller sample of veterans who received diagnostic interviews in both, we had to make a change in one of the two questionnaire items used to define the valence variable. In the NVVRS, the respondent was asked, "Overall, do you feel you personally benefitted in the long run or were set back in the long run by having been involved in the Vietnam War?" but that question was not asked in the Longitudinal Study. However both the NVVRS and the Longitudinal Study asked a parallel question with respect to military service in general: "Overall, do you feel you personally benefitted in the long run or were you set back in the long run by having been in the military service?" so we substituted that item for the one referring to the Vietnam war. The two similar

Table 12.3 VETERANS' APPRAISALS OF THE EFFECT OF MILITARY
SERVICE ON THEIR LIVES ("VALENCE") IN THE NVVRS AND
THE LONGITUDINAL STUDY INTERVIEWS

Effect of Military Service (Valence)*	NVVRS	Longitudinal Study
Positive	61.8% (60)	69.4% (71)
An equal balance of positive and negative	8.9% (13)	15.1% (22)
Negative	29.3% (38)	15.5% (18)
TOTAL	100.0% (111)	100.0% (111)

Note: Percentages are weighted to represent the living population at the time of Longitudinal Study.
Unweighted sample *n*'s are in parentheses.

*Responders who said that military service had either benefitted them or set them back are rated positive or negative accordingly.

Those who had no opinion are rated on the basis of a second question, which asks "What effect has military service had on your life?"

Response choices to that question included "an equal balance of positive and negative effects."

items are fairly highly correlated with each other (r = .66) in the sample of 111 veterans used in the present analysis.

Table 12.3 shows the distribution of valence categories in that sample in both surveys. In the NVVRS, a substantial majority (82%) appraised the impact of their military service as positive or equally balanced, a majority that increased very slightly to 84% by the time of the Longitudinal Study. However, the proportion of "positive" responders decreased between the two surveys, while the proportion seeing "an equal balance" increased markedly from 4.7% to 15.1%.

The equal balance responders had a rate of current PTSD in the Longitudinal Study that was closer to the lower rate among those whose valence was positive. In fact, Table 12.4 shows that, in the sample of 111 veterans who were clinically interviewed in both surveys, the equal balance responders had no current PTSD in the later survey.

We saw in Chapter 11 that, when we combined veterans' assessments of the valence and salience of the impact of the war on their personal lives to define four separate groups based on both variables, the mainly negative/high salience group had an extremely high rate of PTSD, whereas the mainly positive/low salience group had the lowest rate. To analyze these combinations of valence and salience in our sample of 111 veterans, we combined the veterans who said the effect was "entirely or mostly positive" with those who said it was "an equal balance of positive and negative." This latter category of respondent (the "equal balance responders") had been excluded in previous analyses with larger samples. We made this change for two reasons: first, in order to increase the Longitudinal Study sample size; and, second, because the equal balance

Table 12.4 RATES OF CURRENT PTSD BY VALENCE GROUP IN THE NVVRS AND
THE LONGITUDINAL STUDY INTERVIEWS

Effect of Military Service (Valence)*	NVVRS Current PTSD (SCID)	Longitudinal Study Current PTSD (CAPS)
Positive	7.7% (60)	1.7% (71)
An equal balance of positive and negative	0.0% (13)	0.0% (22)
Negative	9.5% (38)	16.6% (18)
TOTAL	10.5% (111)	4.0% (111)

Note: Percentages are weighted to represent the living population at the time of the Longitudinal Study. Unweighted sample n's are in parentheses.

*Responders who said that military service had either benefitted them or set them back are rated positive or negative accordingly.

Those who had no opinion are rated on the basis of a second question, which asks "What effect has military service had on your life?"

Response choices to that question included "an equal balance of positive and negative effects."

responders in the Longitudinal Study were much nearer to the positive valence than to the negative valence responders in rates of PTSD.

Incorporating the revision of the valence variable just explained, Table 12.5 compares the valence/salience appraisal typology at the time of the NVVRS to the same typology at the time of the Longitudinal Study. We see that the negative/high salience group is much smaller at the Longitudinal Study interview (down to 5.1% from 21.1%). The positive or balanced valence/low salience group is essentially unchanged.

Table 12.6 shows that, as in the full, diagnosed subsample described in Chapter 11, the rate of current PTSD in the NVVRS was highest in the negative/high salience group.

Table 12.5 TERTIARY APPRAISALS IN THE NVVRS AND THE LONGITUDINAL
STUDY INTERVIEWS

Tertiary Appraisal	NVVRS	Longitudinal Study	Significance of Difference Between Interviews (p)
Negative/low salience	8.3% (11)	10.3% (6)	.66
Negative/high salience	21.1% (27)	5.1% (12)	.0056
Positive or "balanced"/ low salience	41.3% (40)	54.7% (50)	.21
Positive or "balanced"/ high salience	29.4% (33)	29.8% (43)	.96
TOTAL	100.0% (111)	100.0% (111)	

Note: Percentages are weighted to represent the living population at the time of the Longitudinal Study. Unweighted sample n's are in parentheses.

Statistical tests are performed as described in the note to Figure 12.1.

Table 12.6 RATES OF CURRENT PTSD BY TERTIARY APPRAISAL GROUP IN THE
NVVRS AND THE LONGITUDINAL STUDY INTERVIEWS

Tertiary Appraisal in Each Survey	NVVRS Current PTSD (SCID)	Longitudinal Study Current PTSD (CAPS)
Negative/low salience	4.8% (11)	0.0% (6)
Negative/high salience	25.2% (27)	49.9% (12)
Positive or "balanced"/low salience	6.1% (40)	0.0% (50)
Positive or "balanced"/high salience	7.6% (33)	4.7% (43)
TOTAL	10.5% (111)	4.0% (111)

Note: Percentages are weighted to represent the living population at the time of the Longitudinal Study. Unweighted sample *n*'s are in parentheses.

This finding was repeated in the Longitudinal Study, which revealed an extraordinarily high rate of current PTSD in that group (49.9%).

Most of the Longitudinal Study veterans whose appraisals were negative/high salience were not the same veterans as those who had made that appraisal earlier in the NVVRS. Only three of the 12 men who made that appraisal in the later survey had made the same appraisal in the earlier study.

Table 12.7 and its note on statistical significance indicate that, regardless of the earlier appraisal, it is the current appraisal that is significantly associated with current PTSD. It is possible, perhaps even likely, that many of these 12 men made their appraisals influenced by their persistent PTSD.

Table 12.7 RATES OF CURRENT PTSD IN THE LONGITUDINAL STUDY
INTERVIEW BY THE PRESENCE OR ABSENCE OF NEGATIVE/HIGH
SALIENCE APPRAISALS IN EACH SURVEY

Negative/High Salience in theNVVRS	Negative/High Salience in the Longitudinal Study	Rate of Current PTSD According to the CAPS in the Longitudinal Study
NO	NO	1.9% (76)
	YES	49.4% (8)
YES	NO	0.0% (23)
	YES	51.4% (4)

Note: Percentages are weighted to represent the living population at the time of the Longitudinal Study. Unweighted sample *n*'s are in parentheses.

Significance: effect of NVVRS appraisal *p* = .53, effect of Longitudinal Study appraisal *p* = .02. No significant interaction.

HOW WELL HAVE THE VETERANS READJUSTED AFTER THEIR EXPERIENCES IN VIETNAM?

To answer this question, we investigated education, employment, and marital histories of the Theater veterans. We then compared Theater veterans to an NVVRS sample of veterans who served in the military but not in Vietnam at the time of the Vietnam war (i.e., Era veterans) on these variables.

Theater Veterans

We found that tertiary appraisals at the time of the original NVVRS were strongly re-lated to educational level, employment, and marital status following service in Vietnam (Dohrenwend et al., 2004). Specifically, we found that positive/low salience appraisals tended to be positively related to high attainment in these three variables, whereas neg-ative/high salience appraisals tended to be positively related to low attainment on these three variables. These are the types of appraisals that are associated with the greatest contrast in rates of current PTSD, with lower rates in the positive/low salience type and higher rates in the negative/high salience type.

It seems possible that all three of these variables—employment, educational at-tainment, and marital status—may be related to finding positive meaning in life, with "meaning" defined (as defined by King et al., 2006) as purpose, sense of one's own sig-nificance, and coherence. We looked at how well the veterans scored on these variables.

Table 12.8 compares employment status at the time of the NVVRS (11–12 years after the war ended) to employment status at the time of the Longitudinal Study (close to 40 years after the war ended). As can be seen, most veterans were employed at the time of the NVVRS. The biggest change shown in the Longitudinal Study is the increase

Table 12.8 EMPLOYMENT STATUS IN THE NVVRS AND THE LONGITUDINAL STUDY INTERVIEWS

Employment Status	NVVRS	Longitudinal Study
Employed	93.1% (100)	30.1% (26)
Unemployed	4.3% (8)	2.4% (5)
Retired	1.2% (1)	62.4% (69)
Disabled (unable to work)	0.9% (1)	5.1% (11)
Other	0.4% (1)	— —
TOTAL	100.0% (111)	100.0% (111)

Note: Percentages are weighted to represent the living population at the time of the Longitudinal Study. Unweighted sample *n*'s are in parentheses.

Table 12.9 EDUCATIONAL ATTAINMENT AT ARRIVAL IN VIETNAM, IN THE
NVVRS INTERVIEW, AND IN THE LONGITUDINAL STUDY INTERVIEW

Educational Attainment	At Arrival in Vietnam	NVVRS	Longitudinal Study
Not a high school grad	18.1% (27)	7.4% (10)	4.9% (7)
High school graduate	42.4% (49)	12.1% (17)	17.1% (27)
Some college	25.7% (24)	58.0% (57)	47.3% (46)
College graduate	13.8% (11)	22.5% (27)	30.8% (31)
TOTAL	100.0% (111)	100.0% (111)	100.0% (111)

Note: Percentages are weighted to represent the living population at the time of the Longitudinal Study. Unweighted sample *n*'s are in parentheses.

in retirement status, a status that was not relevant at the earlier time when most of the veterans had not reached retirement age.

Table 12.9 shows that, by the time of the NVVRS survey, the veterans had attained considerably higher levels of education than they had when they arrived in Vietnam. As might be expected, there was a more modest increase in educational attainment in the time between the two surveys.

Table 12.10 focuses on marital status at the time of arrival in Vietnam and at the times of the two surveys. It shows that while only about one-fifth were married when they went to Vietnam, the great majority of veterans were married at the times of the NVVRS and the Longitudinal Study. Roughly the same small proportions were divorced at each

Table 12.10 MARITAL STATUS IN THE NVVRS AND
THE LONGITUDINAL STUDY INTERVIEWS

Marital Status	Arrival in Vietnam	NVVRS	Longitudinal Study
Married*	19.3% (16)	87.6% (90)	81.1% (85)
Separated	—	2.9% (2)	0.2% (2)
Divorced	—	6.3% (13)	6.9% (10)
Widowed	—	0.1% (1)	8.0% (9)
Never married	80.7% (93)	3.7% (5)	3.2% (4)
TOTAL	100.0% (109)	100.0% (111)	100.0% (111)

Note: Percentages are weighted to reflect the living population at the time of the Longitudinal Study. Unweighted sample *n*'s are in parentheses.

*In the NVVRS, "married" includes "common law" if volunteered. In the Longitudinal Study, "married" includes one man (0.6%) who volunteered "living with someone."

Table 12.11 MARITAL STATUS IN THE LONGITUDINAL STUDY INTERVIEW
BY MARITAL STATUS IN THE NVVRS INTERVIEW

	Longitudinal Study					
NVVRS	Married*	Separated	Divorced	Widowed	Never Married	TOTAL
Married*	87.7% (76)	0.2% (2)	3.4% (5)	8.7% (7)		100% (90)
Separated	25.5% (1)		74.5% (1)			100% (2)
Divorced	65.9% (8)		28.4% (4)	5.7% (1)		100% (13)
Widowed				100% (1)		100% (1)
Never Married	13.5% (1)				86.5% (4)	100% (5)
TOTAL	81.1% (85)	0.2% (2)	6.9% (10)	8.0% (9)	3.2% (4)	100% (111)

Note: Percentages are weighted to represent the living population at time of Longitudinal Study. Unweighted sample *n*'s are in parentheses.

*In the NVVRS, one man volunteered "common law" (marriage), and is included here in the married category. In the Longitudinal Study, one man volunteered that he was "living with" someone and has been included here in the "married" category.

survey, and roughly the same, even smaller, proportions had never married. Eight percent of the veterans were widowed at the time of the Longitudinal Study, as opposed to almost none at the time of the NVVRS.

Table 12.11, which looks at marital status in the Longitudinal Study by marital status in the NVVRS interview, tells us that the great majority of veterans who were married at the time of the NVVRS (87.7%) were still married at the time of the Longitudinal Study. Most of the divorced (65.9%) were also now remarried.

Another positive outcome has to do with the veterans' children who were ages 6–16 at the time of the NVVRS. We found that these children were at least as free of serious emotional and behavior problems as their age counterparts in the general population (Chapter 9).

The veterans were also asked at the time of the NVVRS and again at the time of the Longitudinal Study how satisfying they found their current lives.

The large majority (87%), as Table 12.12 shows, said that their way of life was either completely satisfying or pretty satisfying at the time of the NVVRS. Only slightly fewer (83%) gave the same response at the time of the Longitudinal Study.

By and large, most veterans who found their lives pretty or completely satisfying at the time of NVVRS found their lives similarly satisfying at the time of Longitudinal Study, as evidenced in Table 12.13.

As can be seen in Table 12.14, those who changed their NVVRS response to "not very satisfying" in the Longitudinal Study and those who found life not very satisfying at both times had the highest rates of war-related current PTSD. There was almost no

Table 12.12 RESPONSES TO THE QUESTION, "IN GENERAL, HOW SATISFYING DO YOU FIND THE WAY YOU'RE SPENDING YOUR LIFE THESE DAYS?"

Response	NVVRS	Longitudinal Study
Completely satisfying	17.3% (15)	16.9% (17)
Pretty satisfying	69.5% (75)	65.8% (66)
Not very satisfying	13.3% (21)	17.4% (28)
TOTAL	100.0% (111)	100.0% (111)

Note: Percentages are weighted to represent the living population at time of Longitudinal Study. Unweighted sample *n*'s are in parentheses.

Table 12.13 RESPONSES TO THE QUESTION, "IN GENERAL, HOW SATISFYING DO YOU FIND THE WAY YOU'RE SPENDING YOUR LIFE THESE DAYS?" IN THE LONGITUDINAL STUDY BY RESPONSES TO THE SAME QUESTION IN THE NVVRS

NVVRS responses	Longitudinal Study responses			
	Completely satisfying	Pretty satisfying	Not very satisfying	TOTAL
Completely satisfying	19.7% (2)	63.3% (10)	17.0% (3)	100.0% (15)
Pretty satisfying	19.4% (15)	67.0% (45)	13.7% (15)	100.0% (75)
Not very satisfying	—	62.6% (11)	37.4% (10)	100.0% (21)
Total	16.9% (17)	65.8% (66)	17.4% (28)	100.0% (111)

Note: Percentages are weighted to represent the living population at time of Longitudinal Survey. Unweighted sample *n*'s are in parentheses.

Table 12.14 RATES OF CURRENT WAR-RELATED PTSD AT THE LONGITUDINAL STUDY INTERVIEW BY RESPONSES TO THE QUESTION, "IN GENERAL, HOW SATISFYING DO YOU FIND THE WAY YOU'RE SPENDING YOUR LIFE THESE DAYS?" IN THE LONGITUDINAL STUDY AND NVVRS

NVVRS responses	Longitudinal Study responses			
	Completely satisfying	Pretty satisfying	Not very satisfying	Total
Completely satisfying	0.0% (2)	0.0% (10)	53.0% (3)	9.0% (15)
Pretty satisfying	0.0% (15)	0.5% (45)	11.2% (15)	1.9% (75)
Not very satisfying	—	5.9% (11)	12.6% (10)	8.4% (21)
Total	0.0% (17)	1.1% (66)	18.6% (28)	4.0% (111)

Note: Percentages are weighted to represent the living population at time of Longitudinal Study. Unweighted sample *n*'s are in parentheses.

current PTSD among the majorities of the veterans who found their lives satisfying at the times of both surveys.

Comparison with Veterans Who Did Not Serve in Vietnam

The Longitudinal Study included data from an NVVRS sample of Era veterans. To the extent that they were similar to the Theater veterans at the time the latter went to Vietnam, they provide an additional test of the impact of Vietnam service on the readjustment of the Theater veterans. Unfortunately, we do not have Era veteran data in the Longitudinal Study on psychiatric variables including PTSD. We do, however, have data on the marital status, educational attainment, and employment of the Era veterans that correspond with the similar data on the Theater veterans.

We were able to obtain 33 Era veterans to compare with the 111 male Theater veterans. We standardized these Era veterans to the Longitudinal Study sample of Theater veterans on racial/

ethnic background and age. The process for identifying and standardizing this Era sample is described in more detail in Appendix B of this chapter.

We found only one statistically significant difference between Theater and Era veterans on the variables tested. This difference showed a higher rate of unemployment due to disability among Era veterans (20.8%) versus disability among Theater veterans (6.0%). When not statistically significant, the differences between the two groups tended to be very small and, if anything, like unemployment due to disability, to favor Theater veterans over Era veterans. For example, at the time of the Longitudinal Study, 82.7% of the Theater men are married compared to 81.5% of the Era men, and more of the Era men are divorced (17.6%) than Theater men (5.0%). And as far as educational attainment is concerned, 33.4% of Theater veterans are college graduates, compared to 24.8% of the Era veterans.

SUMMARY AND CONCLUSIONS

In answer to our first question, we find that the rate of war-related current PTSD declined by about half in the years between the NVVRS and the Longitudinal Study, furthering the decline of PTSD by almost half from its initial onset before the NVVRS was conducted 10–11 years after the war ended. Clearly, war-related PTSD in this sample of Vietnam veterans was not a lifetime disorder for the vast majority of those who had onsets.

In answer to our second question, the plurality of veterans who made positive/low salience appraisals at the time of the NVVRS increased to a majority at the time of the Longitudinal Study. This suggests a successful transition from the war zone to civilian life, evidenced by their ability to find value in the war experience but also to put the war itself behind them after they returned home.

In answer to our third question, on balance, the results suggest that, for most of the veterans, their readjustment to life after leaving Vietnam was satisfying and productive. However, there are hints that this was not the whole story. A minority of 5.1% still appraised the effects of their experiences in Vietnam as negative/high salience in their lives at the time of the Longitudinal Study. Moreover, although the rate of current PTSD appeared to have declined, there remained a small group of veterans (4%) diagnosed with current PTSD, according to DSM-5, at the time of the Longitudinal Study. In addition, of the veterans who had onsets of the disorder but who no longer met the full set of diagnostic criteria for PTSD at the time of the Longitudinal Study, over three-quarters (77.8%) were experiencing one or more PTSD symptoms—an apparent residue of their experiences in Vietnam. Nevertheless, a comparison with a small sample of Era veterans suggests that the Vietnam veterans' readjustment on such important variables as educational attainment, employment status, and marital history is at least as positive as was the readjustment of contemporary veterans who did not serve in Vietnam.

APPENDIX A: NEW WEIGHTS FOR THE LONGITUDINAL STUDY SUBSAMPLE OF VIETNAM VETERANS

The NVVRS diagnosed subsample ($n = 248$) has sampling strata and weights provided by the original survey research team. These strata and weights are used to adjust for the probabilistic sampling design and to obtain population representative estimates (Kulka et al., 1988, p. B-37). The sample represents the population of 1.26 million male Theater veterans from predominantly urban areas of the U.S.

At the time of the Longitudinal Study, 73% ($n = 182$) of the original subsample were still alive (representing 920,000 male Theater veterans still alive). Of these men, 61% ($n = 111$) responded to the Longitudinal Study, and 39% ($n = 71$) were non-responders to the Longitudinal Study. In order to make the 111 responders representative of the full population of veterans still alive at the time of the Longitudinal Study, a non-response adjustment was made to the original NVVRS sampling weights using non-response propensity score weighting (Chen et al., 2015). Non-response propensity weighting is a straightforward extension of the propensity score theory of Rosenbaum and Rubin (1983) incorporated into survey non-response problems by David et al. (1983).

Specifically, we estimated response propensities by fitting a logistic regression on the sample of 182 men who were still alive with their Longitudinal Study responder status (yes/no) as the outcome. Predictor variables in the logistic regression were taken from the original NVVRS survey. The 11 predictor variables included race/ethnicity, combat exposure, participation in harm to civilians or prisoners, past and present PTSD status, alcohol problems, major depression, tertiary appraisal, pre-war vulnerability, age at entry to the war, and unit cohesion. As Chen et al. (2015) recommend, we estimated parameters in this logistic regression incorporating the original NVVRS sampling weights and strata. Finally, we took the non-response propensity weights for each of the 111 Longitudinal Study responders to be the product of the original NVVRS population sampling weights and the inverse of the response propensity (i.e., predicted probability of response) from the logistic regression. These new weights made the 111 responders representative of the full 920,000 male Theater veterans from the predominantly urban areas who were still alive at the time of the Longitudinal Study. All analyses examining longitudinal associations or trends between NVVRS and the Longitudinal Study incorporated these new weights along with the original strata weights.

APPENDIX B: SELECTING AND STANDARDIZING THE COMPARISON SAMPLE OF ERA VETERANS

We selected a group of Era veterans equivalent to the sample of 111 Vietnam Theater veterans analyzed in this chapter. Because the Theater veteran sample was restricted to those who were given a diagnostic interview in the NVVRS, and because that sample was predominantly urban due to the locations of the interview sites, we limited our comparison sample of Era veterans to men who had likewise been diagnostically interviewed in the NVVRS. Because variables analyzed in this chapter came from both the Longitudinal Study's mail survey and its phone interview, we selected men who had completed both surveys. Among the Era veterans located for the Longitudinal Study, 33 men satisfied these criteria.

Table B-1 compares these 33 men to Era veterans who had died by the time of the Longitudinal Study and to those who were still alive but did not complete the two interviews. It compares these groups with respect to racial/ethnic background and the age at which they began military service. (As we will explain shortly, we chose these two variables because we used them to standardize the sample on the corresponding sample of Vietnam Theater veterans.) Means and proportions are weighted using the original NVVRS full sample weights.

Table B-1 shows that responders' mean age of entry into military service was virtually identical to those of non-responders and of the dead. However, the distribution of racial/ethnic background in the responders differed substantially from that in both the non-responders and the dead. Blacks are heavily under-represented among responders, with the consequence that whites are overrepresented. Hispanics are represented roughly equally in all three groups. However, n's are small. As a result, only one racial/ethnic difference between responders and the other two groups reaches statistical significance—namely, the different proportions of whites among responders and non-responders, with whites more highly represented among responders (90.5% vs. 79.6%).

In order to compare this sample to the sample of 111 Theater veterans, we standardized it on that sample so that the distributions of ethnic/racial group membership and age were similar in each sample. For Theater veterans, "age" is defined as age of arrival in Vietnam. For Era veterans, it is defined as the age at which they began military service. This method is similar but not identical to the standardization method

Table B-1 DISTRIBUTION FOR MALE ERA VETERANS OF RACIAL/ETHNIC BACKGROUND AND AGE OF ENTRY TO MILITARY SERVICE AMONG LONGITUDINAL STUDY RESPONDERS, NON-RESPONDERS, AND NVVRS RESPONDENTS WHO DIED BEFORE THE LONGITUDINAL STUDY

	Alive at time of Longitudinal Study			Dead	TOTAL ALIVE AND DEAD
	Responders	Non-responders	Total		
Variable	% (*n*)	% (*n*)	% (*n*)	% (*n*)	% (*n*)
Sample	100.0 (33)	100.0 (11)	100.0 (44)	100.0 (14)	100.0 (58)
Racial/Ethnic Background					
White	90.5 (16)	79.6 (6)*	88.0 (22)	68.0 (2)	84.4 (24)
Black	4.1 (6)	15.5 (1)	6.7 (7)	27.9 (10)	10.6 (17)
Hispanic	5.4 (11)	4.8 (4)	5.2 (15)	4.1 (2)	5.0 (17)
Mean age when began military service	19.7 (33)	19.7 (11)	19.7 (44)	19.8 (14)	19.7 (58)

Note: Means and proportions are weighted using the original NVVRS full sample weights that correct for over-sampling of racial/ethnic minorities. Subsample weights were unavailable for the diagnostically interviewed Era veterans.

*Differs significantly from value for responders ($p \leq .05$).

used in the NVVRS to compare Theater and Era veterans (Kulka et al., 1988, p. B-38). The NVVRS standardized the Theater sample on the Era sample, whereas we did the reverse for our purpose of comparing Theater and Era samples on readjustment variables. For male veterans, the NVVRS standardized by racial/ethnic group and age *at the time of the interview.* We standardized by age *at entry* to Vietnam or military service because of our earlier finding that arrival in Vietnam at less than 25 years of age was strongly associated with PTSD (see Chapter 5). For that reason, we dichotomized age at that level. As it turns out, none of the 33 Era veterans had entered military service at age 25 or above, so we standardized the Era veterans on a reduced sample of Theater veterans (n = 94) who had arrived in Vietnam at age 25 or under. We standardized the Era veterans on the *weighted* distribution of the 94 Theater veterans, using the weights described in Appendix A and used in most of the tables in this chapter. Because age was taken care of by eliminating the older Theater veterans, the standardization consisted simply of applying a different weight to each Era veteran, depending on his ethnic/racial group (1.5835 for whites, 0.7857 for blacks, and 0.2673 for Hispanics).

REFERENCES

Chen, Q., Gelman, A., Tracy, M., Norris, F., & Galea, S. (2015). Incorporating the sampling design in weighting adjustments for panel attrition. *Statistics in Medicine, 34*(28), 3637–3647.

David, M., Little, R. J. A., Samuhel, M. E., & Triest, R. K. (1983). Nonrandom nonresponse models based on the propensity to respond. *Proceedings of the Business and Economic Statistics Section,* 168–173. Alexandria, VA: American Statistical Association.

Dohrenwend, B. P., Neria, Y., Turner, J. B., Turse, N., Marshall, R., Lewis-Fernández, R., et al. (2004). Positive tertiary appraisals and posttraumatic stress disorder in U.S. male veterans of the war in Vietnam: The roles of positive affirmation, positive reformulation, and defensive denial. *Journal of Consulting and Clinical Psychology, 72,* 417–433.

King, L. A., Hicks, J. A., Krull, J., & Del Gaiso, A. K. (2006). Positive affect and the experience of meaning in life. *Journal of Personality and Social Psychology, 90,* 179–196.

Kulka, R. A., Schlenger, W. E., Fairbank, J. A., Hough, R. L., Jordan, B. K., Marmar, C. R., et al. (1988). *National Vietnam Veterans Readjustment Study (NVVRS): Contractual report of findings from the National Vietnam Veterans Readjustment Study: Draft.* Washington DC: Veterans Administration.

Marmar, C. R., Schlenger, W., Henn-Haase, C., Quian, M., Purchia, E., Li, M., et al. (2015). Course of posttraumatic stress disorder 40 years after the Vietnam war: Findings from the National Vietnam Veterans Longitudinal Study. *JAMA Psychiatry, 72*(9), 875–881.

Nguyen, V.T. (2016). *Nothing ever dies: Vietnam and the memory of war.* Cambridge, MA: Harvard University Press.

Rosenbaum, P. R., & Rubin, D. B. (1983). The central role of the propensity score in observational studies for causal effects. *Biometrika, 70,* 4155.

Schlenger, W. E., Corry, N. H., Kulka, R. A., Williams, C. S., Henn-Haase, C., & Marmar, C. R. (2015). Design and methods of the national Vietnam veterans longitudinal study. *International Journal of Methods in Psychiatric Research 24*(3), 186–203.

Shrout, P. E., Stadler, G., Lane, S. P., McClure, M. J., Jackson, G. L., et al. (2017). Initial elevation bias in subjective reports. Washington, DC: United States National Academy of Sciences. Pnas.org/cgi/doi/10.1073/pnas.1712277115

Spitzer, R., Williams, J., & Gibbon, M. (1987). *Structured Clinical Interview for DSM-III-R, Version NP-V.* New York: New York State Psychiatric Institute, Biometrics Research Department.

Weathers, F. W., Blake, D. D., Schnurr, P. P., Kaloupek, D. G., Marx, B. P., & Keane, T. M. (2013). *The Clinician-Administered PTSD Scale for DSM-5 (CAPS-5).* Interview available from the National Center for PTSD at http://www.ptsd.va.gov.

PART IV

Policy Implications

CHAPTER 13

cら

Some Implications for Policy

BRUCE P. DOHRENWEND

I believe we should care about how soldiers are trained, equipped, led, and welcomed home when they return from war. This is our moral duty toward those we ask to serve on our behalf. (Shay, 1994, p. 195)

[T]here were lessons made available to us . . . during and after the war in Vietnam that we have an obligation to keep in mind—an obligation to those we ask to risk their lives in our name. (Coleman, 2006, p. 163)

Some of the analyses and conclusions in preceding sections of this monograph have policy implications for cohorts of men and women who have followed or will follow Vietnam veterans into U.S. wars. We cannot address here specific implications of significant changes in the U.S. military that have come about post-Vietnam. These include the elimination of the draft, the eligibility of women for increased roles in combat, and the addition of new technological capabilities such as drones, to name a few important examples. However, we suggest that our findings regarding the psychological effects of a range of factors on U.S. veterans of the war in Vietnam may provide a useful background for developing policies aimed at increasing the psychological survival and well-being of veterans of wars fought post-Vietnam.

PRE-WAR VULNERABILITY, SEVERITY OF COMBAT EXPOSURE, AND HARM TO CIVILIANS AND PRISONERS

We examined the roles of pre-Vietnam vulnerability, severity of combat exposure, and personal involvement in harming civilians or prisoners in current post-traumatic stress symptom syndrome (PSS) most intensely in Chapter 5. Though none of these three factors proved sufficient, estimated PSS onset reached 97% for veterans high on all three factors, with harm to civilians or prisoners showing the largest independent contribution.

The implications of these results for the role of involvement in such harm are profound. As we reported in Chapter 6, on the basis of veteran responses to direct, closed questions about personal involvement, we identified 12.8% of the veterans as harmers of civilians or prisoners. Analyses of qualitative information indicate that the figure may be as high as 16%. Other than their much more severe combat exposure, we found very few characteristics of the harmers that differentiated them from veterans who were not directly involved in, or responsible for, inflicting harm on civilians or prisoners.

The human toll on harmers and harmed, and the moral and ethical problems involved, underline the importance of this problem. To the greatest extent possible, the armed forces and government of any country that is involved in any future "war amongst the people" must prioritize the reduction of harm to civilians and prisoners by its military. Vietnam was the first such war for U.S. forces. So, more recently, have been the conflicts in Iraq, Afghanistan, and Syria.

In Vietnam, both the widespread and accepted practice of clearing of villages thought to be under enemy control and the policy of measuring success in terms of body count led directly to the death and injury of large numbers of Vietnamese civilians (see Chapters 1 and 6). It appears that, in wars following the Vietnam war, the U.S. military has abandoned the use of the body count as a measure of success. However, the physical destruction of land and structures in which civilians live and work continues in current wars amongst the people. For humanitarian reasons as well as for the psychological toll on the U.S. war fighters involved, as our research shows, there is strong need to find ways to minimize this devastation.

We also found a strong positive additive interaction between severity of combat exposure and pre-Vietnam vulnerability for current PSS. A veteran's current PSS increased with the severity of combat exposure he experienced. For those with the lowest severity rates of combat exposure, the estimated rate of current PSS is only around 1.0%, regardless of their pre-war vulnerability. By contrast, among those with the highest severity rates of combat exposure, the range is from an estimated current PSS rate of 7% for those with the lowest pre-war vulnerability load, to 83% for those in the most vulnerable group.

These results have implications for policy that need attention. The positive interaction of severity of combat exposure and pre-war vulnerability on current PSS points to the need to keep the more vulnerable soldiers out of the most severe combat situations. Though this may seem obvious, it was not the U.S. policy in Vietnam, where pre-war personal vulnerability showed a modest positive correlation (.28) with severity of exposure.

ELEVATED RATES OF WAR-RELATED PTSD IN BLACK AND HISPANIC MALE VETERANS

As we reported in Chapter 7, both blacks and Hispanics had higher rates of war-related PTSD than majority whites. Because of the major role of severity of combat exposure in the racial/ethnic differences, we investigated the question of why the combat exposure of blacks and, to a lesser degree, Hispanics, was more severe than the combat exposure of majority whites.

The main reason for the group differences in severity of exposure appeared to be the percentages of blacks, Hispanics and majority whites serving in each of the four military branches—some branches (Marines and Army) more likely and others (Navy and Air Force) less likely to send their recruits into combat. However, even within branches of services, there were also racial/ethnic differences in severity of combat exposure.

We recommend that ways be found to equalize rates of recruitment of majority whites, blacks, Hispanics, and members of other racial/ethnic minority groups, as well as their assignments to both combat and other highly stressful roles.

NURSES IN VIETNAM

As we reported in Chapter 8, over 7,000 women served in the American military during the war, an estimated 85% as nurses. Our most striking finding regarding these nurses was the apparent importance of pre-war vulnerabilities in determining which of them actually experienced PTSD onsets—and, even more importantly, which still suffered from the disorder at the time of the Longitudinal Study interviews conducted many years after the war. Having had a childhood in which a family member abused drugs or alcohol was a strong risk factor for PTSD onset, and having had a psychiatric disorder before serving in Vietnam was an extremely potent and highly significant risk factor for both PTSD onset and current PTSD. Nurses with pre-war psychiatric histories were 23 times more likely than their colleagues to suffer an onset of PTSD.

Therefore, it would seem particularly important to limit the exposure of nurses with pre-war disorders to the kinds of stressors that we have found are positively associated with onsets and persistence of war-related PTSD among the nurses. These include their serving on bases and in hospitals subject to enemy attack, being required to assume responsibility for severely wounded soldiers in greater numbers than can be given adequate attention, and exposure to sexual harassment, even rape, by fellow American soldiers.

SECONDARY TRAUMATIZATION

We focused in Chapter 9 on the wives and offspring of 115 clinically interviewed male Vietnam veterans. We found evidence of secondary traumatization in the sons of veterans suffering from current PTSD. Current PTSD in the veterans was also associated with demoralization in their wives or partners, which in turn was associated with behavior problems in their daughters. Even with this evidence of secondary traumatization, however, the veterans' children as a group appeared at least as healthy as their counterparts in the general population. Nevertheless, these associations of veteran PTSD with psychiatric problems found in some of their wives or partners and children underline the importance of policies that make mental health treatment programs readily available for the families of veterans with war-related PTSD or other psychiatric disorders, including the creation of such programs where none exist.

PUBLIC ATTITUDES

As documented in Chapter 1, toward the latter stages of the Vietnam war, following the 1968 Tet Offensive by the North Vietnamese Army and their Vietcong allies throughout South Vietnam, majority public opinion in the U.S. turned against the war. On the basis of analyses reported in Chapter 10, we concluded that changing public attitudes toward U.S. military involvement in Vietnam had a substantial negative effect on veterans' attitudes toward the war they were fighting. This in turn was associated with decreased unit cohesion and increased demoralization among U.S. fighting forces in Vietnam toward the end of the war.

Policy makers have increasingly recognized that negative public attitudes can pose a threat to the mental health of U.S. forces. For example, an initial quote introducing Chapter 10 from President Obama stresses that the public must not blame individual veterans who are sent to fight our wars, even when the wars themselves are unpopular. There is, however, no evidence that maintaining this distinction would be sufficient to eliminate the threat to the well-being of war fighters of negative public attitudes toward an unpopular war. A more effective and comprehensive solution, therefore, would be to commit our military forces to fight only in just wars that merit popular support. We appear to have understood the initial lesson—that is, to respect those who fight our wars—both retroactively for U.S. veterans of the war in Vietnam and currently for the veterans of the wars in Iraq and Afghanistan. But we have done less well in approaching the desired solution of limiting our military engagements to just wars.

VETERANS' APPRAISALS OF THE IMPACT OF WAR ON THEIR CURRENT LIVES

In Chapter 11, we reported our analyses of the appraisals by the veterans of the valence (positive versus negative) and salience (relative importance) of their Vietnam experiences in their present lives. We constructed the following four types of appraisal: positive/high salience, positive/low salience, negative/high salience, and negative/low salience. As expected, negative/high salience was associated with by far the highest rate of PTSD. We had hypothesized that positive/high salience would be associated with the lowest rate of PTSD. Contrary to this expectation, we found that positive/low salience was associated with the lowest rate of PTSD.

The importance of low salience led us to ask the question why that was so. The fact that low salience appraisals, both positive and negative, show less association with PTSD than do high salience appraisals suggests to us that satisfying post-Vietnam activities related to family, education, and work supplied new, or newly reaffirmed, positive meanings that supplanted in importance those veterans' war-zone experiences.

If this is so, programs that increase the relative importance of post-war activities over war-time experiences might have important positive effects on mental health. We note that the G.I. Bill has provided such programs since World War II. Its opportunities, and other comparable opportunities, should be enhanced, especially for veterans of severe combat.

REFERENCES

Coleman, P. (2006). *Flashback: Posttraumatic stress disorder, suicide and the lessons of war.* Boston, MA: Beacon Press.
Shay, J. (2002). *Odysseus in America: Combat trauma and the trials of homecoming.* New York: Scribner.

EPILOGUE

A nticipating his declaration of an official end to the war on May 7, 1975, President Ford said in a speech at Tulane University on April 23, 1975:

> Today, Americans can regain the sense of pride that existed before Vietnam. But it cannot be achieved by refighting a war that is finished. . . . These events, tragic as they are, portend neither the end of the world nor of America's leadership in the world. (Karnow, 1997, pp. 681–682)

Six days later, upon entering Saigon, Colonel Bui Tin, a North Vietnamese colonel said,

> Between Vietnamese, there are no victors and no vanquished. Only the Americans have been beaten. If you are patriots, consider this a moment of joy. The war for our country is over. (Karnow, 1997, p. 684)

But the war did not end for the loved ones of the millions of Vietnamese whose family members died or for those maimed during the war. And the war did not end for the loved ones of the U.S. service members who died in Vietnam and for many of the veterans who fought the war and lived through it.

In the beautiful city of Hanoi, in the former North Vietnam, and in the bustling metropolis of Saigon, now Ho Chi Minh City, in the former South Vietnam, you will find dramatic portrayals of what the Vietnamese call the American War. You can also travel to the preserved tunnels throughout the North built by the Vietnamese for shelter and as hiding places from U.S. bombs.

There are no such museums in the United States. There is, however, the Vietnam Wall in our nation's capital with its 58,000 names—a singular visible atonement our society has made to U.S veterans of the war.

REFERENCE

Karnow, S. (1997). *Vietnam: A history.* New York: Penguin Books.

INDEX

professional football players, draft
    avoidance by, 20
Project 100, 000, 21–22, 182
Projected Probability measure, 93–96
    current PTSD, 135–36
    general distress symptomatology
        measured by, 135–39
    investigation of, 132–34
    onsets of war-related PTSD, 135–36
    overview, 131
    period of war, 136
    time of war entry, 135
protest events, 41–43, 53
    after Cambodian incursion, 62
    Chicano Moratorium antiwar protest, 63
    Kent State shootings, 62–63
    "March Against Death", 61–62
    return of medals by veterans, 64–65
Provincial Reconnaissance Units
    (PRUs), 57–58
Pryor, John, 49
psychiatric disorders, with pre-Vietnam
    onset, 126–27
    risk factor for PTSD, 148–50, 151
    in secondary traumatization analysis, 242
    in women nurses, 218, 227
PTSD. See Post-Traumatic Stress Disorder
PTSD Symptom Checklist (PCL-M), 137
public attitudes, changes in. See changing
    public attitudes

Quang Nam province, Vietnam, 26–27
Quang Tin, Vietnam, 49
Quang Tri City, Vietnam, 67
racial/ethnic minorities
    combat exposure and harming by, 164
    disparities in soldiers, 22
    policy implications, 314–15
    PTSD prevalence rates in, 187, 188, 190
        combat exposure severity, 186, 190–93,
            194, 195
        other risk factors, 189
        prior research reports of higher, 183–84
        subsample composition, 185
        war-zone stress exposure and SCID
            diagnoses, 186–89
    in representative veteran sample, 93
    role in Vietnam War, 182–83
    tertiary appraisals, 282–83

racism, in formal training, 16
Rahe, A. J., 272–73
Ransom, Robert, 37
rape. See sexual trauma
rap groups, 71–73
Readjustment Counseling Service, 73
Reagan, Ronald, 76
recall bias, 184
record-based exposure. See Military-
    Historical Measure
Reh, Donald, 49
Reiland, Dwight, 32
religious affiliation, 280–83
Reporting Vietnam, 162
representative veteran sample
    accuracy of reports, 104
    characteristics of, 92
    current PTSD in, 93–96
    diagnostic histories from
        subsample, 97–98
    percentage exposed to combat, 104–5
    scrutiny of accounts, 107–8
    subsample, 92–93
Rescorla, L., 243
rewards system for body count, 10–11
Rhoads, J., 201, 205
rioting, antiwar, 41
Robins, Lee, 74
Rogers, Bernard, 44
Root, L. P., 215
Rosenheck. R., 185
Rosett, Henry, 71
Ross, David, 44–45
rules of engagement, violations of, 11
Rushton, P., 211

Saar, J., 60
Safer, Morley, 26–27
Saigon, Vietnam, Tet Offensive and, 46–47
Salazar, Ruben, 63
salience, appraisal of, 276–77, 286,
    297–300, 316
Salter, M., 271, 289
sample, in NVVRS
    characteristics of Theater veterans, 92, 94
    comparison sample of male Era
        veterans, 92
    diagnostic histories from
        subsample, 97–98